SS-9

W9-CAL-603

Methods of Group Exercise Instruction

SECOND EDITION

Carol Kennedy-Armbruster, MS

Indiana University, Bloomington, Indiana

Mary M. Yoke, MA, MM

Adelphi University, Garden City, New York

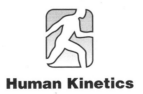

Human Kinetics

Library of Congress Cataloging-in-Publication Data

Kennedy, Carol A., 1958-
    Methods of group exercise instruction / Carol Kennedy-Armbruster, Mary M. Yoke. -- 2nd ed.
        p. cm.
    Includes bibliographical references and index.
    ISBN-13: 978-0-7360-7526-8 (soft cover)
    ISBN-10: 0-7360-7526-7 (soft cover)
  1. Exercise--Study and teaching. 2. Physical education and training--Study and teaching. 3. Exercise personnel--Certification--United States. I. Yoke, Mary M., 1953- II. Title.
    GV481.K416 2009
    613.7'107--dc22

                            2008042662

ISBN-10: 0-7360-7526-7
ISBN-13: 978-0-7360-7526-8

Copyright © 2009, 2005 by Human Kinetics, Inc.

All rights reserved. Except for use in a review, the reproduction or utilization of this work in any form or by any electronic, mechanical, or other means, now known or hereafter invented, including xerography, photocopying, and recording, and in any information storage and retrieval system, is forbidden without the written permission of the publisher.

Notice: Permission to reproduce the following material is granted to instructors and agencies who have purchased *Methods of Group Exercise Instruction, Second Edition:* Appendices A, B, C, D, F, and G. The reproduction of other parts of this book is expressly forbidden by the above copyright notice. Persons or agencies who have not purchased *Methods of Group Exercise Instruction, Second Edition,* may not reproduce any material.

The Web addresses cited in this text were current as of September 2, 2008, unless otherwise noted.

Acquisitions Editor: Judy Patterson Wright, PhD; **Developmental Editor:** Judy Park; **Assistant Editors:** Derek Campbell and Lee Alexander; **Copyeditor:** Jocelyn Engman; **Proofreader:** Sarah Wiseman; **Indexer:** Bobbi Swanson; **Permission Manager:** Dalene Reeder; **Graphic Designer:** Bob Reuther; **Graphic Artist:** Patrick Sandberg; **Cover Designer:** Keith Blomberg; **Photographer (cover):** Neil Bernstein; **Photographers (interior):** Neil Bernstein and Tom Roberts; **Photo Asset Manager:** Laura Fitch; **Visual Production Assistant:** Joyce Brumfield; **Photo Office Assistant:** Jason Allen; **Art Manager:** Kelly Hendren; **Associate Art Manager:** Alan J. Wilborn; **Illustrator:** Bulls Eye Studios, Mic Greenberg, and Jason McAlexander/Interactive Composition Corporation; **Printer:** Sheridan Books

We thank the Student Recreational Sports Center in Bloomington, Indiana, for assistance in providing the location for the photo shoot for this book.

Printed in the United States of America   10 9 8 7 6 5 4 3

The paper in this book is certified under a sustainable forestry program.

Human Kinetics
Web site: www.HumanKinetics.com

United States: Human Kinetics
P.O. Box 5076
Champaign, IL 61825-5076
800-747-4457
e-mail: humank@hkusa.com

Canada: Human Kinetics
475 Devonshire Road, Unit 100
Windsor, ON N8Y 2L5
800-465-7301 (in Canada only)
e-mail: info@hkcanada.com

Europe: Human Kinetics
107 Bradford Road
Stanningley
Leeds LS28 6AT, United Kingdom
+44 (0)113 255 5665
e-mail: hk@hkeurope.com

Australia: Human Kinetics
57A Price Avenue
Lower Mitcham, South Australia 5062
08 8372 0999
e-mail: info@hkaustralia.com

New Zealand: Human Kinetics
Division of Sports Distributors NZ Ltd.
P.O. Box 300 226 Albany
North Shore City, Auckland
0064 9 448 1207
e-mail: info@humankinetics.co.nz

Contents

Preface

Welcome to *Methods of Group Exercise Instruction, Second Edition.* Group exercise is exercise that is performed by a group of individuals led by an instructor. You will notice that we no longer refer to group exercise as *aerobics,* since today there are so many formats of group exercise, many of which do not contain an aerobics segment. The many ways to exercise in a group include traditional cardiorespiratory programs on the floor, step class, stationary indoor cycling, sport conditioning, water exercise, kickboxing, Pilates, yoga, muscular conditioning, and flexibility classes. Group exercise formats, modalities, and trends are constantly evolving. Group exercise classes can be found in a variety of settings such as health clubs, corporate fitness centers, schools, universities, community centers, and hospitals. There is a demand for competent group fitness instructors who have the knowledge and skills to lead dynamic, safe, and effective classes. Further, there is a demand for instructors who can lead more than one type of class. Thus fitness professionals can enhance their marketability by becoming an expert group leader in a variety of class formats. This book will introduce you to the most common group exercise modalities. It is intended for physical education, recreation, fitness, and dance students as well as other fitness professionals who wish to lead group classes. Even if you are not planning to instruct group exercise, you may become a program director responsible for hiring, training, and evaluating group instructors so knowledge of class format, teaching progressions, and safety considerations will enhance your skills whether you are a group exercise leader or a program director.

We believe that this book fills an important gap in the exercise textbook repertory by presenting research-based information on a variety of group exercise modalities while maintaining a strong how-to applied focus. We are extremely pleased that Human Kinetics developed the accompanying DVD and online course that make it even easier for you to learn the practical skills necessary to lead effective group instruction. It is nearly impossible to become a competent instructor simply by reading a book; you must practice and experience the leadership skills with your body as well. To that end, we have incorporated numerous devices to help you apply the information learned in our book, including several practice drills. In many cases, these drills are shown on the DVD as well as described in the text, so you can practice right along with the DVD instructor.

A major distinguishing feature of our book is that the information presented is based on research. Since approximately 1986, a plethora of research has been conducted on group exercise, primarily regarding energy expenditure but also focusing on biomechanics, injury incidence, exercise adherence, and effectiveness of specific exercise programs. Our goal is to present scientific principles and relevant research whenever they are available. Our first edition contained more than 250 research articles. We have added another 200+ articles to this edition, making this the most referenced group exercise textbook on the market. We have also added chapters on sport conditioning, yoga, and Pilates to keep up with the ever-changing group exercise formats that have become staples in the industry.

The purpose of this book is to provide you with the practical skills necessary to teach group exercise classes. Numerous other texts on exercise instruction cover exercise physiology, kinesiology, nutrition, special populations, injury prevention, business matters, behavior modification, and more. Our book focuses on the nuts and bolts of instruction: the specific exercises you'll use and the techniques you'll need for moving to music, choreographing classes, and cueing your students. We'll introduce you to the most popular types of group fitness classes and provide you with the basic skills required to lead them.

Ancillary Material for the Second Edition

For students and course instructors, the practical assignments and practice drills throughout the text reinforce the content while facilitating instruction. In addition, the following ancillary material is available.

- ■ **DVD.** The DVD (found at the end of the book) with over 40 video clips provides invaluable visual and practical information to help students convert the information presented in the text to applied skills necessary for success in their future professions.

- ■ **Instructor Guide**. When used as a course text, *Methods of Group Exercise Instruction, Second Edition*, also includes an updated instructor guide, which offers suggestions for effective use of the book and DVD package, lesson plan outlines, a sample week-by-week syllabus, lab activities, and sample test questions.

- ■ **Test Package**. The updated test package includes a variety of questions, making it easier to create your own tests and quizzes.

- ■ **Online Course**. Online learning options are also available for those instructors and students who prefer the convenience of online learning.

The instructor guide and test package are free to course adopters and can be found at www.HumanKinetics.com/MethodsofGroupExerciseInstruction.

HOW THIS BOOK IS ORGANIZED

This book comprises three parts. Part I (Fundamentals of Group Exercise Instruction) provides a general overview of group exercise: the evolution and advantages of group exercise, the strategies for creating group cohesion within a class, the core concepts in class design, and the use of music, choreography, and cueing methods in designing a class. We introduce an evaluation form that will be used throughout the book to evaluate group classes, providing a template for gauging the effectiveness of the various modalities covered. Additionally, in part I we introduce basic music structure, communication skills, and programming concepts such as exercise progression.

Part II (Primary Components of Group Exercise) offers guidelines leading the four major segments of a group exercise class: warm-up, cardiorespiratory training, muscular conditioning, and flexibility training. The basic concepts covered here pertain to all class modalities. These concepts include intensity, safety, posture and alignment, anatomy, and joint actions. In chapter 7, the muscular conditioning and flexibility chapter, we provide many specific exercises appropriate for group classes. This chapter covers all the major muscle groups and also includes important cues and modifications for each exercise introduced.

Part III (Group Exercise Modalities) focuses on the practical teaching skills required for the most common modalities: step, kickboxing, stationary cycling, sport conditioning, Pilates, yoga, and water exercise. Basic moves, choreography, and training systems are covered for each type of class. Part III is where we get specific, and the drills, routines, and teaching skills covered in this part are addressed on the accompanying DVD as well as in the text. Many of the drills are demonstrated by an experienced instructor on the DVD, so you can practice skills such as anticipatory cueing and teaching to a 32-count phrase. Also in part III you'll find a chapter (chapter 15) on customizing group exercise classes. This final chapter presents the group exercise class evaluation form with practical application ideas and will help you tie all the elements of group exercise together so you can create any new format you would like. Group exercise is ever evolving, and formats we currently have may be retired and replaced by newer and more popular formats. Having the skills to create and customize new formats is important for the future of group exercise.

WHAT'S NEW IN THIS EDITION

Completing the first edition of this text was very taxing, as creating a new book from scratch is difficult. This second edition allowed us to refine and enhance the ideas presented in the initial text. It also reflects the ever-growing need for professionalism in the field of fitness. This need is the reason why we went to great lengths to reference more research and cite more than 200 additional research articles in this edition. This book is not just an opinion of what makes a good group exercise class; it is a reference text based on the scientific findings and observations of prominent researchers who have the same interest we do in learning more about group exercise. In fact, the main reason we both returned to school to obtain our master's degrees in Exercise Science was so we could research and learn more about group exercise. In this second edition we also added a new chapter on sport conditioning in the hopes that physical education curricula may adopt this book and present more fitness concepts in physical education. We made these changes based on the recommendations of several physical education faculty members who reviewed our first edition and gave us feedback on how to make it friendlier to physical educators. This new edition also incorporates new chapters on yoga and Pilates since they are now staples of the group exercise offerings of many facilities. We hope these new additions help you understand more about the ins and outs of group exercise instruction, both from a practical and a professional standpoint. Our purpose in writing this second edition was to continue to bridge the gap between scientific knowledge and the practical implementation of that knowledge.

ABOUT US

We have each taught group exercise for approximately 30 years, and in that time we have seen it evolve from traditional high-impact aerobics to the broad spectrum of classes available today. In addition to our graduate degrees in exercise science, we have accumulated several certifications in group exercise and attended countless continuing education conferences and workshops for high-low impact training, step, kickboxing, stationary indoor cycling, water exercise, Pilates, yoga, slide, dance, sport conditioning, and cardiorespiratory, muscular, and flexibility programming. We have presented to group exercise leaders and personal trainers at numerous fitness conferences around the world, and we continue to teach group exercise classes to the general public, constantly improving our own practical teaching skills. We have each been involved in several research studies, Carol primarily in the area of water exercise and Mary in the areas of high-low impact, step exercise, slide energy expenditures, and the efficacy of exercise on Pilates apparatus—in fact, we first met while speaking about our research at an IDEA research symposium back in 1989! We served together for six years on the credentialing committee of the American College of Sports Medicine, working primarily in the area of group exercise. Carol is currently serving on the national advisory board of the American Council on Exercise and also uses this book in her academic class at Indiana University, where she is a full-time faculty member in the department of kinesiology. Mary serves on the adjunct board of the Aerobics and Fitness Association of America, for which she has authored, coauthored, and edited numerous programs and projects. She is also an adjunct professor in the department of human performance at Adelphi University. Additionally, we have each authored books individually, and we have coauthored another book together. We believe we bring a unique perspective to this text because we are both committed to a hands-on approach yet are thoroughly familiar with the demands of academia and the requirements of science.

As with all formal teaching, skill comes with practice. Teaching group exercise takes courage, perseverance, and energy. It requires continual learning, rehearsal, and discipline. However, the work is worth it because helping others to live more healthful lives by having fun while exercising feels great! There's no better way to help other people than by improving their quality of life. Making a difference by educating, caring for, and motivating your students is a gift both to the participant and to yourself. We hope this book helps you become an agent of change for people wishing to embrace healthy lifestyles. We can't think of a better gift you can give to yourself and others.

Acknowledgments

We are very grateful to the many people who influenced the writing of this book. This book is a tribute to those who have made a difference in our lives. Our parents inspired us to follow our passion and to work hard to make our passion a reality. Thanks to Joan and Bob Caster (Carol's parents) and James and Margaret Yoke (Mary's parents) for their belief in us and continuous support over the years. To our children, Tony and Jessica Kennedy, Nathaniel Yoke, and Zachary Ripka, thank you for keeping us grounded in the fun of day-to-day living. We love the fact that you kept pulling us away from writing to attend your activities. It helped make this book even better. To Marty Armbruster, Carol's husband, thanks for your support and encouragement throughout edition 1 & 2. We also acknowledge and thank all the people we have encountered through the years who have influenced our perception of group exercise. Because the accumulation of knowledge makes for a good book, you all have helped to make this book happen. Thanks to the following people and organizations for their inspiration and input:

ACSM, ACE, AFAA, AEA, Ken Alan, Elisabeth Andrews, Chris Arterberry, Susan Bane, Kim Beetham-Maxwell, Teri Bladen, Jay Blahnik, Penny Black-Steen, Andy Blome, Sharon Bogen, Jane Bradley, Peggy Buchanan, Donna Burch, Can-Fit-Pro, Sharon Cheng, Denise Contessa, Robyn Deterding, Julie Downing, April Durrett, Dr. Ellen Evans, Melinda Flegel, Tere Filer, Dr. Bud Getchell, Nancy Gillette, Laura Gladwin, Maureen Hagan, Lisa Hamlin, Cher Harris, Sara Hillard, Shayla Holtkamp, IDEA Health and Fitness Association, Janet Johnson, Gail Johnston, Graham Melstand, Mindy King, Dr. Len Kravitz, Susan Kundrat, Alison Kyle, Abby Landsman, Karen Leatherman, Deb Legel, Deena Luft-Ellin, Graham Melstrand, Dr. John Shea, Dr. Larry Golding, Pat Maloney, Patti Mantia, Patti McCord, Colleen Curry, , Michelle Miller, Margaret Moore, Ghada Muasher, Maria Nardini, Kris Neely, Greg Niederlander, Charlotte Norton, Tony Ordas, Dr. Bob Otto, Jacque Pedgrift, Dr. Bob Perez, Dr. Jim Peterson, Kelly Pfaffenberger, Linda Pfeffer, Debi Ban-Pillarella, Lauri Reimer, Pat Ryan, Dr. Mary Sanders, Pearlas Sanborn, Holly Schell, Robert Sherman, Linda Shelton, Siri Sitton, Donna Spears, Mike Spezzano, Dixie Stanforth, Kathy Stevens, Lisa Stuppy, Steve Tharrett, Dr. Walt Thompson, Kelly Walker-Haley, John Wygand, and Mandy Zulkoski.

Special thanks to the Indiana University School of Health Physical Education and Recreation for their assistance with the DVD. The use of their facilities and equipment made the DVD and still photos possible. The DVD and still photo instructors include David Auman, Andrew Baer, Allison Berger, Teri Bladen, Erin Brace, Allison Chopra, Chad Coplen, Theresa Collison, Lisandra Cuadrado, Ceceila Fortune, Katie Grove, Malvika Gulati, Alyssa Hinnefeld, Leigh Ann Hoy, Bryan Hurst, Ann Houtoon, April and Michael Jackson, Jake Jones, Jessica Kennedy, Mindy King, Margie Kobow, Tatiana Kolovou, Guo Lei, Kayla Little, Colleen McCracken, Evan McDowell, Cara McGowan, Jessica McIntire, Devin Mcguire, Cherry Merritt-Darriau, Tammy Nichols, Bobby Papariella, Kelly Pfaffenberger, Jill Rensick, Wendi Robinson, Camilla Saulsbury, Misty Schneider, Meagan Shipley, Naima Solomon, Andrew Souder, Jennifer Starr, Will Thornton, Cameron Troxell, Mai Tran, Brock Waller, Jacki Watson, Katie Zukerman and IU Summer One P218 class.

Finally, a great big thanks to the staff at Human Kinetics, especially Judy Patterson Wright, who convinced us to write this book and Judy Park, our faithful developmental editor who possess the patience of a Saint along with wonderful organizational skills to keep us all on track. Thanks also to Tom Roberts and Neil Bernstein for their professionalism and high-quality photos. Special thanks to Doug Fink, Gregg Henness, Roger Francisco, Mark Herman, and Terry Henricks for their wonderful DVD production. We had a blast taping with you guys!

PART I

Fundamentals of Group Exercise Instruction

Introduction to Group Exercise

CHAPTER OBJECTIVES

By the end of this chapter, you will

- understand the evolution of group exercise from aerobic dance,
- know the health-related components of fitness and how group exercise relates to them,
- understand the difference between a student-centered instructor and a teacher-centered instructor,
- be able to list the major professional certifications and continuing education organizations in group fitness instruction, and
- understand group cohesion research in reference to group exercise.

What is the origin of group exercise? A great deal of credit belongs to Jacki Sorensen, who was directly involved with Dr. Kenneth Cooper's early work on aerobic capacity (Schuster 1979). Aerobic dancing was born in 1969 when Jacki was asked to launch an exercise program on closed-circuit TV for the wives of the U.S. Air Force men stationed in Puerto Rico. While preparing for the show, she studied the famed Air Force aerobics program, which was developed by Dr. Cooper. Jacki took Dr. Cooper's 12-minute running test, which evaluates a person's cardiorespiratory fitness based on how far the person can jog or run in 12 minutes. When she scored well on the test even though she had never run before, Jacki figured that her lifetime of dancing had not only kept her figure trim but also kept her heart and lungs in shape. This realization gave her the idea of combining dance with aerobic exercise (Sorenson and Bruns 1983). With this inspiration, she devised specific dance movements to music that others could copy and teach. The intent of the routines was to elevate the heart rate and keep people moving to music to enhance their fitness.

In that same year (1969), Judi Sheppard Missett founded the Jazzercise program and turned her love of jazz dance into a worldwide dance exercise phenomenon. Jazzercise offers a fusion of jazz dance, resistance training, Pilates, yoga, and kickboxing and has improved the health of millions of people worldwide. The program is still going strong and is often offered in churches and community centers, where it can reach the average participant (Jazzercise 2008).

In the 1980s, aerobic dance provided an outlet for many people, especially women, to exercise in a group. The aerobic dance movement brought intentional exercise to the forefront, as before this time, intentional exercise was not in the mainstream. The Aerobics and Fitness Association of America (AFAA) created the first Standards and Guidelines for group exercise in 1983. It also started the first nationally recognized certification for group exercise fitness (which was the first certification both authors of this book took in the industry). In 1984 the IDEA Health and Fitness Association (then called the *International Dance Exercise Association*) held its first international convention. Also during this time the National Sporting Goods Association reported that 24.4 million Americans participated in aerobics (IDEA 2007). Aerobic dance became a pop culture phenomenon—in 1982, *Jane Fonda's Workout Book* (Fonda 1981) topped the best sellers and was followed by her successful high-impact workout video. However, enthusiasm for this new exercise diminished when its injury rates began increasing. Injuries to the shins, feet, and knees were particularly common in high-impact aerobics (Mutoh et al. 1988; Richie et al. 1985). Many variations of aerobic dance, such as low-impact aerobics, were developed to provide more variety and promote a safer way of exercising to music. One study (Brown and O'Neill 1990) found that 66% of participants in high-impact aerobics experienced injuries compared with only 9% of people in low-impact aerobics. Low-impact aerobics became the craze of the late 1980s, and some experts believed it to be a better option than traditional aerobic dance (Koszuta 1986). Less impact produced less jarring on the joints, and thus low-impact aerobics still provided fitness benefits while reducing the risk of injury to the musculoskeletal system. In the late 1980s aerobics participants started to overcome the no pain, no gain experiences that were so prevalent in the early 1980s (Francis and Francis 1988).

Kernodle (1992) believes that step aerobics was invented to cope with a lack of space for activities engaging large muscle groups. He wrote that aerobic dance exercisers became "pioneers in moving in small spaces" (page 68). In 1990 Gin Miller, the developer of Step aerobics, presented step to a large group of instructors at AFAA's APEX convention. She stated her reason for inventing step was to have fun while rehabilitating her knee. In a gym, 20 to 30 people can move effectively in an aerobic dance class. By adding steps that make vertical movement possible, almost twice as many people can participate within the same space. Step was also developed to maximize space and prevent injury (Francis 1990). Step uses gravity to overload the body. It reduces the injury risk because it allows the whole body to work against gravity without subjecting the lower body to the impact forces of high- or low-impact aerobics. Step instructors have figured out ways to add impact into the activity by running on the step or jumping. This activity is mostly low impact but it can become high impact if participants prefer and the instructor gives choices for impact movements.

The step movement of the 1990s led to the development of many forms of group exercise. Water exercise, indoor cycling, trekking, and several other group activities surfaced. Many group classes developed in the 1990s did not require dance skills or even rhythm. Therefore, the term *aerobic dance* was replaced by *group exercise* to better describe the broad scope of activities that had emerged. In 1996, Eller noticed that many clubs had dropped the word *dance* from their schedules. He believed that the dance choreography had become too difficult and was keeping participants from enjoying the activity, and so people were looking for other class options.

Since the 1990s, group exercise has grown into a diverse offering, providing options for almost every ability and preference (see table 1.1). Many classes combine all of the various health-related fitness components into one session. Group exercise classes are the lifelines of many health clubs and fitness centers. They generate enthusiasm and create the connectedness needed to keep people coming back. When group exercise first emerged, many people considered it to be a fad, but by now it has become clear that group exercise is here to stay. The IDEA Health and Fitness Association educates group exercise instructors all over the world. Kathy Davis, the executive director of IDEA, has stated that "fitness instructors are the heart of the health club, for they're the ones who bring the people back to the club every week" (Asp 2007, page 6).

Currently personal training is very popular, but in the same hour a personal trainer spends with one client, a group fitness instructor may reach 40 to 50 participants. Personal trainers who are also group exercise instructors may have many more opportunities to find clients due to their visibility as group instructors. The recent trends in personal training focus on group sessions vs. one on one training as being beneficial to the clients and trainers.

According to the IDEA 2006 survey of fitness trends (Ryan 2006), the average class duration has increased recently, and a greater number of 60-minute classes are being offered. The 2007 IDEA Fitness Trends survey (Ryan 2007) reported that step and high-low impact, while declining slightly, are still staple programs for most facilities. The survey lists core conditioning, indoor cycling, small group, dance, and fusion classes as growing, and describes how the number of classes being offered per week is holding stable at 35. Finally, the 2007 survey found that beginning and intermediate exercisers make up 83% of facility users. Nine percent of facilities had the average length of time for group exercise classes at 90 minutes. As obesity continues to increase and fewer and fewer people participate in physical activity, a person might question why class duration is increasing in group exercise when fewer people are exercising regularly (Jakicic and Otto 2005). As group exercise instructors, we might ask if we are remaining in touch with the general public.

The American College of Sports Medicine (ACSM) recently published its observations on fitness trends (Thompson 2007) in its *Health and Fitness Journal*. The ACSM is attempting to

Table 1.1 Possible Group Exercise Class Choices

Choreograph to music	Stretch and strengthen	Mind and body	Coaching and non-beat driven	Combination/ fusion classes
Step	Stretching	Yoga	Water exercise	Cardio Core
Kickboxing	Group stability ball	Pilates	Stationary cycling	Cycle Strength
Hip-hop	Circuit strength	T'ai chi	Group strength using machines	Step and pump
Latin (dance)	Boot camp	NIA	Trekking	Yogilates

Note. NIA = Neuromuscular Integrative Action.

Health-Related Fitness Components Defined

Cardiorespiratory Endurance

Cardiorespiratory fitness is defined as the ability to perform repetitive, moderate-to-high-intensity, large-muscle movement for a prolonged period of time.

Flexibility

The amount of movement that can be accomplished at a joint.

Muscular Strength

The maximum amount of force a muscle or muscle group can develop during a single contraction.

Body Composition

The percentages of fat, bone, and muscle in a human body.

understand and define a trend versus a fad in the fitness industry. It completed its survey on fitness trends in 2007 and then again in 2008. The 2008 survey was sent to 7,700 fitness professionals certified by the ACSM. The response rate was 24% when including responses from countries outside of the United States. The survey found that the number one fitness trend is that more and more clients are looking for educated and experienced fitness professionals. The limitation of this survey was that the respondents were ACSM certified and thus were educated and experienced. Other interesting findings from this survey were that 10 of the top 20 trends involved instruction of fitness in a group setting. Group exercise is not a fad, as many said it was when it first began. It has become a staple that will be part of the fitness industry for a long time. Thus, as group exercise instructors, we must realize who we are programming to, and how we should direct that programming will be important in making a difference in the overall health and wellness of the population. Let's also not forget that in many clubs group exercise sessions generate a profit (Nogawa-Wasman 2002) on top of providing health benefits for participants.

Group exercise is an exciting field; although it originated in aerobic dance, its current devotees participate in a wide range of activities such as indoor cycling and kickboxing. Given the great variety of group activities, we might ask, how does group exercise work? Are there common features that group exercise classes share? The answer is yes, and this chapter covers general concepts that apply to all group exercise sessions. First, we examine the health benefits of group exercise. Second, we discuss the key teaching skills related to instructing group exercise. Third, we discuss the major certifications available for instructors of group exercise classes. These certifications provide a formal educational framework on which all group exercise classes can be evaluated and taught. Fourth, we cover the advantages of group cohesion.

ENHANCING QUALITY OF LIFE

As instructors, our overarching purpose for offering group classes is to help people live happier and healthier lives through exercise. We want our classes to enhance the quality of life of all our participants. Kravitz (2007) believes that the future of fitness professionals is to develop and endorse programs that are directed toward the enhancement of health for our clients. We do this by incorporating the health-related fitness components into our program design. This book revolves around the health-related components. In fact, in the first four chapters we will review these fitness components and discuss how to accomplish them through group exercise program design. The health-related fitness components include cardiorespiratory endurance, muscular strength and endurance, flexibility, and body composition.

Another important aspect of group exercise is the socialization and connectedness its participants experience. Research confirms that a low level of social support is associated with a two- to threefold increase in risk of cardiovascular disease and mortality (Mookadam and Arthur 2004). A lack of social support is also linked with an increased risk of death from cancer and infectious disease (Uchino 2006). Many of the new forms of group exercise such as stroller babies or organized outdoor walk/run groups increase not only physical activity but also social connectedness (McGonigal 2007). According to Estabrooks (2000), the presence of a highly task-cohesive group has the greatest influence on exercise adherence. For example, many group exercise classes offered at 9 a.m. attract stay-at-home mothers who enjoy exercise and sharing stories about their children. Often, retirees find that their group exercise class is their social outlet. Some exercise classes celebrate birthdays together, go to lunch together, and form their own social network.

As class instructors, we should encourage group cohesion while teaching. In fact, Bray and colleagues (2001) found that the fitness instructor's ability to communicate, teach, and motivate was an important predictor of exercise attendance. Popowych (2005) suggests starting a class with an icebreaker or creating a party atmosphere by tying jingle bells on shoes during the holiday season.

Group cohesion can be accomplished only in a group setting. In strength and conditioning rooms, where the participants are on their own machines and performing their own routines, group cohesion is less likely. Group exercise encourages interaction and can enhance emotional as well

Exercise and Health Research Findings

According to Hedley and colleagues (2004), 66% of adults were either obese or overweight in 2001-02. Among young people aged 6 to 19, 31.5% were at risk for being overweight and 16.5% were overweight. Health experts suggest that if today's youth keep supersizing their meals while downsizing their physical activity, they risk becoming the first generation of Americans to live shorter lives than their parents lived, owing to obesity-related heart disease and diabetes (Weir 2004). In addition, the many health risks associated with obesity are economically costly. According to Bortz (2003), United States citizens ultimately will save money if they are healthy. In fact, Pratt and coworkers (2000) found that the average annual direct medical care cost was $1,019 for physically active people and $1,349 for inactive people. Ostbye and colleagues (2007) documented that obese workers filed double the number of worker compensation claims and lost nearly 184 days due to illness or injury per 100 employees. These statistics are a 13-fold increase over those from nonobese workers.

Exercise is an important part of maintaining a healthy body weight. Jakicic and colleagues (2003) found that a 12-month program combining exercise and diet resulted in significant weight loss and improved cardiorespiratory fitness for various durations and intensities of exercise. The study showed a direct relationship between total weekly energy expenditure and weight loss. Liemohn and Pariser (2002) observed that strengthening the core muscles on a regular basis reduces low-back pain.

So how does group exercise help create healthy lifestyles? Grant and colleagues (2004) studied a group of 26 women in their 60s who were participating in a 12-week group exercise program. The study found that both functional and psychological improvements occurred as a result of participating in a 40-minute group fitness session twice a week. Beginner exercisers are often more comfortable with becoming informed about exercise when they are in the group setting. They like being instructed because they can learn correct exercise techniques and gain motivation to continue working out. Another study on older women and group exercise (Clary et al. 2006) revealed that step and walking programs resulted in better improvements in postural stability or static balance when compared with a program of core stability training (ballates). Any activity that keeps people moving will make a difference in their health. Howley and coworkers (2005) advocate that getting people moving is the first way to control obesity. If group exercise increases energy expenditure, then it will affect the health-related components of fitness.

as physical wellness—especially if the instructor fosters an interactive environment.

As different formats of group exercise continue to be created and studied, the ACSM position stand on fitness for healthy adults continues to evolve (American College of Sports Medicine 2006). It is interesting to note that the current guidelines validate a typical group exercise class format dating back to the inception of group exercise in the 1970s. The guidelines include cardiorespiratory, muscular strength and endurance, and flexibility training, all of which have been a part of the group exercise experience for a very long time. Today, many group exercise classes are also incorporating balance exercises into their experiences. Balance and agility exercises are recommended in the current ACSM guidelines for older adults (Nelson et al. 2007). The authors of these important guidelines refer to balance and agility exercises as *neuromuscular exercises.* Incorporating balance exercises into the group experience not only helps prevent falls in older adults but also enhances the neuromuscular system in order to prevent the deterioration of balance that occurs with age.

Table 1.2 summarizes the 2006 ACSM position stand on fitness for healthy adults. The recommended duration for cardiorespiratory exercise continues to be 20 to 60 continuous minutes or 10-minute bouts accumulated throughout the day to equal 20-60 minutes for 3 to 5 days per week. Including 30-minute group classes in programming is a good way to attract participants who may be new to group exercise and to help them meet the guidelines for exercise participation. Many facilities are finding success with 30-minute or shorter classes; Lofshult (2002) suggested that the most popular class length is 30 minutes because it accommodates the busy lives of today's participants.

Offering a variety of class times and activities is important for successful fitness programs. At the beginning of the decade, public health experts (Hooker 2003) predicted that fitness professionals would begin collaborating to expand movement experiences, especially at the community level. This has come to fruition; one example is the way the group exercise experience is being moved outdoors in the form of boot camps, neighborhood walking groups, and stroller baby classes.

The *Surgeon General's Report on Physical Activity and Health* (Pate et al. 1995) focuses on the importance of activity within daily living, such as walking the dog or taking the stairs. It states that every U.S. adult should accumulate 30 minutes or more of moderate-intensity physical activity on most, preferably all, days of the week. Recently, the U.S. Health and Human Services Department (HHS) expanded this report into the *Guidelines for Physical Activity* (2008), advocating for 150 minutes of physical activity per week with less emphasis on frequency of exercise. Group exercise instructors cannot assume that people are getting 150 weekly minutes of physical activity due to the conveniences of daily living. In the '70s and '80s we could assume most American participated in 30 minutes of daily physical activity. Now we can no longer assume this is the case. Clapp and Little (1994) studied the physiological effects of participants and instructors who were performing three types of group exercise routines (low impact, high impact, and step). These researchers concluded that the participants consistently underestimated their level of performance. It is clear that neither instructors nor participants are clear about the intensity of exercise in a group setting.

As instructors, we need to stress the guidelines for exercise as well as activities of daily living. For instance, a hip-hop class may involve only moderate cardiorespiratory intensity movement and may not contain the other class elements such as muscular strength and flexibility. The HHS report would support the fact that the participants are getting their weekly physical activity regardless of what fitness component is being focused on. Therefore knowing where participants are with their physical activity and fitness levels will be important in terms of meeting their healthy lifestyle goals.

The challenge for group exercise instructors is to apply current research and information from the ACSM 2006 position stand (see table 1.2) and the HHS Guidelines for Physical Activity (2008) report to develop safe, effective, and highly motivating workouts that make a difference in participants' health and wellness. Enhancing quality of life is a theme we need to carry throughout our group exercise class. Franco

Table 1.2 2006 ACSM Position Stand on Fitness for Healthy Adults

Training	Mode	Frequency	Intensity	Duration
Cardiorespiratory	Large muscle groups; dynamic activity	3-5 days/week	40-85% of HRR or $\dot{V}O_2R$; 55-90% of HRmax; 12-16 RPE	20-60 continuous minutes or 10-min bouts accumulated throughout the day to equal 20-60 min
Resistance	8-10 exercises to include all muscle groups	3-5 days/week	Volitional Fatigue (19-20 RPE); stop 2-3 reps before volitional fatigue (16 RPE)	One set of 3-20 repetitions
Flexibility	Static stretch all major muscle groups	*Minimal*: 3-5 days/week *Ideal*: 5-7 days/week	Stretch to tightness but not to pain. No bouncing!	15-30 seconds, 2-4x/stretch

and colleagues (2005) found that 30 minutes of walking gave older adults aged 50 years or older 3.5 more years of disease-free life. In addition, researchers at the University of Illinois reported that participating in 12 weeks of aerobic exercise for 3 hours a week significantly increased brain volume in older adults (Begley 2006). If we can provide these benefits to our group exercise participants, then we are giving them a very valuable gift. The gift of health and life is more precious than any other gift a person can receive.

An effective class begins with the attitude and atmosphere established by the instructor. A wide range of factors can influence a class environment. In the following discussion we focus on the professionalism of the group exercise instructor, who needs to be both a motivator and an educator (Claxton and Lacy 1991; Francis 1991; Kennedy and Legel 1992).

STUDENT-CENTERED VERSUS TEACHER-CENTERED INSTRUCTION

The motivational and inspirational aspect of instructing group exercise includes having new moves, catchy music, and state-of-the-art equipment as well as communicating and cueing movements effectively. The educational part of instructing group exercise involves knowing why certain moves are selected, incorporating current research and knowledge within a session, and

making educated decisions about the information given to participants. It is important to be both a teacher-centered and a student-centered instructor at the same time.

Let's compare and contrast a teacher-centered instructor with a student-centered instructor. The teacher-centered instructor focuses on developing relationships with students that are anchored in intellectual explorations of material; in group exercise, this means learning the movements and following along. They focus more on content than on student processing, and their approach is associated with the transmission of knowledge. Your focus while wearing the teacher-centered hat is to help students imitate your movements successfully. The student-centered instructor, on the other hand, strives to establish an atmosphere of independence, encouragement, attainable goals, and reality. A student-centered instructor places the learning characteristics of all learners under the microscope and pays special attention to low-performing learners. Your goal when acting as a student-centered instructor is to clarify and individualize what is needed to create positive learning experiences to help your students enjoy success and the overall experience.

Learning to take responsibility for the health and well-being of participants starts with establishing a positive and professional attitude and atmosphere. Kandarian (2006) believes a group exercise instructor needs to be an instructor and not a performer. He advocates for instructors to "leave their post up" positions from the front of the class and move around the room so they can get to know their participants (page 87). A purely student-centered instructor is often perceived as being there to make a difference in people's lives. A purely teacher-centered instructor can be mistaken as being there for their own personal workout. Following are examples of how a teacher-centered instructor and a student-centered instructor perceive the learning experience. Possessing attributes from both of these styles will enhance the learning experience of students in a group exercise class. Recent observations of online learning experiences are beginning to demonstrate the importance of having both teacher-centered and student-centered learning experiences (Edmundson 2007).

PROFESSIONAL CERTIFICATION AND CONTINUING EDUCATION

A group exercise class must be built on the foundation of participant safety. An important aspect of safety is becoming certified by a national organiza-

tion. You do not necessarily have to be certified in order to teach group exercise, but certification proves that you have content knowledge and are serious about your role as a professional fitness instructor. Malek and colleagues (2002) confirmed the value of formal education when they found that a bachelor's degree in exercise science and possession of ACSM or National Strength and Conditioning Association (NSCA) certification as opposed to other certifications were strong predictors of a personal trainer's knowledge. We suggest that similar credentials might be strong predictors of a group exercise instructor's knowledge. A recent ACSM article on credentialing (Whaley 2003) discussed the importance of formal academic education in creating fitness professionals. Many universities are now offering degree programs for fitness professionals. This was not the case when the fitness profession was just starting in the 1970s. We encourage you to continue your formal education, especially if you want to manage a fitness center and enhance healthy living for your participants. Fitness instructors who desire to place their participants' health and well-being at the forefront of group exercise

Teacher-Centered Instruction

- Instructor's role is to give information.
- Emphasis is on getting the movement right and performing the correct patterns.
- Students are the only learners.
- Instructor teaches from a stage and does not leave the front of the room.
- Students passively reflect on the information and movements that are given to them.
- The overall class atmosphere is competitive and individualistic.

Student-Centered Instruction

- Instructor's role is to coach and facilitate the experience.
- The instructor and the students learn together.
- The instructor moves around the room and makes contact with all participants during the class.
- Emphasis is on moving and learning from errors rather than performing perfectly.
- Students are actively involved in the learning process, and the instructor carefully observes the students' progress before moving on to more difficult movements.
- The culture is cooperative, relaxed, and supportive.
- Partner exercises or countdowns of exercises bring the group together and make it less competitive.

need to gain as much knowledge about how the body works as possible. The International Health, Racquet and Sportsclub Association (IHRSA) recommends that club owners hire fitness instructors with certifications from agencies accredited through the National Commission for Certifying Agencies (NCCA). IHRSA believes that doing so will help fitness professionals take a legitimate place on the health care continuum because accreditation of a credentialing organization by NCCA is the standard for many other allied health professionals (nurses, athletic trainers, and so on). According to the American Council on Exercise (ACE 2005), certification is the hardware of the fitness business and education is the software. We recommend getting certified and attending continuing education offerings so that you can be the best fitness professional you can be.

Many national certifications involve written and practical exams for which an instructor must demonstrate basic skills in exercise leadership and its related components (e.g., anatomy and physiology, heart rate monitoring). We recommend taking nationally recognized certifications because these tests are designed by many professionals who agree on pertinent knowledge in the field of exercise instruction. Local or club certifications or training programs are always a good place to start getting the education you need to take a national certification exam. Most nationally recognized certifications require you to have cardiopulmonary resuscitation (CPR) certification before sitting for the exam. The ACE Group Fitness Instructor certification is the only national exam in group exercise that is NCCA approved. There are many personal training certifications that are NCCA approved. At the end of this section is a list of organizations that provide fitness training and certification. We have been involved with many of these organizations and know that they all have good training programs for group exercise instructors.

Many organizations and universities train group exercise leaders, and it is good to experience different kinds of training; however, when it comes to certification, make sure the organizations you choose are credible and their tests are professional. Many fitness professionals have more than one certification depending on what skills they need and use. Usually a group-focused certification and a one-on-one certification are good to have. We recommend taking more than one certification exam, because completing each is a learning experience in itself. It is our hope that more and more universities will offer exercise leadership classes so that certification will become simply a verification of knowledge. We also hope that this book will prompt faculty and staff within universities to provide academic training for group leadership. Currently many academic institutions offer degrees in kinesiology (the study of movement), but often these degrees do not include a group exercise leadership component. There is a difference between a fitness professional and an instructor who works part time leading fitness classes. The fitness professional often has had formal training and education in exercise prescription and fitness assessment.

Some companies, recreation departments, and health clubs insist that their instructors be nationally certified. Others set up their own training or coursework that must be completed. Either method is a step toward elevating exercise instruction and ensuring a certain level of knowledge and expertise. But having a certification does not automatically mean that you will be a wonderful instructor. It just means that you are serious and willing to increase your knowledge and experience. We have attended many workshops, lectures, and seminars from the organizations mentioned in this chapter. We keep our national certifications current but also continually update and improve our teaching skills through continuing education events held by many of these organizations. Certification is important but continuing education is equally important.

■ American College of Sports Medicine—ACSM certification is recommended for the professional who has a degree in a health-related field and supervises a program in a facility. A bachelor's degree is required for most ACSM exams. The exam is administered online and requires knowledge of exercise science, fitness assessment skills, and leadership principles.

■ American Council on Exercise—ACE offers the only NCCA-credentialed group exercise exam. A four-year degree is not necessary for taking the ACE Group Fitness Instructor certification exam. ACE has other certifications for personal trainers and has developed a new Advanced Health and Fitness Specialist Certification exam for the

Group Fitness Certification and Continuing Education Organizations

Aerobics and Fitness Association of America (AFAA)

15250 Ventura Blvd., Ste. 200
Sherman Oaks, CA 91403
877-968-7263
www.afaa.com

Alberta Fitness Leadership Certification Association (AFLCA)

c/o Provincial Fitness Unit
University of Alberta
Edmonton, Alberta T6G 2H9
780-492-4435
www.provincialfitnessunit.ca

American College of Sports Medicine (ACSM)

401 W. Michigan St.
Indianapolis, IN 46202-3233
317-637-9200
www.acsm.org

American Council on Exercise (ACE)

4851 Paramount Dr.
San Diego, CA 92123
800-825-3636
www.acefitness.org

Can-Fit-Pro

110-225 Consumers Road
Toronto, ON M2J 1RA
800-667-5622
www.canfitpro.com

SCW Fitness Education

1618 Orrington Ave., Ste. 202
Evanston, IL 60201
877-SCW-FITT
www.scwfitness.com

World Instructor Training Schools (WITS)

206 76th St.
Virginia Beach, VA 23451-1915
888-330-9487
www.witseducation.com

IDEA Health and Fitness Association

10455 Pacific Center Ct.
San Diego, CA 92121-4339
800-999-4332
www.ideafit.com

YMCA of the USA

101 N. Wacker Dr.
Chicago, IL 60606
800-872-9622
www.ymca.net

fitness professional who possesses a four-year degree in a health-related field.

■ Aerobics and Fitness Association of America—AFAA does not require a four-year degree to take its exam. The exam includes both a written and a practical component. AFAA offers some of the most specific certifications in the group exercise industry, such as certifications in primary group exercise, step, kickboxing, and emergency response. AFAA also offers many continuing education workshops such as Practical Skills and Choreography; Perinatal Fitness, Senior Fitness, Floor, Core, and More for Personal Trainers; Practical Pilates; Practical Yoga Instructor Train-

ing; Midlife Fitness for Women; and Mechanics of Injury Prevention.

■ The Alberta Fitness Leadership Certification Association—AFLCA is a not-for-profit organization dedicated to creating, promoting, and implementing national standards for the training and certification of group exercise leaders. The AFLCA provides a minimum of 44 hours of training involving a written theory exam, specialty training courses, and assessment of practical skills. AFLCA approved trainers currently offer a wide variety of Certification and Accreditation training, including the following: exercise theory, group exercise fundamentals, resistance training, aquatic exercise, fitness for the older adult, choreography, cycle, step, portable exercise equipment, and mind/body group exercise training.

■ Can-Fit-Pro—Can-Fit-Pro offers a variety of certifications in group exercise, personal training, nutrition, pre- and postnatal exercise, older adult exercise, mind–body exercise, and sport conditioning. Program courses are delivered in person and range from 16 to 25 hours in length. Most certification exams consist of a written theory exam and an assessment of practical skills. Can-Fit-Pro courses and exams are delivered nationally by a team of trainers and master trainers.

■ SCW Fitness Education—SCW certification blends practical, theoretical, and physiological knowledge of successful teaching techniques for group exercise. The emphasis is on class sequencing, warming up, proper progressions, creative delivery, musical phrasing, proper cueing, and choreography development. This certification focuses on leading in front of others and demonstrating proper teaching skills.

■ World Instructor Training Schools—WITS has schools nationwide in colleges and universities to meet the needs of serious students entering the fitness field. WITS provides a 6-week course that is 36 hours long and includes a final written and practical skills exam. Half of the course is theoretical and the other half is hands on and practical. Students must develop actual group exercise routines, which they then lead in the final exam.

■ IDEA Health and Fitness Association—IDEA holds several conferences for fitness instructor education throughout the year, including an international conference, a personal training conference, and several others that are filled with group exercise ideas and education on fitness and health concepts. IDEA also publishes the *IDEA Fitness Journal,* which is an excellent resource for group exercise instructors, as every edition has a section devoted to improving group exercise instruction.

■ YMCA of the USA—Each YMCA operates independently and therefore has different certifications and training procedures. Overall the various YMCAs offer certifications both in group exercise and in personal training. Their trainings involve hands-on and practical skills for teaching group exercise.

GROUP COHESION RESEARCH

The major emphasis of training programs for group exercise instructors has been on class content. What has been lacking is guidance on connecting the participants so that a sense of community develops within the group class. Alan (2003) believes that this connection is often what brings older adults to a group exercise experience. Teaching group classes from a student-centered perspective with an emphasis on developing group cohesion can enhance adherence. According to Carron and colleagues (1988), group cohesiveness is related to individual adherence behavior. For example, when participants meet and socialize with others in the class, they are more likely to keep coming and therefore keep exercising. Carron and colleagues suggest that we all should examine how to keep groups of participants coming back to class so that we can enhance the health and wellness of the overall population. Therefore, investing resources in improving group exercise classes and creating a sense of community within a fitness facility is a logical step in improving national health.

Heinzelmann and Bagley (1970) reported that 90% of adult participants in an exercise program prefer to exercise in group settings. Similarly, Stephens and Craig (1990) reported that 65% of participants prefer to exercise in groups rather than alone. Group exercise programs also appear to produce higher rates of exercise maintenance than individual-based programs produce (Massie and Sheperd 1971). Spink and Carron (1992) found that group cohesion in female exercise participants played a role in adherence behaviors. Finally, Carron and colleagues (1988) had class participants, both those who dropped out and those who stayed with the program, assess the cohesiveness of their classes. Participants who stayed with the program held higher perceptions of cohesiveness.

Spink and Carron (1994) stated that while the university setting provides greater perceptions of task cohesion, the health club setting relies more on social factors for adherence. For example, when students are graded on attendance, their attendance improves. In clubs, creating social opportunities allows fitness classes to build cohesion and improve attendance.

Seniors tend to have a better exercise experience when the experience includes social activities outside of the exercise class. Estabrooks and Carron (1999) found that elderly exercisers who have stronger beliefs in the social cohesiveness of their exercise class have more positive attitudes about exercise. In a study by Spink and Carron (1993), an exercise class that participated in a team-building intervention program had significantly fewer dropouts than a similar class that did not undergo the team-building program. Finally, Carron and colleagues (1996) have shown that developing a highly cohesive group that is focused on the exercise task and its possible outcomes is likely to have a strong effect on compliance.

All of this research tells us that as group exercise instructors, we need to do more than stand in front of a class and lead exercises. We need to engage in exercise together. By focusing on being student-centered teachers, we can make a difference in the cohesiveness of our classes and ultimately this difference will improve the health and wellness of our participants. The following suggestions are practical ways for facilitating cohesion in a group exercise class:

- Learn your participants' names and have them learn one another's names.
- Schedule social outings.
- Share personal stories—be human with your participants!
- Use partner exercises and have participants introduce themselves while doing exercises.
- Discuss current health topics with participants.
- Have participants count down or up with you when performing exercises.
- Name movements after participants.
- Keep track of attendance and connect with participants who are not coming to class.
- Celebrate birthdays, anniversaries, and any other important dates.

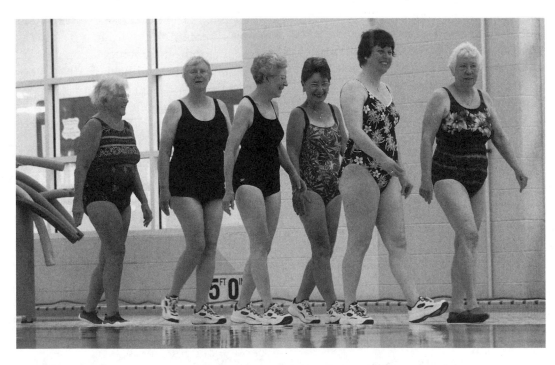

▶ A focus on healthy lifestyle brings many seniors to group exercise classes, where they enjoy socialization benefits as well.

- Have holiday themes or tie jingle bells on participants' shoes.

CHAPTER WRAP-UP

Group exercise can be very powerful if participants feel welcome, learn new things, get to know others, are taught safely, and believe that their time is being well spent. The experience can not only make a positive change in their emotional outlook but also improve their health and quality of living. One of the biggest challenges for the group exercise instructor is to balance all of the health and emotional elements of the group exercise experience—this is, perhaps, the most difficult skill a fitness professional can master.

Once we move beyond emphasizing quantized fitness gains and aesthetics, we can understand that the real power of exercise lies in the experience itself. Group exercise is definitely an experience, and the instructor makes or breaks that experience.

▶ Assignment

Part 1: Attend a group exercise class and evaluate whether the instructor has a student-centered or teacher-centered style. Give a minimum of three specific examples that support your analysis.

Part 2: Interview the class participants about the level of group cohesiveness. Ask whether they have met people through the experience and if that has helped their adherence. Write a one-page paper on your findings.

Evolution of Group Fitness

CHAPTER OBJECTIVES

By the end of this chapter, you will

- understand the evolution of fitness from body image to health,
- be able to give examples of marketing tactics for group exercise,
- understand why group exercise instructors are role models,
- know how to create a healthy emotional environment, and
- understand basic business practices for group exercise programming.

The gluteus medius muscle abducts the hip, but why does a participant need to strengthen this muscle, and what exercises work the muscle effectively? During the aesthetic movement of the 1970s through the 2000s, the main purpose for exercising was to lose weight and look better, and many of us still select exercises based on cultural influences that dictate what our bodies should look like. You can't turn on a TV without seeing an advertisement about how some exercise video helped Susie look "like this." Today, our looks are still important to us, but we also want more out of fitness: We want to feel better. We want to have more energy to enjoy life regardless of our age, and we want to maintain our independence as long as possible by performing daily tasks with vigor. It is estimated that the average American loses 13 to 15 years to dysfunction: While we may live a long life, we spend the last few years of that life unable to function independently. Thus each of us will fight for our independence in our later years.

The shift from aesthetics to health is a result of the baby boomers experiencing a lack of function in their later years. A 70-year-old client signed up for personal training because he could no longer open jars. Another one could not pick up a bar of soap dropped in the shower and so sought help to improve his ability to perform adult daily living (ADL) tasks. The inability to perform ADL tasks often leads people to a group exercise setting. The number of Americans aged 65 years and older will increase from 35 million in 2000 to 40 million in 2010 (a 15% increase) and then to 55 million in 2020 (a 36% increase). This age group has helped to coin the term *functional training*.

The baby boomers started the fitness movement, and they continue to dictate its direction. Table 2.1 outlines the effects the baby boomers have had on group exercise instruction and how the functional training movement has developed. Astrand's (1992) article titled "Why Exercise?" contained the first hints of the functional training movement. In this article he stated, "If animals are built reasonably, they should build and maintain just enough, but not more, structure than they need to meet functional requirements" (154). Wolf (2001)

suggested that "training movements and not muscles may be the paradigm shift needed for today's functional conditioning" (23). Santana (2002) defined functional training as "a specific duty or purpose of a person or thing" (22). Functional training develops the muscles to make the performance of everyday activities easier, smoother, safer, and more efficient. Functional exercises improve a person's ability to function independently or perform a sport more effectively. This focus underlies what is perhaps the most important benefit of attaining fitness: Everyday activities become easier and quality of life improves. Other research (Flegal et al. 2005) looking at the estimated number of deaths in the United States associated with being underweight, overweight, and obese found that being overweight alone is not associated with excess mortality. Overweight individuals can improve their health by attending group exercise in the same way that leaner individuals can. Slowly society is moving away from a focus on aesthetics to one that emphasizes purposeful movement and enhanced quality of life. However, another study linked obesity to an increased risk for dementia (Whitmer 2005). This study indicated that obesity in middle age is an independent risk factor for future dementia. Thus staying active and maintaining a normal weight may not be important for overall increased length of life but may be important for being free from other diseases that limit functional capacity.

Much of the 1970s exercise equipment was designed to enhance aesthetics and not for improving functional abilities. For example, a seated biceps curl variable resistance machine improves the strength of the biceps, but if you lift with your arms and your lower back gets injured while lifting, you have not trained the whole system but instead have trained the individual parts. Recently researchers have begun to acknowledge that the body works as a system and so we need to train it as a system if we wish for our strength training to enhance our lives. DeVreede and colleagues (2005) studied 98 healthy women aged 70 years and older. One group was assigned to an exercise program based on functional tasks (e.g., performing sit-to-stand exercises) and another group was assigned a traditional resistance exercise pro-

Table 2.1 Baby Boomers' Influence on Fitness Trends

Decade	Baby boomers' age	Trend
1970s	20s	High-impact aerobics, running 10K races
1980s	30s	Low-impact aerobics, walking, running 5K races
1990s	40s	Step, slide, water exercise, indoor cycling, yoga
2000s	50s	Functional fitness, stability balls, balance devices
2010s	60s	Core strength, neuromuscular/proprioceptive emphasis—preventing falls

gram (using variable resistance machines in a circuit). Both groups exercised three times per week for 12 weeks. The results showed that the functional exercises were more effective than the resistance exercises when it came to improving functional task performance. Ginis and colleagues (2003) found that regardless of body image concern, women who worked out in front of mirrors felt worse after exercising than women who exercised without mirrors. A study on body image among women who were strength training confirmed that the training improved not only strength but also body image (Ahmed et al. 2002). Fitness is becoming a prominent part of people's lives as they find a sense of purpose in working out that goes deeper than how they look. We may have started the fitness movement based on appearance, but this focus is certainly changing as we move into the functional training era of physical activity. Some people believe that soon we will no longer be discussing *exercise* and *fitness*. We will remove the *E* and *F* words for good and instead begin discussing the importance of physical activity in our lives. The terms *exercise* and *fitness* have turned away some potential participants from enjoying movement experiences. Group exercise is more than a movement experience—it also has a very social component.

We need to emphasize both and promote the fun and social atmosphere of group exercise in order to bring back past participants who have had a bad experience with exercise and fitness.

Over the past few years, the quantum theory of physics has gained acceptance (Capra 1982). One aspect of this theory is the idea that the world should not be analyzed into independent, isolated elements—the system should be considered as a whole. For example, a person may develop arteriosclerosis, a narrowing and hardening of the arteries, as the result of an unhealthy lifestyle that involves improper diet, lack of exercise, and excessive smoking. Surgical treatment of a blocked artery may temporarily alleviate the resulting chest pain, but it does not make the person well. The surgical intervention merely treats a local effect of a systemic disorder that will continue until the underlying problems are identified and resolved. An analogous scenario in the fitness setting is training individual muscle groups without training the core that houses those muscle groups. We cannot use the strength we gain by doing a bench press unless we also work on total-body strengthening. This concept is the essence of the new fitness movement. Pilates, yoga, and tai chi are types of group exercise classes that have gained popularity because of this trend.

CULTURAL INFLUENCES ON BODY IMAGE AND EXERCISE

By looking back at the Reebok advertisements promoting aerobic shoes for group exercise, we can witness the aesthetic movement in action. Many of the ads from athletic shoe companies in the 1970s, 1980s, and 1990s showed a small picture of the shoe and a very large picture of a very fit body (usually a female body). These ads contained two messages. The first was that if you bought the shoes, you would get the body in the picture. The second was that

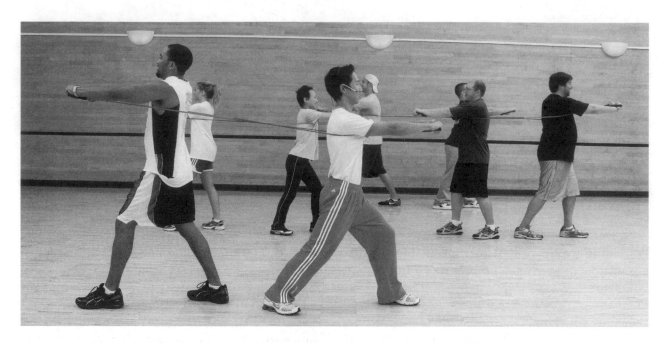

▶ Group exercise classes continue to be a prominent part of fitness center offerings, as they provide the structured activities that help increase adherence in all participants, from beginners to advanced exercisers.

participating in group exercise would help you get the body in the picture. Several studies on exercise and weight loss conducted during the 1990s (Gaesser 1999; Miller 1999) encouraged people to place a greater emphasis on lifestyle change and pay less attention to aesthetics. Nike was one of the first companies to change its focus from aesthetics to promoting healthy lifestyles. According to Bednarski (1993), who was a marketing executive for Nike at the time, it was difficult to convince male managers that women needed a different marketing strategy, but eventually Nike created an empowering campaign for women that featured shoe ads about how it felt to be fit through sports and exercise. The focus was more on all the things people could do with this newfound energy than on what they looked like. Many of the ads did not feature any people; instead, they touted the health benefits of exercise. Enhancing self-esteem was seen as more important than changing body shape.

Health clubs and workout videos also used body image to market programs and products. The *Buns of Steel* video campaign is one example. Naming group exercise sessions by body parts is another example. Classes like Ultimate Abs,

Butts and Guts, and Absolute Arms all played on the aesthetics message. One way you can move your program into the new functional fitness era is by naming your classes in a positive, educational way. One fitness center uses time to describe its classes. For example, it calls a class *Step 45* instead of *Ultimate Step* so that participants will know that the class lasts 45 minutes. The more hard core the class name sounds, the fewer beginners the class will attract.

Although we have come a long way in changing the message from aesthetics to function, we still have a long way to go. In an article on triathlon training, Kahlkoetter (2002) stated that "women often begin training for the purpose of losing weight and looking better, rather than for inner satisfaction and health" (48). Hollywood, television, magazines, and movies are often to blame for the unrealistic images put before us. However, one example of an attempt to set things straight is that of Jamie Lee Curtis. After being featured in the fitness movie *Perfect,* she admitted to engaging in many unhealthy practices in an effort to keep her perfect body. In a *More* magazine article (Wallace 2002), she posed for a picture with no makeup or body touch-ups so that people could see her true self. Hopefully her example will lead others to unveil the Hollywood myth of the perfect body. Men are not immune to the body image issue. According to Beals (2003), muscle dysmorphia (a form of body image disturbance found among male weightlifters) is on the rise; half of those with this disorder have tried anabolic steroids.

GROUP EXERCISE INSTRUCTORS AS ROLE MODELS

According to Westcott (1991), participants rate knowledge as the most important characteristic of their fitness instructor. Most participants also look up to their fitness instructor as a role model. This puts a lot of pressure on instructors: What kind of role models are we? In an article by Evans and Kennedy (1993), results of an informal research study of female fitness instructors showed that while their average body fat was 20% (which is quite low, because the average in the United States is 32%), 46% of the fitness instructors believed they were very or somewhat overweight. A study (Nardini et al. 1999) of 148 female fitness instructors found that 64% perceived an ideal body as one that was thinner than their current body. Olson and colleagues (1996) studied female aerobics instructors and found that 40% of the instructors indicated a previous experience with eating disorders. The aerobic dance instructors in this study had Eating Disorder Inventory scores that suggested behaviors and attitudes consistent with those of female athletes whose sports emphasize leanness and of women who have eating disorders such as anorexia and bulimia. A survey conducted at a large national conference on water fitness (Evans and Connor 1995) revealed that 48% of water fitness instructors agreed that they constantly worry about being or becoming fat. Another study (Krane et al. 2001) looking at female athletes and regular exercisers suggested that concern about excessive exercise in these women was warranted.

Fitness professionals experience a myriad of intrinsic and external pressures to achieve the coveted lean and toned appearance. These pressures may lead us to engage in dangerous exercise behaviors and weight loss techniques. We must take care of ourselves as well as take care of our participants who may have body image problems. Yager and Jennifer (2005) identified the important role that educators play in preventing eating disorders. In order to screen potential instructors and create healthy environments, we must be healthy ourselves. If you are teaching group exercise classes but do not have a good body image, consider talking to a counselor or stepping down as a fitness instructor until you resolve your personal issues. You cannot be an effective role model if you cannot walk the talk. The good news is that several of the new group exercise formats are improving body image self-acceptance through increased body awareness. Impett and coworkers (2006) found that frequent yoga practice is associated with greater body awareness, positive affect, and satisfaction with life as well as decreased negative affect.

Davis (1994) studied physical activity in the development and maintenance of eating disorders and found that, for a number of anorexic women, sport or exercise is an integral part of the progression toward self-starvation. She suggests that overactivity be viewed as a primary and not a secondary symptom of eating disorders. As instructors, we should not teach several classes in one day, as by doing so we will be telling our participants that overexercising is healthy. We also ought to role model healthy behaviors such as taking the stairs instead of the elevator or parking our car farther away from the building so that we have a longer walk in. Modeling daily activities to our participants is as important as modeling healthy intentional exercise patterns.

Freeman (1988) reminds us that body image is independent of physical characteristics. An attractive person can feel plain or unattractive. Because body image and self-esteem are perceptions, changing our bodies will not improve our image or self-esteem unless the physical changes are accompanied by changed perceptions. Improving body image involves changing how we think about our bodies. Taking charge of our own body image perceptions and educating our participants about body image are important if we are to be positive role models.

> ### Resources for Disordered Eating and Body Image
>
> www.nationaleatingdisorders.org—National Eating Disorders Organization
>
> www.eatright.org—American Dietetic Association
>
> www.4woman.gov—National Women's Health Information Center

CREATING A HEALTHY EMOTIONAL ENVIRONMENT

In addition to being positive role models, group exercise instructors need to establish a comfortable emotional environment for their participants. Education, motivation, and creative class content are not the only factors that keep participants coming back to group exercise. It is necessary to tap into participants' feelings to affect adherence. Bain and colleagues (1989) performed a research study on overweight women taking part in an organized exercise program. The authors found that 35% of the participants who were overweight dropped out, while only 7% of the participants who were at their recommended weight quit the program. Although factors such as safety, comfort, and quality of instruction affected the women's exercise behaviors, the most powerful influences seemed to be the social circumstances of the exercise setting, especially concerns about visibility, embarrassment, and judgment by others. As the instructor, you should acknowledge all the participants—from the ones you know to the ones who always hide at the back of the room. What you do and say can affect class atmosphere, and a simple hello can make all the difference to a newcomer in group exercise. Ornish (1998) believes that interpersonal interaction might be the single most important ingredient for creating an accepting environment in a group exercise experience. Goleman (1998) suggests that having emotional intelligence in any group setting dictates the success of the group experience. Goleman

believes that "the emotional economy is the sum total of the exchanges of feeling among us. In subtle (or not so subtle) ways, we all make each other feel a bit better (or a lot worse) as part of any contact we have; every encounter can be weighted along a scale from emotionally toxic to nourishing" (1998, 165). A specific example of supporting others within a group exercise setting is announcing before class how great it feels to be in a group exercise class to improve overall health and well-being. Contrast this with telling the class how you ate two desserts the night before that you intend to work off during the session. The first statement leaves participants with a health-related sense of purpose for the workout. The second statement can send a message that punishment through exercise is recommended after overindulging.

In another study on group dynamics in physical activity, Fox and colleagues (2000) found that enjoyment during physical activity is optimized when a positive and supportive leadership style is coupled with an enriched and supportive group environment. Instructors affect adherence and may be an important predictor of exercise behavior. We help create a sense of community that is often what brings adults to a group exercise experience. Using social intelligence (Goleman 2006) as well as emotional intelligence in any group setting dictates the success of the group experience. A specific example of failing to apply social intelligence in a group exercise setting is staying in the front of the room and talking only to participants in the front row. The participants in the middle and back rows may feel unacknowledged by you. If instead, you know the names of everyone, greet all the participants when they come into class, and move around the room to encourage them throughout the workout, you will be creating a healthier emotional and social atmosphere. Social intelligence is another key ingredient for being a positive role model.

An environment where instructors present a body beautiful can also intimidate participants. Eklund and Crawford (1994) compared two similar video exercise routines that differed in the apparel of the instructor—in one, the instructor wore a thong-style exercise leotard while in the other the same instructor wore shorts and a

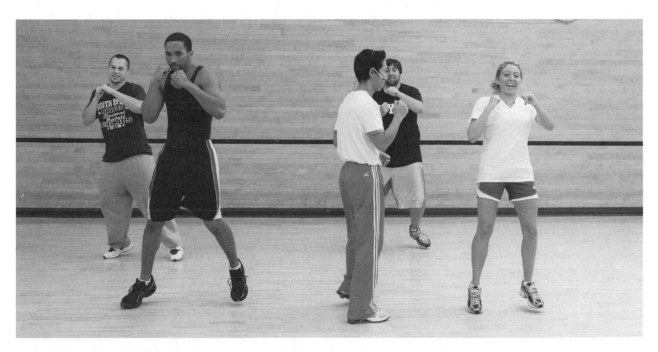

▶ A group exercise instructor dressed professionally and socializing with participants.

T-shirt. Physique-anxious participants rated the thong leotard video more unfavorably than the shorts and T-shirt video. Thus instructors can help participants become more comfortable with their own bodies and keep them exercising by wearing modest exercise clothing. We live in a culture in which a thin and toned body is seen as the ideal. According to Ibbetson (1996), the idea that thinness is beauty is so well accepted that body image dissatisfaction is remarkably high. Some researchers indicate that body image disturbance is so prevalent that it can be considered a normal part of the female experience (Silberstein et al. 1987). Evans (1993) makes the following recommendations for enhancing participant and instructor body image perceptions:

- Wear professional attire that is not too revealing and will make all participants comfortable.
- Display educational materials on body image acceptance at strategic locations.
- Use positive motivational strategies. For example, encourage activity outside of class.
- Choose music that sends a positive message.

BASIC BUSINESS PRACTICES FOR GROUP EXERCISE PROGRAMMING

Teaching group exercise requires a very unique set of skills. Instructors must be able to entertain, educate, role model, and think on their feet. In his bestselling book *Blink: The Power of Thinking Without Thinking,* Malcolm Gladwell (2005) suggests that falling back on involuntary subconscious processes can be more effective than using higher-level cognitive functions when completing certain tasks. In many ways his book describes and appreciates the skill set needed to teach group exercise. An instructor has little time to process all that needs to be processed. Decisions must be made within a blink of an eye. A qualified leader is essential for a high-quality group exercise program, and hiring appropriate instructors saves a lot of time and money with initial training.

Group fitness instructors make an average of $23.75 U.S. per hour, specialty instructors make an average of $27.50 U.S. per hour, and yoga or Pilates instructors make an average of $29.50 U.S. per hour (Gavin 2007). Since a program that offers group exercise has a large financial investment, let's review practices that will enhance both the instructor's and the supervisor's knowledge of the business of group exercise.

Fostering Teamwork

Excellence begins with teamwork. Instructors who are part of a good exercise staff cooperate by doing their job and covering their classes, while instructors who are part of an excellent group exercise staff feel like everyone is part of a team and work to support the team. Griffith (2005) made some excellent suggestions for team-building activities that foster fun and enthusiasm within a group exercise staff:

- Divide your staff members into teams based on their specialty areas and assign them tasks.
- Create a choreography notebook of step moves developed by all step instructors on staff.
- Create an overall schedule for group strength classes so instructors and participants know which muscles will be worked in which class.
- Have the mind–body class instructors develop a flier that describes the differences between yoga and Pilates.

Whenever it is possible, have the instructors work together to solve problems. This creates a sense of ownership for instructors, and their loyalty to the program will skyrocket. Instructors who do not feel a part of the team often seek employment at another facility, so keeping group exercise instructors happy is important. Remember that group exercise is often the heart of the club. If the heart of the club is happy, then so are the club members. Fostering teamwork is a good business practice.

Recruiting and Retaining Group Exercise Instructors

Gregor (2006) suggests that all prospective instructors be put through a detailed hiring and auditioning process before being offered a job. A personal interview, an audition, shadow teach-ing, and a final evaluation make up the standard process for hiring and preparing an instructor to teach. Several examples of how to recruit and train instructors are available (Brathwaite et al. 2006; Davidson et al. 2006).

As an instructor, you are a consumer of the industry. Strive to find a program that will be the best experience for you. A good experience often occurs because of sound business practices. Check the facility group exercise schedule. Is the program diverse? Are 30-minute classes offered so you know health and wellness are a priority for the owners? If the class schedule contains mostly hour to hour-and-a-half classes they are not catering to the average population and thus may have fewer participants overall in their program. The management's priority is often the bottom line. It can become the job of the staff and instructors to keep the health and wellness of the club members at the forefront. Hagan (2005) suggests that facility schedules should have a start and finish date for classes, offer multilevel classes, offer fusion classes, and highlight a new specialty class in order to enhance adherence of participants. If you find such a schedule, then you have found a good club or facility that you will want to check into further. Look at the mission statement of the organization you are considering. If the mission focuses on enhancing the health and wellness of participants and the organization demonstrates sound business practices, you will enjoy being a group exercise instructor at its facility. Always check into business practices before auditioning to be an instructor for a given organization.

Continuing Education

An excellent group exercise program requires and provides continuing education that keeps its instructors stimulated and updated. Often facilities bring in speakers or pay a stipend for instructors to attend conferences. An excellent organization not only retains instructors via incentives to perform continuing education but also evaluates its instructors. Feedback is the breakfast of champions (Tharrett 2008) and the way to grow as a professional. When applying with an organization, it is important to find out if you will be evaluated as a group exercise instructor. Ask for an evaluation of your class or videotape it yourself and watch yourself teaching. This is a wonderful way to learn about your abilities as a group exercise instructor. There are many tools that help evaluate the effectiveness of a class. One is the group exercise class evaluation form, discussed in chapter 3 and provided in appendix A; there are others that have been introduced in the professional literature (Eickhoff-Shemek and Selde 2006). Learning and growing as a professional is an important aspect of teaching group exercise. Always check to make sure the organization you are working for has sound business practices that you are proud to represent.

CHAPTER WRAP-UP

Fitness professionals need to be leaders in moving the industry from the aesthetic era of exercise to a more purposeful reason to improve our health and wellbeing. We can choose to buy into the ideal body image presented to us by the media and society at large or to portray a normal, healthy example to our participants. A healthy body image is not something that we can take for granted as exercise instructors, as many of us are affected by our own body image perceptions. However, feeling good about ourselves and projecting this confidence to our participants could be the most important health message that we have to offer them. Representing health and wellness for the participants is an essential component of enjoying who you are working for as an instructor for group exercise. That is why it is also important to work for an organization that has sound business practices and supports the health and wellness of its members.

▶ Assignment

Part 1: Write a 250-word story that examines your physical activity from the time you started exercising until now. Describe how your exercise experience has changed for you over the years.

Part 2: Look up the Web site of a fitness facility that offers group exercise classes. Write down the Web site, the facility name, and the mission statement and look over the group exercise schedule. Check to see if the Web site outlines the facility's hiring process for group exercise instructors. Write a brief 200-word paragraph on your findings.

Core Concepts in Class Design

CHAPTER OBJECTIVES

By the end of this chapter, you will

- be able to integrate the components of health into group exercise class design,
- understand how to create a positive preclass atmosphere,
- understand basic health screening for group exercise leaders,
- know important principles of muscle balance and muscle action terminology,
- understand range of motion,
- comprehend a six-step exercise progression model, and
- review a structural evaluation tool for group exercise instructors.

Integrating the components of health into the group exercise program requires a look into the overall class format. There is no single class format that fits every type of group exercise class. In a step class, it is very appropriate to warm up using a step; however, in a kickboxing class, practicing boxing moves is more appropriate than using a bench during the warm-up segment. In a water exercise class thermoregulation is important, so performing static stretches to enhance flexibility at the end of the workout may not be recommended. Static stretching may be beneficial in the warm-up and stretching segment of a low-impact class for seniors, but a 15-minute abdominal class may forego stretching because the purpose of the class is abdominal strengthening. All are examples of why the same class format may not be suitable for all group exercise classes.

Let's take a closer look at the basic segments of a group exercise session:

1. Warm-up
2. Cardiorespiratory activity
3. Muscular conditioning
4. Flexibility and cool-down

These segments apply to most types of group exercise, including high- and low-impact programs, step classes, water exercise, indoor cycling, and sport conditioning. Most group classes begin with a preclass preparation followed by a warm-up that includes specific rehearsal movements to prepare for cardiorespiratory activity. These movements are performed at a low to moderate speed and range of motion; they are designed to warm up the body for activity and increase blood flow to the muscles. A cardiorespiratory segment follows the warm-up and is aimed at improving cardiorespiratory endurance and body composition and keeping the heart rate elevated for 10 to 45 minutes. After the cardiorespiratory workout, a gradual cool-down returns the heart rate to resting levels and prevents excessive pooling of blood in the lower extremities. A muscular conditioning segment might be included before or after the cardiorespiratory segment, depending on the activity. The class then ends with a flexibility and cool-down component that includes stretching and relaxation exercises designed to further lower the heart rate, help prevent muscle soreness, and enhance overall flexibility.

HEALTH-RELATED COMPONENTS OF FITNESS

Chapters 5 through 7 review in detail how to incorporate the health-related fitness components into a group exercise class. These components are the warm-up and stretch, cardiorespi-

---

Muscular Conditioning Terminology

- **muscle strength**—The maximum force a muscle or muscle group can produce at one time.
- **muscle endurance**—The ability to perform repeated muscle actions, as in push-ups or sit-ups, or to maintain a static muscle action for a prolonged duration.
- **muscle power**—The ability of a muscle or muscle group to move a force quickly. Power = force × distance ÷ time.
- **muscle stability**—The ability of a muscle or muscle group to stabilize a joint and maintain a desired position. This is particularly important for postural muscles that stabilize the spine, pelvis, and shoulder girdle.
- **overload**—Giving the body a challenge greater than it has had in the past. Overload may be accomplished by increasing the exercise frequency (number of days per week), duration (number of sets or repetitions), intensity (amount of weight lifted), or mode (type of exercise). The exercise mode can be modified by switching to a new exercise for the same muscle group; adding an unstable surface such as a stability ball, BOSU balance trainer, or foam roller; or changing from dumbbell to elastic resistance.

ratory conditioning, muscular conditioning, and flexibility and cool-down. Before delving into formats designed for specific classes, this chapter reviews the common principles that apply to all group exercise classes. The principles of muscle balance apply to all aspects of a group exercise class; selecting proper exercise progressions is also important. Learning the range of motion of different muscles and understanding how to select exercises for a group exercise setting are also critical to promoting healthy lifestyles for your participants. Finally, having an evaluation form that lists and reviews these concepts allows the group exercise program director and instructor to be on the same page with how to implement these principles in a class.

Notice that three of the four main segments of a group exercise class are aligned with the health-related fitness components listed in the 2006 ACSM position stand on exercise (see table 1.2 in chapter 1). When the first ACSM position statement was published in 1978 (ACSM 1978), it contained only cardiorespiratory guidelines. At that time there was very little research on strengthening the musculoskeletal system. As clinicians and researchers began to realize that many people were experiencing back pain, the research focus turned to the musculoskeletal system. In the 1990 ACSM position stand, muscular strength and endurance were included along with cardiorespiratory fitness, but there was still no mention of flexibility. Clinicians and researchers then discovered the importance of having flexible as well as strong muscles, and the 2006 ACSM position stand included flexibility. Group exercise classes have long included all these fitness components even though ACSM guidelines were limited in the past. The current ACSM position stand (ACSM 2006) focuses on all the health-related fitness components, and these components are usually included in a general group exercise class. As the fitness field moves toward functional fitness, it is speculated that balance and proprioception training soon will be included in the list of fitness components, because good balance and proprioception are necessary for efficient movement.

The degree to which each of the health-related fitness components is developed in any particular individual can vary widely. For example, a person may be strong but lack flexibility or may have great cardiorespiratory endurance but lack muscular strength. Each component of fitness should be included in a program. We should understand the definitions of muscular strength and endurance and flexibility so that we know that they're being properly included (see "Muscular Conditioning Terminology" on page 28).

The 2006 ACSM position stand was reviewed briefly in chapter 1. The emphasis that a group exercise class gives to each fitness component will vary depending on the objective of the class as well as the fitness level, age, health, and physical skill of the participants. Our goal as fitness

Various Roles of Muscles

Muscles can play different roles depending on the action they are performing. For example, in a triceps kickback, the triceps extends the elbow and is therefore the prime mover (agonist). In a biceps curl, the triceps acts as the antagonist while the biceps flexes the elbow (the biceps muscle is the agonist). And in a bent-over row, the triceps is only an assistor, assisting the action of shoulder extension (the latissimus dorsi are the prime movers). The triceps can also act as a stabilizer. Consider its role in maintaining the plank position—the triceps stabilizes the elbow joint, maintaining elbow extension. So, as you can see, one muscle—the triceps—can play several different roles depending on the exercise.

- **agonist**—The prime mover, which is the muscle that is responsible for the movement that you see.
- **antagonist**—The muscle acting opposite the agonist; it elongates and allows the agonist to contract and move the joint.
- **assistor**—A muscle that assists in performing a movement but is not the prime mover.
- **stabilizer**—A muscle that stabilizes a joint and helps to keep it from moving. When muscles perform a stabilizing role, they contract isometrically.

Muscle Action Terminology

■ **isometric movement**—A static muscle action in which there is no change in the muscle length or the affected joint angle. Breathing is important when performing an isometric action; breath holding and straining, known as the *Valsalva maneuver,* can increase blood pressure.

■ **isotonic or dynamic movement**—A muscle action that is not held but instead involves movement. This is the most common type of muscle action for nonpostural muscles. There are two types of isotonic actions:

- **concentric action**—The shortening contraction of the muscle as it develops tension against a resistance (often called the *positive phase).*

- **eccentric action**—The lengthening action of the muscle as it develops tension against a resistance (often called the *negative phase).*

■ **isokinetic movement**—A muscle action performed using special equipment not generally found in fitness facilities. In this type of action, the speed of the movement is controlled, and any action applied against the machine results in an equal reaction force.

professionals is to include all the components of fitness in our program but not necessarily all in one class. For example, a stretching class will enhance flexibility, and a hip-hop class will provide cardiorespiratory conditioning. Because our participants have busy schedules, we need to make the most of exercise time by emphasizing the health-related fitness components in our programming.

PRECLASS PREPARATION

An effective group exercise class starts with appropriate preclass preparation. Most group exercise instructors arrive at least 15 minutes before a class starts in order to prepare equipment, set up the stereo system, greet participants as they begin to arrive, and have some mental preparation time. Preclass preparation also involves getting to know your participants so you can design the class to improve their health and well-being.

A few common points must be considered when preparing for any group exercise class. As the instructor, you should know your returning participants and orient new participants, create a positive atmosphere, and begin class on time with equipment ready for use.

Teaching a Mixed-Level Class

Teaching a class with both beginner and advanced participants can be challenging. A mixed class is usually the norm rather than the exception because of scheduling conflicts. Describing classes by duration is one way to help participants find a class at the appropriate level. An example is offering a step class that lasts 30 minutes, one that lasts 45 minutes, and another that lasts 60 minutes. The participants can then choose a step class based on their fitness level. The 30-minute step classes should contain simpler movements to provide beginners with basic cardiorespiratory training and introduce them to basic moves on the step. Kennedy (2004) reported that members of a focus group who attended group exercise classes stated that they stayed away from classes that included the words *turbo, ultimate,* or *extreme* in their titles. These names do not always appeal to the beginner. More descriptive names such as Step 30, Cycling 45, or Kickboxing 60 may appeal to a broader range of participants and will allow participants to choose their preferred duration. Offering 20- to 30-minute classes focusing on stretching or muscular conditioning will also help prepare some of the more sedentary participants for the longer classes that contain all the fitness components. Some participants, such as those who walk to work every day, may need only a flexibility or a muscular strength and conditioning class. Offering different class options and venturing beyond the typical hour-long format that encompasses all the fitness components will help you meet the health goals of a greater number of people.

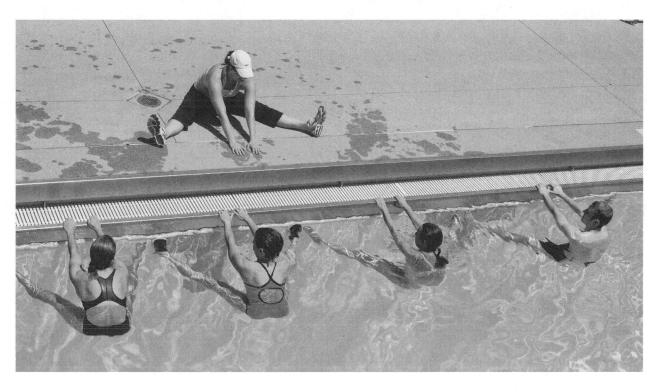

▶ A water exercise class may emphasize the flexibility component of fitness.

Know Your Participants

How do we individualize programs and protect participants during a group exercise class? By knowing the participants! You must know where people have been and what they want and need in order to lead them successfully. Knowing a participant's personal health is an essential part of providing excellent customer service and safety as well as decreasing professional liability.

Although there are many ways of obtaining information, the ideal is to have the participants fill out a written medical history form that you can review before they arrive to class. Unfortunately, a completed medical history is often the exception rather than the rule. All of us have been in the situation where our class is just getting underway when a new participant appears. Using a short medical history form can help solve this problem. You can have a new participant fill out the short form upon arrival. Then you can quickly review the contents, clarify any vague information, and make a mental note of areas needing emphasis during class.

An example of a completed short form is included for your reference (see figure 3.1). Short and long health history forms and an informed consent form are located in appendixes B through D. These forms have been adapted from many sources and can be changed to fit your specific needs. The format is not really important. What you need is a great deal of information in a small space.

The British Columbia Ministry of Health designed the Physical Activity Readiness Questionnaire (PAR-Q) to help identify individuals for whom exercise may pose a hazard. The PAR-Q can be used as a short form or can be conducted verbally. The developers of the PAR-Q suggest that participants who answer *yes* to any of the questions may need to postpone vigorous exercise or exercise testing and seek medical clearance. The PAR-Q is found in appendix E.

Orienting New Participants

A health information form is the beginning of building a shared responsibility for an exercise class and one way to integrate new participants into your class. On this form you also can ask

SHORT HEALTH HISTORY AND CONSENT FORM

Name: _John Smith_   Date: _8-15-08_

The following information will be kept strictly confidential and will be utilized only to help make your workout safe. Please check any conditions that may apply to you.

Have you ever been told by a physician that you have or have had the following?

	YES	NO
Heart attack		✓
High cholesterol (>200)	✓	
Cancer		✓
Arthritis		✓
Seizures		✓
High blood pressure	✓	
Diabetes		✓
Osteoporosis		✓
Stroke		✓
Abnormal EKG		✓
Lung problems		✓
Gout		✓

If you are currently taking any prescription or over-the-counter medications, please list them here:

Beta-blockers

_____

_____

	YES	NO
Do you smoke?		✓
Can you swim?		✓
Do you exercise, aerobically, at least 3 to 4 times a week?		✓

Do you have any past injuries to, or current problems with, any of the following areas?

	YES	NO
Irregular heartbeat		✓
Dizziness		✓
Neck		✓

Low back	☐	☑
Feet	☐	☑
Chest pain	☐	☑
Fainting	☐	☑
Hands	☐	☑
Midback	☐	☑
Ankles	☐	☑
Loss of coordination	☐	☑
Cramping	☐	☑
Hips	☐	☑
Shoulders	☐	☑
Knees	☐	☑
Heat intolerance	☐	☑
Shin splints	☐	☑
Calves	☐	☑

I realize that there are risks, including injury and possible death, to all exercise. While every effort will be made to decrease any risk of injury, I take full responsibility for my participation in this class. Knowing that I may participate at my own pace and that I am free to discontinue participation at any time, I will inform the instructor of any problems—immediately.

Signature: _John Smith_

Date: _8-15-08_

▶ **Figure 3.1** As an instructor, what would you consider if you received this completed short history form from a new participant?

participants when their birthday is, what their favorite reward is, and any other pertinent information that might enhance their performance. To further assist them, you can provide written information about exercise, the facility schedule, or the program in general.

As exercise instructors, we want our participants to feel that they are responsible for their workout and to inform us of their personal physical limitations so we can assist them as much as possible. We can accomplish this by having the participants read and sign an informed consent form. A sample of an informed consent form is in appendix D. Obtaining informed consent ensures that we have met an individual's right to know that there are risks associated with exercise.

Participants also have the right to know how potential injuries may manifest themselves, how the risk of injury will be minimized, and what responsibility they have in reducing their risk.

You must use some type of medical history or informed consent sheet, as it is a critical ingredient in demonstrating care for participants. Also, these forms help establish the foundations of safety, responsibility, and communication, which are necessary elements of the group exercise experience.

Creating a Positive Atmosphere

In chapter 2 we discussed many aspects of being a model instructor, from wearing appropriate attire to creating a healthy emotional environment.

These points are all part of being an effective instructor and therefore need to be included in the evaluation process.

The following are ways to create a positive class atmosphere:

- Introduce yourself to the participants and have them introduce themselves to others in the class.
- Wear attire and footwear that fit the population, and tell participants what gear they need for the class.
- Explain the class format and review what participants can expect from the class.
- Smile, give positive motivational cues, and be energetic with body language cues.

Creating a positive atmosphere begins with introducing yourself and having students introduce themselves before class begins, especially when you are teaching in a facility where different people come to class every week. These introductions help to establish an attitude of "We're in this together." Also, if participants know your name and the names of others in the class, they will be more likely to ask questions and talk to one another. New people coming into a group exercise class are often afraid to ask questions and often feel out of place. Understanding this and asking for class communication will create a more open and safe environment for all involved.

The instructor's attire must be appropriate for the specific group exercise class. For example, when you are teaching a class for seniors, wearing a midriff-baring spandex outfit is inappropriate because it might be intimidating. Observe what participants wear to class and try to match their clothing so they will feel more comfortable. Ask what attire they prefer. At the same time, balance the comfort level of the class with functionality. Your spinal alignment and form should be visible with each movement you demonstrate. Make sure to notice what participants are wearing and discuss appropriate footwear and attire for the various group exercise classes you teach. For example, some indoor cycles have special clipless pedals that require a specific type of cycling shoe. Likewise, water exercise requires a swimming suit that can give the support needed to exercise effectively.

Finally, give an overview of the class format after introducing yourself. Because so many different classes are being offered and so many unique instructional techniques are being used, the participants need to know your class expectations. Tell them about water breaks, heart rate checks, expected intensity levels, and any other pertinent information that might help make the class a student-centered experience. For example, you might begin your class by saying, "This is a 30-minute stretching class. There will not be an aerobic component. The only equipment you will need is a mat. Please take your shoes off for the class." In some fitness centers, participants enter the class and see a dry erase board that contains the instructor's name, a welcome note, and a list of equipment needed for the session. The board informs participants about class expectations if they miss the verbal announcements. After previewing the class format, the instructor should explain to participants their individual responsibilities. One such responsibility is exercising at the desired intensity. There is nothing worse than having a participant come to you after class and say, "This class was too easy for me." Intensity is the responsibility of the participant, not the instructor. You must suggest modifications that allow participants to pick an appropriate intensity level, but you are not responsible for choosing that intensity level.

 See the DVD for a demonstration of creating a positive atmosphere.

MUSCLE BALANCE

Instructors usually include base moves (moves that appear over and over again during the routine) within the cardiorespiratory segment. These base moves often work the quadriceps and hip flexor muscles. Examples include the basic march in place in basic cardio segments, the basic step in step, the cross-country skier in water exercise, and the flat-road medium resistance in cycling. The problem with these base moves is that many participants use the quadriceps and hip flexors extensively in activities of daily living; therefore, exercise routines that continue to use these muscles repeatedly can create muscle imbalance. Balancing daily flexion with other movements is important. Understanding how the body functions in daily movement can help you determine which muscles are naturally stronger and which muscles need extra attention during the group exercise session. For example, walking forward works the hip flexors, and so focusing on movements that use the buttocks and the hamstrings (the muscle groups opposing the hip flexors) helps participants achieve muscle balance. Also, the abductors are important stabilizer muscles for the hips. Thus incorporating abductor moves into the cardiorespiratory segment is recommended (see figure 3.2).

Water exercise is the exception to the need to focus on muscle balance. In water exercise, muscle balance is achieved automatically because there is no gravity. When we flex the hip in water, the iliopsoas and rectus femoris perform the work assisted by buoyancy. When we extend the hip, the hamstrings and buttocks perform the work. This is why in the water there is automatic muscle balance. With the exception of water exercise, it is important to analyze what movements work which muscle group and vary the selection to promote overall muscle balance as well as minimize repetitive movements.

Make the most of your floor space to minimize repetitive motions and select movements that work the muscle groups in opposing ways. Use different geometric configurations when using floor space (i.e., move in circles, diagonally, up and back) during the aerobic segment to help increase safety and interest. Try performing figure eights, walking in circles, walking around the step, and making letters like an A or a T either on the floor or on a step to add variety and fun to your cardiorespiratory segment.

To ensure that your routines balance the muscles properly, let's take a moment to review where the major muscles are and what they actually do. Each joint has several muscles attaching to it, and these muscles act in opposition to each other (see figure 3.3). Maintaining a balance of strength and flexibility in the muscles around your joints is an excellent way to prevent injuries and promote smooth functioning.

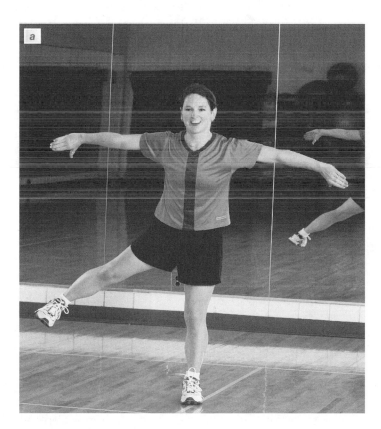
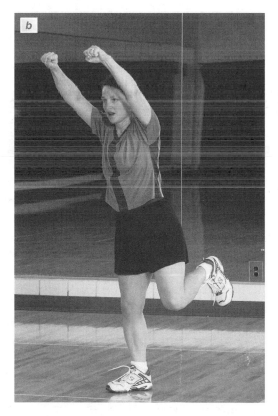

▶ **Figure 3.2** Working these muscle groups helps balance the movements of daily living: *(a)* abductors and *(b)* hamstrings.

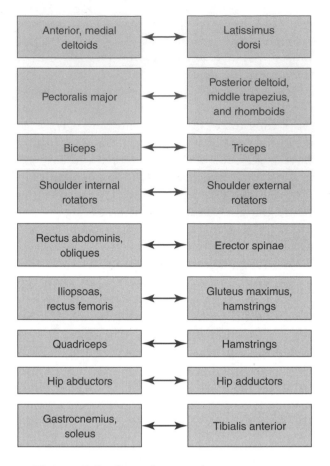

▶ **Figure 3.3** Opposing muscle groups.

You will notice that many of your students possess typical muscle imbalances attributable to activities of daily living, sedentary lifestyle, obesity, poor posture, or simply the natural tendency to perform activities in a forward direction. You need to know what these common muscle imbalances are and how you can help correct them by incorporating appropriate strengthening or stretching exercises into your class. Muscle imbalances left unchecked often lead to injury, especially when participants increase their frequency, intensity, or duration of exercise. Table 3.1 lists the most common muscle imbalances.

Because most muscle imbalances arise from a lack of muscular balance in activities of daily living, we need to keep in mind what participants do when they are not in an exercise class. Then we can analyze which muscle groups participants need to develop to counterbalance the muscles they use most often in daily activities. Think of the group exercise class as

an opportunity to balance the work of daily living. Stretching and strengthening muscles that are not regularly used can help participants improve overall muscle balance. This approach brings the role of the group fitness instructor closer to that of an individualized trainer (Kennedy 1997). For a summary of which muscles generally need strengthening and stretching for improved health, see table 3.2.

Table 3.2 was created by conceptualizing the muscles we use for routine living. For example, we normally pick up an object by using elbow flexion, which works the biceps concentrically. We then put the object down by working the biceps eccentrically against gravity. Because of the direction of gravity, we often do not need to work the triceps in daily living. The list in table 3.2 is designed to help enhance functional daily living skills for participants who are exercising for health and fitness. It is not meant to suggest that the stronger muscles should not be worked in a group exercise setting; however, we need to focus on balancing the weaker muscle groups and the stronger muscle groups, especially if our goal is to create workouts that will benefit participants in their daily lives.

The strategy for dealing with muscle imbalances is to strengthen the weak, loose, or small muscles and stretch the tight, short, or strong muscles. For example, since the abdominals typically are weak or loose, it makes sense to include strengthening and shortening exercises such as abdominal crunches in your class. Conversely, since the low-back muscles (the erector spinae) are commonly tight and tense, it makes sense to incorporate feel-good stretches such as the angry cat stretch on hands and knees to lengthen and relax the lower back. If this muscle imbalance between the abdominals and the erector spinae isn't addressed, the spine will gradually be pulled out of alignment, and this misalignment leads to excessive lordosis, or swayback. Excessive lordosis is a contributing factor in low-back pain, a chronic disorder that 8 of 10 people in developed countries will experience at some point in their lives (Frymoyer and Cats-Baril 1991).

The abdominals can be trained dynamically through their full range of motion as spinal flexors. This type of training is especially important when the abdominals are weak and

Table 3.1 Common Muscle Imbalances

Muscle	Problem	Typical cause	Correction
Pectoralis major	Tight	Poor posture when sitting and standing	Stretch
Posterior deltoids, middle trapezius, rhomboids	Weak, overstretched	Poor posture when sitting and standing	Strengthen
Shoulder internal rotators	Tight	Poor posture, carrying and holding objects close to body	Stretch
Shoulder external rotators	Weak	Poor posture	Strengthen
Abdominals	Weak	Poor posture, obesity	Strengthen
Erector spinae	Tight (and often weak)	Poor posture, obesity	Stretch (and strengthen)
Hip flexors	Tight	Poor posture, sedentary lifestyle	Stretch
Hamstrings	Tight	Sedentary lifestyle	Stretch
Calves	Tight	Wearing high heels	Stretch
Shin	Weak	Not enough use in daily activities	Strengthen

Table 3.2 Muscle Balance for Functional Training

Muscles that need strengthening	Stabilizers that need strengthening	Muscles that need stretching
Anterior tibialis	Erector spinae	Gastrocnemius and soleus
Quadriceps and hamstrings	Abductors	Quadriceps and iliopsoas
Rhomboids and middle trapezius	Adductors	Upper trapezius
Pectoralis minor and lower trapezius	Abdominals	Pectoralis major
Shoulder external rotators (teres minor and infraspinatus)		Hamstrings
Triceps		Erector spinae
Gluteals		Anterior and medial deltoids
Posterior deltoid		

overstretched and are contributing to excessive lordosis. The abdominals also can be trained isometrically as stabilizers of the spine. In stabilization or core-strengthening exercises, a primary focus is contraction of the transverse abdominis to cause a hollowing or a sensation of navel to spine. Some practitioners use the term *bracing* to help describe the action needed to keep the spine in a neutral position. In stabilization exercises, other joints and muscles may be moving, creating the challenge of maintaining a motionless spine throughout the duration of the exercise. A system of exercises designed to build a strong core is known as *Pilates* (developed in the 1920s by Joseph Pilates). This type of exercise has become very popular and promotes core strength, endurance, and flexibility. See chapter 14 for more information on Pilates.

Rounded shoulders and a hunched upper back (known as *excessive kyphosis*) can also become habitual over time, leading to neck, shoulder, and upper-back pain. Help your students prevent this problem by leading them in more posterior deltoid, middle trapezius, and rhomboid exercises than chest exercises and by emphasizing chest and anterior deltoid stretching.

 See the DVD for a demonstration of using opposing muscle groups for balance.

BALANCING STRENGTH AND FLEXIBILITY

Another aspect of balance is the relative balance that exists between the strength and the flexibility of a particular muscle group. If participants have a great deal of flexibility in a particular muscle group, you may need to emphasize strength exercises rather than stretching to avoid injury to joint structures and ligamentous tissues. If the participants have greater strength than flexibility in a particular muscle group, you may need to perform flexibility exercises to avoid strains to the muscles and tendons. Many people believe the misconception that more flexibility and more strength are always beneficial. In fact, it is the relative balance between flexibility and strength that creates a healthy system.

Both the athlete and the average adult with back problems require an appropriate emphasis on stretching or strengthening. Gymnasts, who are often the epitome of flexibility (especially of the spine), have high rates of back pain and injury. Their back pain can be associated with hyperflexible joint structures caused by overstretching of the spinal ligaments, as well as with the impact forces experienced in dismounting and hyperextending in the spine. Strong muscles may be able to compensate for hyperflexibility, but without strengthening exercises, pain and injury continue to weaken the spinal structure. Thus the extreme flexibility required in gymnastics makes lifelong back and abdominal strength exercises essential to any gymnast's program. After gymnasts leave the sport, they still must continue these strengthening exercises to maintain adequate function, because the damage done while practicing the sport is very likely irreversible.

People whose spinal ligaments might be overstretched due to a back injury from an accident or from repetitive motion of the spine have similar problems. As long as they perform their strengthening exercises, they can control pain and maintain a reasonable level of function. When they stop their strengthening exercises, the pain increases and reinjury may result. Much of low-back pain is caused by improper body mechanics often related to sedentary living. Fitness instructors can make a huge difference in back pain by educating clients about proper posture in everyday tasks. A study (Kellett et al. 1991) on the effects of an exercise program on sick leave caused by back pain found that the number of sick leave days attributable to back pain decreased by 50% in the exercising group. Telling a person with back pain to rest may cause even more back problems, because the muscle weakness and joint flexibility caused by inactivity are often the reasons for the onset of back pain. Literature on back pain (Cinque 1989) reminds us that a number of physicians recommend getting out of bed and into the gym. In the final analysis, you as the instructor need to recognize what muscle or muscle group is responsible for a specific action and what muscle group works in opposition to that action. You need to consider what exercises you will choose to enable your participants to function optimally during exercise and daily life.

RANGE OF MOTION

Understanding joint range of motion (ROM) for each muscle group is another part of teaching safe and effective exercise technique. Why is understanding joint ROM important? Imagine you are teaching a standing hip abduction exercise. ROM for hip abduction is approximately 45°. If participants are abducting beyond 45°, then they are probably using the hip flexor muscle group to perform the action since hip flexion has a ROM of 120° (the hip flexor group is a strong muscle group and has the largest ROM). If you do not know that ROM for the hip abductors is 45°, you will not be able to recognize when participants need to correct their technique (so that they can get the most out of their workout). The highlight box illustrates joint ROMs for the major muscle groups. Note that ROM is a *range* and not an absolute number.

Some participants will have greater ROM in a joint than others have due to their overall flexibility. This is an important concept to teach when discussing ROM.

PROGRESSIVE FUNCTIONAL TRAINING CONTINUUM

Used in the traditional sense, *progression* refers to progressively overloading the body's systems

Joint Range of Motion

Hips and Knees

- Knee extension: 90°
- Hip flexion: 120°
- Hip flexion with knee flexion: 120°
- Knee flexion: 125°
- Hip hyperextension: 10-15°
- Hip abduction: 45°
- Hip adduction: 40°

Spine

- Spinal lateral bending: 30°
- Spinal rotation: 40°
- Spinal flexion from standing: 70°
- Spinal flexion from lying down: 70°
- Spinal hyperextension: 70°

Arms and Shoulders

- Arm flexion: 135°
- Shoulder adduction: 50°
- Shoulder hyperextension: 45°
- Shoulder abduction: 90-180°

Neck

- Neck abduction and adduction: 40°
- Neck hyperextension: 50°
- Neck flexion: 40°
- Neck rotation: 55°

Foot

- Plantar flexion of foot: 45°
- Dorsiflexion of foot: 10-15°

and increasing the training stimulus over time to gradually increase fitness adaptations. In resistance training, the muscles gradually become stronger or gain endurance as well as enhanced neuromuscular control, coordination, and balance. Gradual adaptation can be achieved by changing the variables of exercise frequency, intensity, duration, and mode. Our progressive functional training continuum addresses mode, or type of exercise. Addressing this issue is very important to group exercise because instructors have to decide what exercises they are going to teach in their classes. The progressive functional training continuum (Kennedy 2003; Yoke and Kennedy 2004) helps instructors make better decisions for their participants. Figure 3.4 outlines the continuum.

At one end of the continuum are less-skilled exercises that require less balance, stability, proprioceptive activity, and motor control. Such exercises are safe for almost everyone and require the least amount of instructor cueing. Many of these exercises are performed in a supine or prone position, require isolation movements rather than total-body movements, and strengthen individual muscle groups. A few examples are the supine triceps extension, prone scapular retraction for the middle trapezius and rhomboids, and prone hip extension for the hamstrings and gluteus maximus. These exercises are low risk, easy to cue, and relatively safe for almost all populations.

At the other end of the continuum are exercises that need a great deal of skill and require an ability to maintain joint integrity, including integrity of the spinal joints and the joints involved in core stability (which is the ability to maintain ideal alignment in the neck, spine, scapulae, and pelvis no matter how difficult the exercise). These challenging exercises also place a high demand on proprioceptors and on the neuromuscular system for smooth coordination. As a result, the ability to perform these exercises safely depends on the exerciser's specific experience and overall fitness level. Many sport-specific exercises are categorized at this end of the continuum. A few examples of difficult and controversial exercises include deadlifts, plyometric lunges, handstand shoulder presses, and

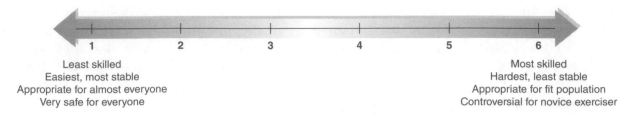

> ▶ **Figure 3.4** Progressive functional training continuum.

V-sits. Although these exercises are considered difficult and higher risk, a very fit person with excellent core stability might be able to perform them safely and appropriately. As a group exercise leader, you have to choose which exercises will be safe for your whole class. We recommend also selecting exercises that allow all participants to be successful. Exercises ranging from 1 to 4 on the continuum are most appropriate for group classes. Exercises in the 5 and 6 portion of the continuum ought to be reserved for advanced classes or personal training. Let's look at the six levels of the progressive functional training continuum in more detail.

Level 1

Isolate and educate. This level focuses on muscle isolation and trains participants to contract individual muscle groups. This helps them build confidence and body awareness and improve their basic muscle functioning. Exercises at this level are often performed in the supine or prone position, with as much of the body in contact with the floor or bench as possible, lessening the need for stabilizer muscle involvement. As a result, these exercises are generally quite safe; just about everyone can learn to do them effectively with minimal risk of injury. Gravity is usually the main form of resistance applied at this level. This level is perfect for almost all group exercise classes because all participants would be successful with these choices.

Level 2

Add external resistance by adding weights, increasing lever length, or using elastic bands or tubes. In many cases, the actual exer-

cise performed at this level is the same exercise performed at level 1—the difference is the added resistance. Notice that in both levels 1 and 2, the instructor needs minimal safety and alignment cueing; it's relatively easy for exercisers to perform these types of exercises safely and effectively while maintaining proper form because of the decreased stabilizer involvement.

Level 3

Add functional training positions. Level 3 progresses the body position to sitting or standing, both of which are more functional positions for most people. Sitting or standing reduces the base of support and increases the stabilizer challenge. In most progressions, the targeted muscle group is still isolated as a primary mover and the stabilizers are merely assisting. This is often the stage in which standing dumbbell exercises or standing exercises using tubing are introduced.

Level 4

Combine increased function with resistance. At this level, resistance from gravity, external weights, or bands and tubes is maximized and overload is increased on the core stabilizer muscles. The exercises at this level are performed in functional positions; most are performed in a standing position to use the core stabilizer muscles. These exercises begin the process of overloading the muscles for the stresses of daily living.

Level 5

Work multiple muscle groups with increased resistance and core challenge. At level 5, the exercises use multiple muscle groups and joint actions simultaneously or in combination with one another. Resistance, balance, coordination, and torso stability are progressed to an even higher level. The emphasis at this level is on challenging the core stabilizers even more. For example, completing an overhead press with dumbbells while simultaneously squatting challenges the core more than simply performing a squat or an overhead press.

Level 6

Add balance, speed, and rotational movements. Exercises at this level may require balancing on one leg, balancing on a stability ball, plyometric movements, spinal rotation while lifting, or some other life skill or sport-specific maneuver. For example, training to clean your house requires power and rotation—not movements that work just a single muscle group. The risk of injury is increased at this level, so instructors must be cautious when introducing these exercises to a group. Although including speed and rotation is not as safe as performing simpler movements, it is how we live. Sensible progression to this level will transition into enhanced life skills. A sample progression is outlined in figure 3.5.

 See the DVD for an application of the progressive functional training continuum.

GROUP EXERCISE CLASS EVALUATION

The group exercise class evaluation form can be found in appendix A. This form covers the principles that apply to most group exercise classes. We will review these principles here and in chapters 5, 6, and 7. You can use this form as an evaluation tool when you are observing classes and as a checklist to enhance your teaching and evaluating skills. Although it is difficult to generalize all group exercise classes to one evaluation tool, we feel the principles included on this evaluation form apply to most group exercise classes. However, if you are teaching a 30-minute muscular conditioning and flexibility class, the warm-up segment and the muscular conditioning and flexibility segment may be the only ones you will use off the form. On the other hand, if you are teaching a 60-minute kickboxing class, then you can use all the components of the evaluation form. This form reflects the health-related fitness components, the ACSM guidelines for exercise, and the basic research-based concepts of exercise physiology. As instructors, we need to keep these in mind when we are teaching group exercise classes so that we can make a difference in the health and wellness of our participants.

Safe, effective, and purposeful class design requires a specific knowledge of fitness in order to provide the appropriate overload needed to achieve the desired gains. Therefore, one of the purposes of the group exercise class evaluation form is to put instructors on the same page and to give them a common language for discussing class format. We recommend that you use this form to evaluate a class and look for the different components of a group exercise class before you attempt to teach. When you complete this chapter and chapters 5, 6, and 7, you will have a general understanding of what is needed to create a safe and effective group exercise experience. In an academic setting, the group exercise class evaluation form in appendix A can be used to grade how well a student applies theory to application. In other settings, this form can be used to set expectations on what should be implemented into all group exercise classes regardless of the selected format (e.g., step, kickboxing, or sport conditioning). Our hope is that program managers require instructors to put thought into how they can deliver the important principles of exercise science that apply to a group exercise setting. The group exercise class evaluation form seeks to summarize these principles and help instructors put them into action. Following is a sample evaluation form completed by a group exercise leader in preparation for an evaluation and audition (figure 3.6). It is our hope that sharing this form with you here, before we discuss all the concepts it covers, will help you understand the big picture of where we are going with putting application into practice.

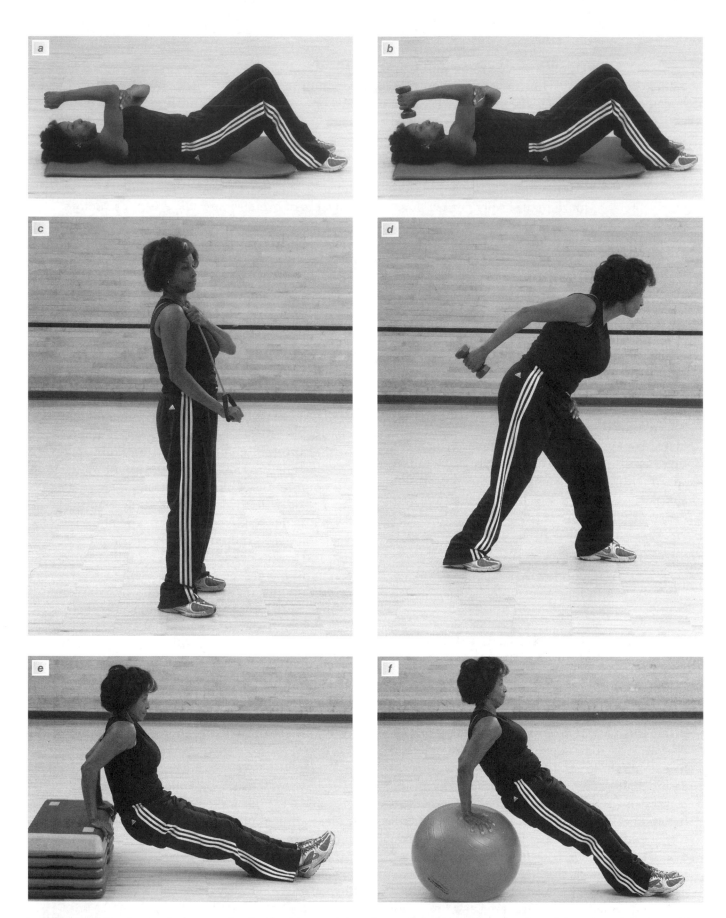

▶ **Figure 3.5** A sample progression for the triceps: *(a)* supine unilateral triceps extension, *(b)* supine extension with weights, *(c)* standing press-down with tube, *(d)* triceps kickback, *(e)* dips off a bench, and *(f)* dips off a stability ball.

GROUP EXERCISE CLASS EVALUATION

Instructor: _Sally Smith_

Evaluator: _____

Date: _____

Class: _Step-10_

Time: _11:15_

Scoring System: 2 = Proficient, 1 = Adequate, 0 = Inadequate

Pre-Class Organization

Begins class on time .... | 1 |

Has equipment and music ready for use.. | 0 |

Acknowledges class .... | 2 |

Comments: _Check CD to see if it works properly_

Warm-Up

Includes appropriate amount of dynamic movement..................................... | 2 |

Provides rehearsal moves.. | 2 |

Stretches major muscle groups in a biomechanically sound manner with appropriate instructions............. | 2 |

Gives clear cues and verbal directions .... | 2 |

Uses an appropriate music tempo (120-136 beats per minute) or motivating music that inspires movement ..... | 1 |

Comments: _Begin stepping in place; grapevine right; tap up, tap down on step; grapevine left; tap up, tap down; right foot march; march up on bench, wave arms; march down, push-down; grapevine left; step up; squat; squat, roll up; right foot on step, toe up on bench, reach out; reverse it, lift back foot; up and down on toes; march right; march bench; step touch; hamstring curls; grapevine left; tap up on left; squat, shoulder press; left foot tap up and reach out; reverse lift back foot; hip hinge (round forward); march; music below tempo (116bpm)_

▶ **Figure 3.6** A completed group exercise class evaluation form.

Warm-Up

Muscle groups	Warm-up	Stretch
Quadriceps and hip flexors	Squat on the floor	Standing hip hinge—keep arms moving—biceps curls
Hamstrings	Hamstring curls on the bench	Front foot on bench, toe up; reach out
Calves	Up and down on toes on the floor	Lift back foot with front foot on bench; bring back foot in slightly and repeat
Shoulder joint muscles	Large arm circles	Shoulder press
Low-back muscles	When doing hip hinge, round arms forward	When squatting, roll up back

Cardiorespiratory Training

Gradually increases intensity 2

Uses a variety of muscle groups (especially hamstrings and abductors) 2

Minimizes repetitive movements 1

Promotes participant interaction and encourages fun 2

Demonstrates movement options and gives clear verbal cues 2

Gradually decreases impact and intensity during cool-down following the cardiorespiratory session 2

Uses music volume and tempo (134-158 beats per minute) appropriate for biomechanical movement 1

Comments: _Repeat combo in 8-count increments after teaching movements; music below tempo (124bpm); use basic moves where the intensity can be increased or decreased based on the energy placed into each movement and the use of arms to get the heart rate up_

Intensity Monitoring

Pulse Rate (PR) or Rate of Perceived Exertion (RPE) application

Takes pulse rate (PR) or RPE at middle of activity 2

Keeps participants moving during PR counts 2

Gives modifications based on PR or RPE results and encourages participants to work at their own levels 2

Comments: _These comments you made during the session were great: "Your rating of perceived exertion should be around 7 because we are halfway through the session." "If you are not at a 7, jump up more on your step, make each move count, move your arms more. If you are around 9, decrease your arm movements to prevent injury."_

▶ **Figure 3.6** _continued_

Muscular Conditioning and Flexibility Training

Gives verbal cues on posture and alignment. 2

Encourages and demonstrates good body mechanics. 1

Observes participants' form and suggests modifications for participants
with injuries or special needs as well as progressions for advanced participants 2

Gives clear verbal directions and uses appropriate music volume 2

Uses appropriate music tempo for biomechanical movement 2

Chooses appropriate music for flexibility training. 2

Includes static stretching 1

Appropriately emphasizes relaxation and visualization 2

Comments: _Strengthening only the rectus abdominis due to time. To complete the entire torso, the obliques (spinal flexion_
with rotation and lateral flexion) and transverse abdominis (compression) must also be strengthened. In addition, the stretch
for the obliques (which would be stretched with the spine rotated and extended—a supine spinal twist) is being skipped.

Muscle group worked	Position/exercise for strengthening	Comments
Upper body	_Triceps dip (on step)_	_Place hands on step with fingers pointed forward. Press shoulder blades down and away from ears. Straighten and flex elbows. Avoid flexing elbows greater than 90° because of shoulder injury. If too difficult on step, just perform on the floor._
Lower body	_Calf exercise (ankle plantar flexion)_	_Stand with proper alignment, knees soft, abdominals contracted, and feet hip-width apart. Stand on edge of step and lower heels as far off the step as possible. Return to starting. If too difficult on step, just perform on the ground._
Torso	_Basic crunch_	_Lie supine with knees bent. Place feet on step. Exhale and flex spine, pulling ribs toward hips. Bring shoulder blades off floor and avoid arching lower back. If too difficult, take feet off step._

▶ **Figure 3.6** *continued*

Muscle group worked	Position/exercise for stretching	Comments
Upper body	*Triceps stretch*	*Stand with feet shoulder-width apart, knees flexed, abdominals in. Point one elbow toward the ceiling and reach your hand down your back. Gently support the stretch with your other hand and press your elbow down. Avoid hunching the shoulders and keep the head forward.*
Lower body	*Calf stretch and soleus stretch*	*Stand with feet staggered and point all the joints forward. Place both hands on your front thighs, keep back heels down, contract your abdominals, and keep the chest slightly lifted, shoulders back and down. Bring back foot in slightly and perform same movement; this stretches the soleus.*
Torso	*Rectus abdominis stretch*	*Lie prone and prop yourself up on your elbows, stretching the spine up and away from your hips. Lengthen the neck and allow it to continue as a natural extension of the spine. Press down against the floor with your forearms to lower the shoulders away from the ears. Slide shoulder blades down your back.*

Overall Summary

Your verbal cues, positive energy, and exercise choices are your strong points. Overall this was a very solid class!

_____

_____

_____

_____

_____

_____

_____

_____

▶ **Figure 3.6** *continued*

CHAPTER WRAP-UP

The general concepts outlined in this chapter apply to all group exercise classes. As instructors, we need to integrate the health-related fitness components into our classes, include preclass introductions and screenings, observe the principles of muscle balance, and learn proper progressions of exercises and appropriate ROMs for movements. This chapter also provided a general overview of the group exercise class evaluation form (found in appendix A), which is an outline of the general principles applying to group exercise classes. You will be referring to this form throughout this book. You will also be using it for assignments and for your final presentations.

▶ **Assignment**

Write down the main headings on the group exercise class evaluation form (preclass organization, warm-up, cardiorespiratory training, intensity monitoring, muscular conditioning and flexibility training). Leave space after each to make notes. Attend a group exercise class and record five observations for each segment. Turn your observations into a 2,000- to 2,500-word paper on what you saw being taught from each segment that refers to the general principles reviewed in this chapter (muscle balance, ROM, and so on). List specific movements and methods you observed being taught by the instructor in each of the main segments.

Music, Fundamental Choreography, and Cueing Methods

CHAPTER OBJECTIVES

By the end of this chapter, you will

- understand issues of using music in a group exercise class,
- understand safety issues and good alignment and technique for cardiorespiratory classes,
- understand the elements of variation,
- know how to create smooth transitions,
- be able to build basic cardio combinations,
- know how to use different choreographic techniques,
- be familiar with different training systems for high/low impact classes,
- be able to cue basic moves in a cardio class, and
- be able to teach a 2-minute cardio routine with at least two 32-count blocks and proper cueing.

In this chapter we'll cover the elements you need to know in order to lead a great music- and choreography-driven class. We'll also discuss legal issues regarding music use and information about sound systems. Then we'll cover basic choreography issues, including performing the common moves, building combinations, teaching freestyle, and transitioning smoothly from one move to another. After that, we'll discuss cueing to music as well as various other types of cues. Finally, we'll describe how to give participants feedback in a nonthreatening way. Most of this information is important for leading any choreography-based class that is taught to music (on the beat), including cardio workouts, step, kickboxing, Zumba, and more. If you practice the drills we suggest and follow along with the DVD accompanying this text, you'll be leading a class like a pro in no time!

MUSIC FOR GROUP EXERCISE

Music is a vital part of almost all group exercise classes. Subjects regularly report that they believe their exercise performance is better with music accompaniment (Kravitz 1994). Music also appears to provide a motivational construct to exercise, buoying participants' mental state. In one study, students who listened to their favorite music while exercising reported feeling more comfortable and experiencing less fatigue (Yamashita et al. 2006). Numerous studies have revealed music's effects on mood, activity level, heart rate, blood pressure, and more (Hallam 2001). In cardio programs, step classes, and several other modalities, participants time their moves to coincide with the beat of the music. In Pilates, yoga, water exercise, sport conditioning, indoor cycling, and some equipment-based classes, participants use music to motivate themselves and make the movement experience enjoyable even if they don't necessarily move on the beat. Therefore, you can use music to provide structure to your class or simply to set the mood.

You must understand and work with the music you use in your group exercise classes. Especially in a cardio class, it feels good to move on the beat, and your students will feel more successful, positive, and energized when you lead them to move with the music. Additionally, because many people hear or feel the beat of the music, they unconsciously feel clumsy or uncoordinated when taking a class with an instructor who is off the beat. Participants in cardio and step classes especially expect their movements to flow with the music. Also, by using the music structure appropriately, you can reduce the need for constant cueing.

The next sections outline the basic elements of teaching to popular music. Practice the suggested drills until you can automatically hear the musical components. Most skilled instructors have the beat, the downbeat, the 4-count measure, and the 8- and 32-count phrases in their heads at all times when leading class; hearing the music simply becomes second nature with practice. Note that there are certain tempos that fit well with the various segments and types of group exercise (see the special section titled "Recommended Beats per Minute" on this page).

Beat

The beat is the smallest musical division of a phrase. Each regular rhythmic pulse is a beat, also known as a *count*. Beats are further organized into downbeats and upbeats. The downbeat is the stronger, more important or emphatic beat. The upbeat is the weaker, less important beat that immediately follows each downbeat.

Recommended Beats per Minute

Warm-up: 120 to 136 beats per minute

High/low impact cardio segment: 134 to 158 beats per minute

Step: 118 to 128 beats per minute

Muscle conditioning: Less than 132 beats per minute

Flexibility work, yoga, and Pilates: Less than 100 beats per minute or music without a strong beat

For example, figure 4.1 illustrates the downbeats and the upbeats in the song "Jingle Bells."

The downbeat falls on the most accented part of a word and usually on the most important words in a phrase, whereas the upbeat falls on the unaccented part of a word or the less important words. Also, when you are counting the beats forward in a measure, the downbeats are on the odd numbers (1 and 3) and the upbeats are on the even numbers (2 and 4).

Measure

The measure is the basic organizational unit in music; it contains a series of downbeats and upbeats. In almost all popular music used in step and cardio classes, each measure holds four beats: downbeat, upbeat, downbeat, upbeat. Such music is said to be in *4/4 metered time,* which technically means that there are four quarter notes in each measure. In the example given in figure 4.1, the words *jingle bells* take up one measure.

Phrase

A phrase consists of at least two measures of music. Hence, it is common to speak of an 8-count phrase (two measures), a 16-count phrase (four measures), and a 32-count phrase (eight measures) in step or cardio music. A 32-count phrase contains four 8-count phrases grouped together and is ideal for building routines and choreographic combinations. Participants usually feel more successful and energized when new movement patterns are initiated at the beginning of each 32-count phrase; the first downbeat of the 32-count phrase is sometimes called the *top of the phrase.* Listen for the drumroll or other increase in musical momentum that comes at the end of each 32-count phrase

(technically the 7th and 8th counts of the last, or fourth, 8-count phrase) and signifies the new 32-count phrase to follow.

Typically, the 8-count phrases within each 32-count phrase are divided into dominant and less-dominant phrases, such as the following:

- First 8-count phrase: dominant
- Second 8-count phrase: less dominant
- Third 8-count phrase: dominant
- Fourth 8-count phrase: less dominant but with drum roll or other musical momentum during 7th and 8th counts

 See the DVD for the practice drill on counting out the beat (4 counts and 8 counts at 120 beats per minute and 132 beats per minute).

Make this learning process easier on yourself by selecting music that has a strong, easy-to-hear beat. You can also try commercial music that has been professionally premixed for step, kickboxing, and cardio classes. This music is blended (metered) into continuous 32-count phrases and is preferable to music found in music stores, which is not metered for group exercise and contains extra beats and bridges, making counting, choreography, and cueing much more difficult. See "Music Resource List" on page 52 for contact information.

Half Time and Double Time

When a movement is performed in half time, it is performed twice as slowly as normal. In other words, a box step (making a square pattern with your feet) usually takes 4 counts, but when performed in half time, it takes 8 counts. Performing in double time, then, means to perform a move twice as fast as usual.

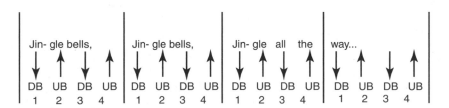

▶ **Figure 4.1** In simple songs such as "Jingle Bells," the upbeats (UB) and downbeats (DB) are easily identified.

Music Resource List

Burntrax Fitness Music	www.burntrax.com	800-672-8729
CardioMixes	www.cardiomixes.com	866-322-6868
Dynamix	www.dynamixmusic.com	800-843-6499
GF Mix	www.gfmix.com	702-938-1700
Kimbo Educational	www.kimboed.com	800-631-2187
MusicFlex	www.musicflex.com	800-430-3539
Muscle Mixes Music	www.musclemixesmusic.com	800-833-1224
Power Music	www.powermusic.com	800-777-2328

■ Practice Drill

Using popular music with a strong beat, listen for the 8-count division within the music. Find the 8-count grouping with the strongest initial downbeat; this is the beginning of the 32-count phrase. To help integrate this information into movement, try this simple drill: (1) Leading with your right foot, walk eight steps to the right on the first 8-count phrase. (2) Make a sharp 90° turn to your right and walk eight more steps on the second 8-count phrase (always leading right). (3) Make another sharp 90° turn to your right and walk eight more steps on the third 8-count phrase. (4) Make another sharp 90° turn to your right and walk eight more steps on the fourth 8-count phrase, returning to your starting point. You should have made a large square pattern with your feet. Repeat to the right or try the same drill to your left, leading always with the left foot. Keep practicing this drill with different speeds and styles of music.

Music Styles

One of the most enjoyable aspects of teaching to music is the availability of so many different styles of music. Adapting the music to your participants' interests and ages will enhance their enjoyment and willingness to keep exercising. Dwyer (1995) found that when participants had a choice of music, they reported higher intrinsic motivation than did the participants who were not asked for input. Ask your participants what they like to listen to. Try new musical styles to stimulate creative energy and open up new opportunities for choreography. Keep an open mind and have a sense of play as you experiment with the different music styles:

- Rock, pop, Top 40
- House, techno, club
- Oldies, Motown
- Funk, rap
- Latin, salsa
- Reggae
- Big band, swing
- Country
- Mind–body
- World beat (Irish, Peruvian, African, Middle Eastern)
- Holiday (Halloween, Valentine's Day, Fourth of July)
- Theme (beach, girl power, rainy day music)

■ Practice Drill

Listening to any piece of popular music, close your eyes and tap your feet, pat your knees, or clap your hands to the regular continuous beat. Write a list of 20 songs and their beats per minute and describe which portion of the workout each song would fit best.

Responsibilities for Using Exercise Music

The 1976 revision of the Copyright Law of the United States, which went into effect in 1978, made clear statements about the responsibilities of fitness instructors, studios, and centers regarding the music they use. Tested throughout the judicial system and upheld by the U.S. Supreme Court, the law states that copyright owners have the right to charge a fee for the use of their music in a public performance. A public performance is defined as a performance made in a place open to the public or any place where a substantial number of persons outside a normal circle of family and friends are gathered.

All exercise classes—whether they take place in a private club, public hall, exercise gym, or corporate fitness center—fall into the category of public performance. Because music is a copyrighted entity, corporations, studios, fitness centers, and instructors who use music during their exercise classes place themselves in jeopardy of violating the U.S. Copyright Law if they do not pay royalties to the people who write, publish, and distribute the music.

The American Society of Composers, Authors and Publishers (ASCAP); Broadcast Music, Inc. (BMI); and the Society of European Stage Authors and Composers (SESAC) are the main organizations that represent the artists who record the music used in group exercise classes. Together, these organizations represent more than 100,000 composers, lyricists, and publishers. They ensure that their members receive royalties and that the U.S. Copyright Law is enforced.

The ASCAP and BMI both vigorously pursue violators and potential violators of the law. ACE (2000) recommends that clubs and studios obtain a blanket license for their instructors. The license fees for clubs are determined by the number of students who attend classes each week, by the number of speakers used in the club, and by whether the club uses single or multiple floors. Independent instructors who teach in several locations may need to obtain their own personal music performance license. Be sure to check with each club where you teach regarding music licensure. Also, know that you are much more likely to be protected from copyright infringement if you buy CDs or download songs that were specifically created and prelicensed for group exercise classes (see "Music Resource List" on page 52). For more information on the costs of licensing and for further clarification of the U.S. Copyright Law, check out www.bmi.com, www.ascap.com, and www.copyright.gov. It is an instructor's responsibility to stay up to date on issues surrounding the U.S. Copyright Law, as opportunities for playing music increase with technological advances.

More and more fitness music companies are making it possible for customers to download prelicensed music directly onto an iPod or MP3 player. Doing so allows you to create your own playlist. Other new avenues for playing music include the music-editing software programs that let instructors mix songs, tracks, sounds, and music speeds. All these technological advances mean that an instructor's individual music style and selections may become increasingly important in class popularity and exercise adherence.

Sound System Fundamentals

A good sound system is essential for most group exercise classes. A basic sound system consists of one or more sound sources (microphone, CD player, radio tuner, cassette player, iPod docking station, or digital music controller) connected to an amplifier and speakers. All systems, whether portable or fixed, contain these basic elements.

The more self-contained systems (portable and ministereo systems) have no capacity for adding extra speakers or source devices such as wireless microphones (Goodman 1997). These systems also have no provisions for mixing sounds from more than one source, such as a wireless microphone and a CD player. More accessible systems, such as karaoke systems, keyboard amplifier and speaker systems, and professional portable sound systems, allow you to add external sound sources and speakers, as do music-editing software and digital music controllers. Products change so quickly that making specific recommendations for a sound system is unfeasible. It is worth your time to research a product that will sound good and also be easy to

Music Volume in Fitness Classes

The IDEA Health and Fitness Association makes the following recommendations regarding safe volume levels for music played during group exercise classes (Goodman 1997). These recommendations are based on the standards established by the U.S. Occupational Safety and Health Administration (OSHA). Fitness professionals who work outside of the United States are urged to refer to the official volume guidelines established for their particular countries.

1. Because hearing loss is slow, cumulative, and often painless (loud music does sometimes hurt!), group exercise instructors need to be aware that the intensity of their music and accompanying voice can put them and their students at risk without causing any apparent symptoms.
2. Health facilities and instructors have an obligation to their members and students to ensure safe music intensities during group exercise classes.
3. Music intensity during group exercise classes should measure no more than 90 decibels (dB).
4. Because the instructor's voice needs to be about 10 decibels louder than the music in order to be heard, the instructor's voice should measure no more than 100 decibels.
5. Fitness facilities are urged to place a Class 1 or 2 sound level meter (available from many electronics stores for less than $100 U.S.) on a stand near the center of the front of the room in order to measure sound levels during classes. Instructors or other staff members should check the meter regularly to make sure volume levels are safe. The volume control on the music amplifier is not an accurate means of measuring sound intensity.

maintain. Try calling other fitness organizations to see what they have found to be successful.

Voice Care

Long and colleagues (1998) conducted a study on voice problems experienced by aerobic instructors. Of the instructors who were surveyed, 44% experienced partial or complete voice loss during and after instructing. They also experienced increased episodes of voice loss, hoarseness, and sore throat unrelated to illness since they began instructing. Heidel and Torgerson (1993) found that instructors experience a higher prevalence of vocal problems compared with individuals participating in group exercise. If you are instructing on a regular basis, using a microphone is essential to your vocal health. Other recommendations for voice care include the following:

- Keep your head, jaw, neck, and shoulders relaxed when teaching.
- Face your class whenever possible; project your voice out rather than down or up.
- Use visual cueing as much as you can.
- Develop good breathing habits; learn to perform abdominal breathing.
- Keep your throat hydrated.
- Avoid irritants such as smoke, smog, or certain foods.
- Avoid clearing your throat frequently, as doing so creates even more phlegm.
- Avoid screaming, yelling, or shouting when teaching—use that microphone.

The technology of sound systems advances as quickly as computer technology advances. The bottom line is that you need a good sound system, a microphone with a headset and receiver, and high-quality speakers. These products will create a big difference in the quality of your group exercise instruction. After all, music is one of the main reasons why participants venture into the group exercise setting versus exercising alone on a stair-climber or an elliptical machine. According to Harmon and Kravitz (2007), music facilitates exercise performance by reducing the feeling of fatigue, increasing psychological arousal, creating a physiological relaxation response, and enhancing motor coordination. Monroe (1999) stated that music (along with the creative use of silence) is the heart of movement. She said, "If you love your music and have a passion for it, it will move you—and it will move the people you teach" (37).

FUNDAMENTAL CHOREOGRAPHY

In a cardio class, participants perform movements that work the large muscle groups to promote cardiorespiratory fitness and its benefits. These movements are traditionally dancelike and can be executed while jumping (high impact) or while keeping one foot on the floor at all times (low impact). Classes mixing high- and low-impact movements may be labeled as *cardio conditioning, aerobic dance,* or simply *high-low.* Learning the skills necessary to teach cardio classes forms the foundation of group exercise instruction for many group leaders. The basic skills described in this chapter, such as anticipatory cueing, smooth transitioning, and choreography building, also apply to most other forms of group exercise, including step, kickboxing, muscular conditioning, water exercise, slide, Zumba, and NIA. The elements on the group exercise class evaluation form (appendix A) that pertain to cardiorespiratory programs are listed on this page.

To minimize repetitive stress on the joints and to prevent boredom (for both the leader and the participants), the best group instructors constantly vary their moves and movement patterns. Too much of any one move can create excessive wear on the joints. Movements must be balanced. You must balance forward moves with backward moves, balance right and left sides, and right and left leads. To protect the joints, you should avoid using too many high-impact movements, too many repetitive jumps on one leg (no more than eight in a row), and too many repetitive moves that stress the musculoskeletal system. Moves such as jumping jacks, ski jumps, and scissors deliver large impact forces to the joints. To create the safest class, you should combine these types of moves with a totally different move, such as a march.

Demonstrate proper technique at all times to help prevent injuries. When performing high-impact moves, roll through the entire foot with each jump, bringing first the toes and then the heels to the floor. This toe-ball-heel landing pattern distributes the impact forces over the whole foot. Be careful with lateral foot movements such as grapevines and shuffles, especially on a carpeted surface. They increase the risk of a lateral ankle sprain, especially if participants perform them while fatigued. When performing lunges, keep the heel of the back foot up to prevent excessive eccentric loading of the calf muscles (potentially leading to Achilles tendinitis). It is also wise to avoid wearing ankle weights during cardio classes, as doing so increases the risk of injury. If you use light hand weights, chose a reduced music speed (such as 138 beats per minute) to minimize the risk of upper-body injuries. Hand weights less than 3 pounds (1.36 kilograms) have not been shown to significantly affect caloric expenditure in cardio activities (Yoke et al. 1988). Hand weights greater than 3 pounds (1.36 kilograms) are not recommended during cardio activities because of the increased potential for upper-body injury. Avoid keeping the arms overhead for prolonged durations; in addition to increasing the risk of injuring the shoulder joint, keeping the arms

Group Exercise Class Evaluation Form Essentials

- Gradually increases intensity
- Uses a variety of muscle groups
- Minimizes repetitive movements
- Promotes participant interaction and encourages fun
- Demonstrates movement options and gives clear verbal cues and directions
- Gradually decreases intensity during postcardio cool-down
- Uses music volume and tempo (134-158 beats per minute) appropriate for biomechanical movement

up can elicit the pressor response by elevating the heart rate without creating a corresponding increase in oxygen consumption. Avoid knee and elbow hyperextension, both of which can result from excessive momentum during kicks or rapid press-outs.

In addition to considering joint health and injury prevention, good instructors are aware of potential safety issues caused by the difficulty of a move or the participant's ability. Keep all movements fluid and under control. Be careful with sudden changes in direction; always provide clear, advance cueing to prevent falls and collisions. Finally, always provide an alternative to turning steps such as pivot turns. Some participants become dizzy and disoriented with this type of move.

■ Technique and Safety Check

To keep your classes safe, observe the following recommendations.

Remember to

- provide a variety of moves (front to back, side to side, and right to left),
- roll through the entire foot with each jump,
- be careful with lateral foot movements,
- keep the back heel up when performing lunges,
- be careful with sudden changes in direction, and
- give an alternative to turning steps.

Avoid

- too much high impact,
- too many repetitive jumps on one leg (no more than eight in a row),
- too many repetitive moves that stress the musculoskeletal system,
- excessive momentum,
- knee and elbow hyperextension,
- keeping the arms overhead for prolonged durations, and
- using ankle weights.

BASIC MOVES

A skilled cardio instructor has a large repertoire of moves that allows for endless variety and creativity. Most of these moves can be performed at low to moderate impact (one foot stays on the floor during the move) or high impact (both feet leave the floor during the move). For example, a grapevine can be performed by always having one foot on the ground (low impact) or by jumping from foot to foot (high impact). Research has shown that low- to moderate-impact cardio routines, when performed with full ROM and appropriate choreography, can provide a cardiorespiratory stimulus similar to that of high-impact routines (Clapp and Little 1994; Otto et al. 1986, 1988; Parker et al. 1989; Williford, Blessing et al. 1989; Williford, Scharff-Olson et al. 1989; Yoke et al. 1988, 1989). Instructors may choose to lead routines or classes that are entirely high impact, entirely low impact, or a combination of both. Following is an introduction to basic lower-body and upper-body moves for cardio classes.

Lower-Body Moves

Lower-body moves and patterns can be divided into 2-count moves and 4-count moves, which are listed on page 57 and demonstrated on the accompanying DVD. These moves have many variations, as you will see in the next section.

 See the DVD for a demonstration of basic 2-count and 4-count moves for the lower body.

An aerobic or cardiorespiratory exercise is one in which large, major muscle groups move repetitively through full ROM for a prolonged duration. Therefore, you should keep the lower body moving at all times during a cardio class. Lower-body muscles contain more muscle mass than upper-body muscles and will consume more oxygen, thus providing a stronger cardiorespiratory stimulus. Studies have shown that simply staying in one place with minimal lower body involvement while vigorously pumping the arms brings up the heart rate but does not significantly increase oxygen consumption or caloric expenditure (Parker et al. 1989).

2-Count and 4-Count Moves for the Lower Body

2-Count Moves

- Walk, march, jog
- Step touch
- Hamstring curl
- Knee lift (front or side)
- Kick (front, side, or back)
- Heel dig (front or side)
- Toe tap (front or side)
- Jumping jack
- Heel jack
- Twist
- Pony
- Kick, ball change
- Lunge
- Pendulum (ticktock)
- Scissors
- Ski jump
- Plié

4-Count Moves

- Grapevine
- Walk front for 3, tap on 4 (also known as a hustle)
- V-step (also known as *out, out, in, in*)
- Mambo
- Box step (also known as a *jazz square*)
- Charleston
- Shuffle
- Power squat
- Cha-cha
- Rocking horse
- Jig

Upper-Body Moves

In many group exercise activities, the arms can move bilaterally (right and left sides perform the same movement simultaneously, as when performing biceps curls with both arms) or unilaterally (right and left sides move individually or perform different movements simultaneously, as when performing alternating biceps curls). In addition to being bilateral or unilateral, upper-body moves can complement or oppose the lower-body moves. For example, when you are performing knee lifts, your right arm can reach up when the right knee lifts (complementary arms), or it can reach up when the left knee lifts (opposition arms). Upper-body moves also can be categorized as low-range, midrange, and high-range movements. Examples are biceps curls (arms at sides), front raises to shoulder height, and overhead presses, respectively.

 See the DVD for a demonstration of high/low arm patterns. These patterns can be used in other group exercise modalities as well.

ELEMENTS OF VARIATION

Variation can help you get more mileage out of your basic moves. Almost every basic move can be altered in numerous ways to create interest, additional challenge, and fun! Variations give the illusion of new moves and choreography, when in fact you are only tweaking moves that are already familiar to your participants. The primary elements of variation are the lever, plane, directional, rhythm, intensity, and style variations.

Performing a lever variation simply means moving from a move with a short lever to a move with a long lever, or vice versa. For example, progressing from a knee lift to a kick is a lower-body lever change; similarly, moving from a bilateral front raise to a bilateral biceps curl is an upper-body lever change. This element of variation does not work for all moves.

■ Practice Drill

Practice both the low- and the high-impact variations of the lower-body moves listed in this chapter. Then try adding different arm movements: Try low-, mid-, and high-range movements; unilateral and bilateral movements; and opposition and complementary movements. See the accompanying DVD for a demonstration of this drill.

A plane variation is changing the plane of movement while performing essentially the same action. When you change a front kick to a side kick or change a front raise to a lateral raise, you are executing a plane variation. The basic planes are the frontal (abduction and adduction movements), sagittal (flexion and extension movements), horizontal (horizontal shoulder adduction and abduction or twisting movements), and diagonal planes. This variation does not work for all moves (see figure 4.2).

A directional variation can mean changing the direction of the movement. If you are facing front, you can perform the same move while facing the side or back, or if you are traveling forward (e.g., as in a hustle), you can travel diagonally instead. A directional variation can also mean traveling with the move instead of performing it in place. For example, you can move while performing alternating knee lifts instead of remaining in one place. Varying the direction is an excellent strategy for increasing intensity and energy expenditure. It's amazing how familiar moves such as knee lifts can feel completely different when the direction changes! Some moves will naturally feel better when you are moving in a certain direction; jumping jacks, for instance, feel much more comfortable when moving backward rather than forward. A simple traveling combination might be four jumping jacks backward (8 counts) followed by a march or jog forward (8 counts). Repeat for a complete 32-count phrase.

Rhythm variations involve changing the rhythm of the move or adding sound to the move. An example of a rhythmic change is switching from alternating single knee lifts (a 2-count move) to alternating double knee lifts (a 4-count move). Other moves that go easily from single to double and back again are hamstring curls, step touches, and lunges. Experiment with rhythmic sound variations: Try adding single and then double or triple claps to some moves. Snaps and stomps are also fun. Or, ask participants to yell, whoop, or grunt at various points in the song; this technique has the potential to totally energize your class! Just keep your group's demo-

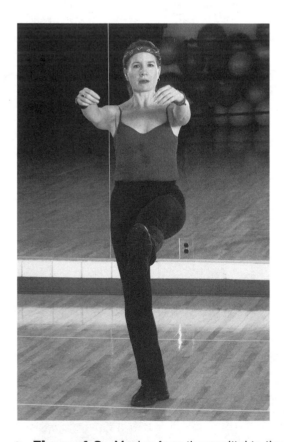 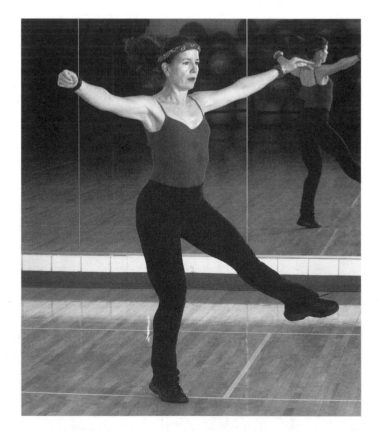

▶ **Figure 4.2** Moving from the sagittal to the frontal plane.

graphics and individual characteristics in mind; some people may be uncomfortable with making sounds, whereas others will enjoy it.

You can create a physiological intensity variation in a number of ways, including

- increasing the lever length of the move,
- increasing the ROM of the move,
- increasing the speed of the move (or of the music itself),
- taking bigger steps when traveling as well as taking wider steps in stationary moves such as step touches, or
- changing the literal level of the move, which is also known as *vertical displacement.*

An example of vertical displacement occurs when a low-impact move is changed into a high-impact move. During a low-impact move such as a step touch, the center of gravity remains on the same level as the person steps side to side. However, in a high-impact move such as a side-to-side pony or triple step, the center of gravity moves up and down and the movement involves more muscle mass, thus increasing the intensity. Vertical displacement can also occur in a downward direction, such as when bending the knees deeper during a low-impact step touch so that the emphasis is *down,* up (instead of *up,* down). A deeper bend shifts the center of gravity downward and requires more muscle mass activation without jumping. Many low-impact moves lend themselves to this type of intensity variation, including hamstring curls, knee lifts, kicks, and lunges. Conversely, of course, you can lessen the intensity of these moves by decreasing any of these variables (see figure 4.3).

Physiological intensity is not necessarily the same as complexity or psychological intensity. A combination built with simple choreography can be quite intense in terms of heart rate, oxygen consumption, and caloric expenditure. Ironically, a very technical or complex combination involving many intricate foot and arm patterns can actually lower the exercise intensity, because participants must focus on remembering what comes next and on not appearing clumsy. Later in this chapter we discuss sequencing and choreographic issues in greater depth.

 See the DVD for a practice drill demonstrating the elements of variation (lever, plane, directional, rhythmic, intensity, and style variations).

One of the most enjoyable ways to alter your moves is by playing with the style variation. A grapevine, for instance, can look and feel completely different when performed with a funky style versus a sporty style, even though it's essentially the same move! Other styles include Latin (salsa), hip-hop, dance, martial arts, country, jazz, Irish, or African. Expand your repertoire of styles and increase your fun potential!

SMOOTH TRANSITIONS

When skilled instructors teach, their moves flow seamlessly from one to the other, making the choreography easier to cue and easier for participants to follow, thus enhancing participant success. Spend some time on the drills in this section to build your skill at connecting moves. For the smoothest transitions, keep it

■ Practice Drill

Play your favorite music (pick a song with a strong beat) and perform a basic move such as a march, step touch, or grapevine. Add upper-body movements. On every 8th or 16th beat, change your move slightly by varying the lever, plane, direction, rhythm, intensity, or style. For example, go from a basic step-touch with lateral arm raise to a front raise. Then try a direction change: Move the step touch (with front raises) diagonally to the front of the room and back again. Hold the basic move and then try changing the rhythm: Take two step touches to the right and then two to the left. Add an additional rhythm change by clapping on the 4th count each time. Return to the basic move. Have fun with a style change: Emphasize the upbeat by stomping the inside foot on the step touch while loosening the arms (allowing the elbows to flex slightly on the upbeat) and popping the torso slightly with an upbeat hip-hop style. When you feel you've exhausted the possibilities, go to another move and try more elements of variation.

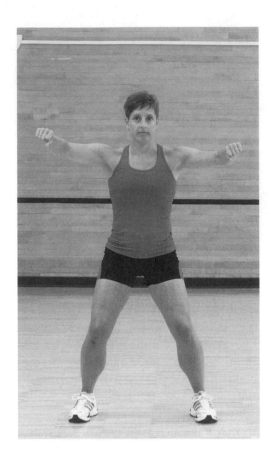
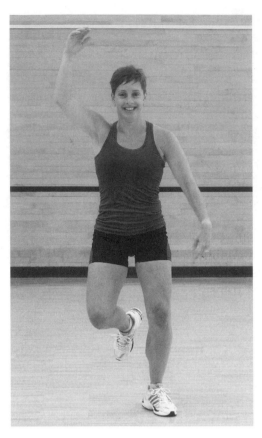
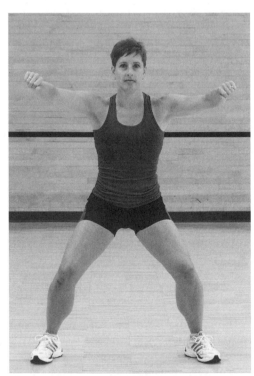
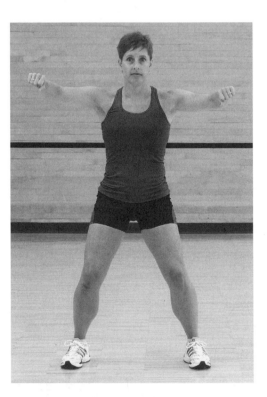

▶ **Figure 4.3** Intensity variations of the same move: *(top left)* basic step touch, *(top right)* high-impact step touch, *(bottom left)* low-impact step touch with knees flexed, and *(bottom right)* deep flexed knee for more intense low-impact variation.

simple. It's best if you change only one thing at a time—change only the arms or only the legs or only the lead foot.

Connecting End Points

Some moves just naturally transition into other moves. Most of the elements of variation provide for smooth transitions: Executing a plane change from a front kick to a side kick is an example of a smooth lower-body transition. The subtle change from a front kick with a front raise to a side kick with a lateral raise is easy for almost every participant to grasp and requires a minimum of cueing. Notice that each move has a starting point and an end point. The smoothest transitions connect moves that have one of these points in common. For example, a bilateral front raise (a 2-count move) starts with the arms down and ends with the arms up at shoulder height in the sagittal plane. A lateral raise (another 2-count move) also starts with the arms down but ends with the arms up at shoulder height in the frontal plane. These two moves flow together well because they share a common starting point: arms down. It's easy and natural to go back and forth between these two moves; in fact, you could even create a combination 4-count upper-body move by putting these two moves together. You could then repeat the 4 counts over and over.

 See the DVD for a drill demonstrating smooth transitions.

■ Practice Drill

Keeping your feet stationary, practice transitioning from one upper-body 2-count move to another, making sure that the two moves have a common denominator (starting point or end point). Perform each 2 count move at least 4 to 8 times (for a total of 8-16 counts), and challenge yourself by connecting at least eight different upper-body moves sequentially. If necessary, pause briefly between moves to find a move with a common end point, but keep practicing until you eventually eliminate the pause. See the accompanying DVD for an example of this drill.

■ Practice Drill

Start with a simple lower-body move (e.g., a march) and add a simple upper-body move such as bilateral biceps curls. After 8 or 16 counts, change the upper-body move but maintain the lower-body move, experimenting until you find upper-body movements that share a common connecting point and flow smoothly and naturally (as in the previous drill). Notice if the transition feels right to your body. Continue for 8 or 16 more counts and then, maintaining your new upper-body move, smoothly transition to a new lower-body move. In this drill, only half the body changes at a time. Remember, you are working for smoothness; think of it as finding moves that flow so naturally that cueing is completely unnecessary. As you improve your skill, increase the speed of your transitions and switch to a new upper-body move or a new lower-body move every 4 counts.

Leading Foot

Another factor in creating smooth transitions and easy-to-follow choreography is to maintain an awareness of which foot is leading at all times (this is important!). In other words, you'll enhance your participants' success if you always lead with the same foot in each move throughout a combination. So, if you start with a step touch to the right (right foot leads off on the 1st count, or downbeat), then you should also start your grapevine to the right, if that's your next move. Starting a grapevine to the left after leading right in a step touch will confuse your participants and make the combination harder to follow. In addition to constantly hearing the downbeat in the back of your mind, stay aware of your lead foot and make sure it contacts the floor on the downbeats of the music. After performing a combination all the way through with the right foot leading, balance your body's neuromuscular and biomechanical systems by performing the entire combo with the left foot leading.

Connector Moves

You may have noticed that in some lower-body moves, both feet do the same thing at the same time; examples include pliés, jumping jacks, and double-time bouncy heel lifts (see figure 4.4). These symmetrical moves are valuable as filler moves and can help you switch your leading foot if you haven't built a lead change into your combination. Because both feet are doing the same thing at the same time, it's easy to start the next move on either the right foot or the left foot.

Other types of moves are so basic that they can be used over and over as fillers to ease transitions between other moves and to create participant security. A walk, march, or jog is a good filler. A good beginner combo might be walk 8 counts, perform four knee lifts (8 counts), walk 8 counts, step touch four times (8 counts), walk 8 counts, perform four hamstring curls (8 counts), walk 8 counts, perform four kicks (8 counts). This adds up to two 32-count phrases, or 64 counts. The 8-count walk interspersed between all the other moves can enhance participant confidence and provide a psychological break from complex choreography. (Incidentally, these 8-count walks could be made more interesting by traveling, adding impact, changing the style,

or adding arm variations.) Once participants become comfortable with the combination, try removing all the filler moves (the walks). What you'll have left is a 32-count combination that is more complex: four knee lifts, four step touches, four hamstring curls, and four kicks.

Every instructor needs filler moves as reliable standbys for those times when the brain seems to stop working and you simply can't remember what's supposed to come next! If this happens, you can always return to the safety of a walk, march, or jog.

Moves That Don't Fit Easily

Some moves simply don't fit well together. When designing a combination, you may have to incorporate one or two transition moves to make the choreography smoother and easier to follow. For example, moving from a plié to a front kick is awkward; transition moves are needed for a more natural flow. A possible solution could be plié (8 counts), step toe touch side (8 counts), step toe touch front (8 counts), and then step kick front (8 counts).

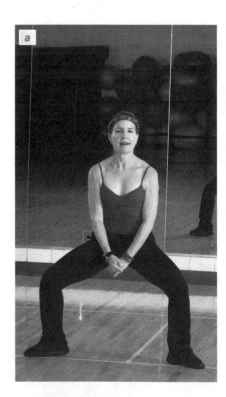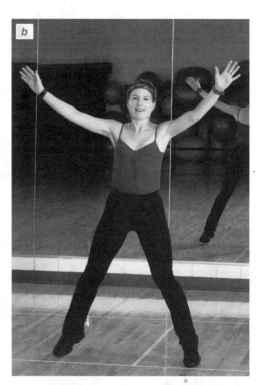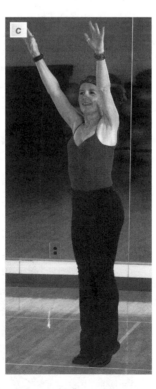

▶ **Figure 4.4** Connector moves: *(a)* plié (flex knees down, up, down, up), *(b)* jumping jack, and *(c)* bouncy heel lifts (flex knees down, up, down, up—may add a jump-shot action with the upper body).

BUILDING BASIC COMBINATIONS

Many instructors prefer to teach cardio classes with 32-count combinations of moves, sometimes referred to as *blocks.* Usually these combinations have been designed and practiced before class. Here are the typical steps used in designing a cardio combination:

1. Start with four lower-body moves that flow together. Make sure each move fills 8 counts for a total of 32 counts. Practice to find the smoothest arrangement of the four moves. Add transitional moves when necessary and eliminate moves that don't fit well but stay within the 32-count framework.

2. Find upper-body movements that go with the lower-body combination.

3. Check to see that your combination
   - provides a balance of complex and simple moves,
   - can be modified with appropriate intensity and complexity variations,
   - flows smoothly,
   - is easy to cue (see cueing section on page 67), and
   - can be broken down easily (more about this later).

4. Repeat this process with another 32-count combination (sometimes referred to as a block). If you plan to link several blocks of 32-count combos together, you will need to see that they have common end points and starting points for smooth transitions between blocks.

 See the DVD for a demonstration of building a basic combination.

Showing Modifications

Skilled instructors are adept at providing intensity and complexity modifications to accommodate different skill and fitness levels among the participants. Generally, instructors should teach at an intermediate level and demonstrate intensity variations for exercisers who are above or below that level. For recommendations on ways to vary intensity, see the practice drill on this page. A group instructor should also occasionally incorporate an intensity drill into the class routine; with an intensity drill, participants will be more likely to take responsibility for themselves and modify moves to fit their own needs. For an example of an intensity drill, see the practice drill on this page.

The more complex your choreography is, the more important your ability to show modifications and break down your routines. This is particularly true with choreography that includes pivots or turns, as some participants tend to get dizzy or disoriented when turning. Always provide alternatives for pivots and turns. For example, a 4-count pivot turn can always be modified to a 4-count mambo or even a march.

Breaking Down and Building Combinations

A combination is broken down when an instructor takes the finished choreography and essentially works backward. In other words, many participants won't be able to grasp the final, most complex, most intense version of your routine the first time you show it. So instead of beginning with the final combination, you can start with the most basic, simplest moves of the

■ Practice Drill

To begin an intensity drill, show a basic move such as a hamstring curl and cue, "Show me this move at low intensity." Watch the participants do the move for a moment and then say, "Now show me the same move at medium intensity." Finally, ask the participants, "Can you show me this move at high intensity?" It helps build participant confidence if you call out suggestions for increasing and decreasing intensity during the drill. Once the participants have demonstrated high intensity, have them show both medium intensity and low intensity again so that they know how to both increase and decrease the intensity of the hamstring curl. Repeat with other simple moves such as knee lifts, grapevines, or even a basic march.

combination and gradually build in intensity and complexity until participants are performing the final product. Breaking down a combination may take quite a while, depending on your choreography and your participants' skill levels. Design all your routines so that you can easily break them down into their basic components. Some practitioners call this the *part-to-whole method.* Practice teaching your routines as if you were leading novice participants through your combinations for the first time. Let's look at an example of how to break down a 32-count combination that contains a rather complex move. The final version of this combination is as follows:

1. Facing the left corner, perform two kick-ball-changes (right leg performs full ROM kick while right foot is leading) followed by one box step (jazz square). This is the complex move. The upper body performs alternating punches on the kick-ball-change and the arms sweep backward on the box step—8 counts altogether. See the accompanying DVD for a demonstration.

2. Repeat for another 8 counts.

3. Facing front, step touch right and left, and then repeat. The upper body performs a lateral raise through its full ROM—this move takes 8 counts.

4. Perform four jumping jacks, turning so that the last jack faces the right corner. The upper body performs overhead presses—this move requires 8 counts. You have now completed 32 counts altogether.

5. Repeat the entire combination on the other side, leading with the left foot.

Here's how to break down this combination:

1. Start by repeating the kick-ball-change over and over again, right foot leading. Drill this move without arms until the majority of your class can perform it correctly. You could even break this move down further by teaching it in half time.

2. Now drill the box step, continuing to repeat the move until it appears that most of your participants are comfortable with it.

3. Next, combine the two moves: two kick-ball-changes with one box step. Again, repeat this two-move pattern over and over until participants have it.

4. Adding on, perform four sets of right and left step touches for a count of 16.

5. Perform eight jumping jacks for a count of 16.

6. Now that your participants know the four movement patterns you'll be using, return to the beginning of the combo. At the top of the next 32-count phrase, lead your group in an expanded version of the final combination (still leading right): four sets of the two kick-ball-changes followed by a box step (32 counts), four sets of right and left step touches (16 counts), and eight jumping jacks (16 counts).

7. Repeat this expanded version; this time, add the upper-body movements.

8. Repeat the combination again, asking for more energy and greater ROM during the kick part of the kick-ball-change.

9. Finally, reduce the combination to its intended version: two sets of the two kick-ball-changes followed by a box step (16 counts), two sets of right and left step touches (8 counts), and four jumping jacks (8 counts).

By this time, the participants should be familiar enough with the routine that they are ready to try it with the left foot leading. Because this routine is complex and it's best to balance left with right, it's probably wise to go through all nine steps of the breakdown on the left side.

The combination we've just broken down illustrates the concept of balancing complex with simple moves. Because the kick-ball-change requires agility and feels complex to most participants, the simple step touches and jumping jacks provide a nice physiological and psychological balance. In addition, any decrease in intensity required by the complex footwork in the first moves can be balanced with the jacks at the end of the combination.

The teaching techniques used in this example include adding on and repetition reduction.

Adding on is just like it sounds: After the class has learned a move, pattern, or short sequence, the instructor adds a new move or pattern to the existing sequence, gradually putting together the final product. Repetition reduction is useful because most participants need to repeat a move in order to learn it (particularly if it is complex). Thus skilled instructors teach combinations in expanded versions that include many repetitions of each move. In other words, a combo that is intended to be 32 counts is drilled in a 64-count or 128-count version. In beginner classes, the combo might remain expanded; it is not always necessary to reduce a combination to its most complex form. Repetition reduction, the process of reducing the number of repetitions to the most complex, 32-count version of a combination, is also called *pyramid building:* You start the sequence with large numbers of repetitions and gradually eliminate repetitions until the desired combination is achieved.

 See the DVD for a choreography overview of high-low impact moves.

ADDITIONAL CHOREOGRAPHY TECHNIQUES

Although combination building is the most common way to teach cardio classes, it is not the only way. Other choreographic teaching techniques (in addition to breaking down a combination, adding on, and repetition reduction) include layering, using building blocks, and playing flip-flop. All of these techniques are usually planned and practiced in advance of the actual class. Another choreographic technique, called *freestyle* or *linear choreography,* is extemporaneous.

Freestyle Choreography

The freestyle method, also known as using *linear progressions,* is a valid and effective technique. Whereas combination-style choreography is usually planned and organized into patterns, freestyle choreography is spontaneous and delivered on the spot, without an emphasis on pattern development. In freestyle, one move flows smoothly into the next move, which flows into the next move, and on and on. There is little repetition.

 See the DVD for a practice drill on freestyle choreography.

Although freestyle demands skill on the part of the instructor, it is psychologically easier for participants, who don't have to remember complex moves and patterns. In well-led freestyle, exercisers don't have to worry as much about appearing clumsy or inept, because they are always at least half right! This is because, ideally, the instructor changes only one thing at a time, either changing the upper-body movement while keeping the lower-body movement the same or changing the lower-body movement while maintaining the upper-body movement. This kind of linear progression allows participants to commit more fully to the moves and perform with greater intensity, which can result in a better training effect and higher caloric expenditure than might be achieved with combination choreography.

The best way to improve your skill at freestyle is, of course, to practice it. The drills described previously in the sections on variation and combining end points in smooth transitions are particularly useful for freestyle. Here's an example of freestyle choreography:

1. Start with a basic march.
2. Add arms pressing front.
3. Keeping the arm movement, change the march to a heel dig front.
4. Keeping the lower-body movement, change the arms to an overhead press.
5. Maintaining the upper-body movement, change the legs to a toe touch side.
6. Staying with the leg movement, change the arms to side press-outs.
7. Keeping the arm movements, change the lower body to heel digs to the side.
8. Keeping the heel digs, change the arms to long-lever lateral raises.
9. Maintaining the lateral raises, change the legs to a high-impact heel jack.

10. Maintaining the upper-body raises, change to a jumping jack.

11. Change the legs once more to a step touch (with same upper-body lateral raises).

12. Keeping the step touch, change the arms to unilateral overhead presses.

This example generally alternates upper-body changes with lower-body changes, but you may sequence your changes however you like as long as you provide variety and muscle balance and avoid excessive repetitions of moves that stress the musculoskeletal system. Each move can be performed for 4, 8, 16, or even 32 counts, depending on your class (be sure to begin the cardio session on the 1st count of an 8-count phrase). As always, you must maintain an appropriate intensity level: Performing too many low-intensity moves in a row results in a low-intensity progression.

Notice that each move in the freestyle example transitions smoothly into the next. Not only is this easier for participants to follow—it's also much easier for you to cue! In fact, good freestyle requires a minimum of cueing; participants simply have to keep watching as they move and they will naturally move with you. Freestyle choreography provides an ideal format for those times when you want to promote group interaction and sociability while working out or when you want to make class announcements or educational points. Because it's not as necessary to give anticipatory cues (cues that let exercisers know what move is coming next), you can talk about other subjects. Freestyle is especially useful during the warm-up and at any point in the routine when you sense that participants are experiencing brain strain from too much concentration or memorization of complex choreography. Many instructors intentionally intersperse freestyle between choreographed routines to give their class psychological breaks and to help boost intensity levels. The freestyle technique is also great for participants with less experience or coordination because they don't have to remember specific sequences.

Layering

The layering technique is used to add more and more complexity to a move or combination. Each layer is repeated until participants appear confident, and then another layer of complexity is added. See the following example of layering:

1. Perform 3 counts of walking in place with a knee lift on the 4th count. Repeat to the other side.

2. Layer with a directional variation: Travel forward, repeating the move twice for a total of 8 counts, and then travel backward, repeating the move twice for 8 counts.

3. Increase the complexity by keeping the pattern only on the 8 counts forward; walk for 8 counts backward without any knee lifts.

4. Layer by adding a hop on the 4th and 8th counts forward (on the knee lifts) while abducting the arms to shoulder height.

5. Layer by adding jazz style to the forward movements. While hopping and lifting the left knee, twist the spine and adduct the knee across the body, showing the left hip; while hopping and lifting the right knee, twist the spine and adduct the knee across the body, showing the right hip.

6. Layer the backward walk by performing a pivot turn on counts 5, 6, 7, and 8 (finish facing forward).

As you can see, the example repeated the same 16 counts over and over, but gradually the patterns became more interesting, stylistic, and complex.

 See the DVD for a demonstration of moving from basic to complex choreography.

Building Blocks and Linking

A block is a 32-count combination of moves. Instructors can create several blocks and then link them together for one long combination (e.g., A + B + C + D). When linking several blocks together, try naming them or associating them with key words or numbers to help your students recall the different blocks. For example, you could cue your class with "Now let's do Carol's combo" (named after Carol) followed by "Next the shuffle routine" (this routine has a shuffle in it) followed by "It's time for the traveler" (a combo with large traveling moves).

Flip-Flop

The flip-flop works well for combinations that have clearly defined elements such as high-impact and low-impact or stationary and traveling moves. After participants have become very familiar with the initial combination, flip-flop the key elements; for example, change all the low-impact moves to high impact and all the high-impact moves to low impact. By using the flip-flop, you gain more mileage from existing combos.

TRAINING SYSTEMS

The major training systems used in cardio classes are continuous training (also known as *steady-state training*); interval intensity training, which may be timed or sporadic; interval training using different cardio modalities (usually timed); and interval cardiorespiratory and strength training.

In continuous, or steady-state, training, different choreographic techniques are used to produce one long, continuous endurance workout with few intensity variations. Even though low-impact and high-impact moves may be used throughout, the overall effect is steady; participants are encouraged to work in their target heart rate zone without major fluctuations (see figure 4.5).

In interval intensity training, intensity levels fluctuate among high, low, and moderate. The instructor provides high-intensity patterns or short, intense combos for an anaerobic (power) interval. During this interval, which may last for 15, 30, or 60 seconds, participants are encouraged to challenge themselves, perhaps pushing into the top range of their target heart rate zone (or even beyond, for advanced participants). Patterns used during the intervals may include plyometric, bounding, or power moves. The cardiorespiratory conditioning segment can be organized into regular timed intervals (e.g., a 4-minute song with a typical high-low combination followed by a 1-minute power interval, with this sequence repeated five times), or the intervals can be interspersed randomly throughout the cardio portion of the class.

Interval training with varying cardiorespiratory modalities is a great way to incorporate cross-training and alleviate boredom. A typical format might be 4 minutes of cardio followed by 4 minutes of step, repeated for 32 minutes. Other modalities to consider include kickboxing, slide, gliding, and jumping rope.

Another popular system for overall class organization is to alternate timed intervals of cardiorespiratory training with strength training. For example, you might lead the class in 4 minutes of cardio, 4 minutes of squats and lunges, 4 minutes of cardio, and 4 minutes of biceps and deltoid exercises.

CUEING METHODS

Proper cueing is essential for a successful high-low cardio class. Class members will have different learning styles. Most will learn best by watching you, others will learn by hearing your verbal instruction, and still others will learn by doing the moves (visual, auditory, and kinesthetic styles, respectively). Use as many styles as possible, and expand your teaching

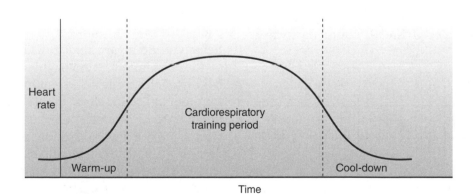

▶ **Figure 4.5** Steady-state training.

vocabulary so that you can say the same thing in multiple ways. Several types of cues are necessary, including anticipatory, movement, motivational, educational, alignment, and safety verbal cues, plus visual cues. In this section we describe these different types of cues as well as discuss the advantages and disadvantages of mirroring your class.

Anticipatory Cueing

An anticipatory cue tells your participants when to do the next movement and what that next movement will be. Learning to deliver timely and appropriate anticipatory cues often takes considerable practice, so be patient and practice the drills given in this book, and eventually you will become an instructor who is easy to follow. To give good anticipatory cues, you must understand music structure and be able to hear the beat, the downbeat, and the 4-, 8-, and 32-count phrases, as discussed earlier in this chapter.

It's easiest for your class if you count backward when cueing an upcoming new move or transition. If you count, "4, 3, 2, and _____," your participants know that after "_____" (where the 1 would be) there will be a new move. This helps them to pay attention and be ready to change and move with the rest of the class. If your anticipatory cue is short (e.g., "step touch"), only one beat might be needed, as in, "4, 3, 2, step touch." Longer cues (e.g., "grapevine right, arms up") take more time to say and therefore will need more beats: "4, 3, grapevine right, arms up."

Instructors don't usually speak on every single beat for anticipatory cueing; not only is doing so too wordy and confusing—it's also hard on your voice! Instead, count backward

Counts	8	7	6	5	4	3		2	1	8
Footstrike	(March) R	L	R	L	R	L		R	L	(Step-touch) R
Cue	"4,			3,			2,	step	touch"	

▶ **Figure 4.6**   Practice transitioning from the march to the step touch while cueing.

on every other beat of your 8-count phrase, as shown in figure 4.6. Practice this example by clapping your hands on every beat while you speak in rhythm at the suggested times. This method of counting on every other beat works very well when you are performing 2-count moves.

Cueing 2-Count Moves

Starting without music, march, feeling your lead foot (e.g., right foot) coming down on every other beat (a march is a 2-count move). Begin to practice the cue given in figure 4.6 ("4, 3, 2, step touch"), saying "4" when your lead foot strikes the floor (this is a downbeat and the first beat of an 8-count phrase). If all goes well, you will be ready to step touch to the right at the end of the 8 counts, beginning the new move (step touch) with your right foot (lead foot) on the downbeat. Notice the paradox: You are saying one thing while your body is doing something else. This probably won't feel natural at first, but keep practicing—it's a skill worth acquiring if you want your participants to all do the same thing at the same time and feel satisfied with your class!

After mastering the transition from march to step touch while cueing, see if you can continue the step touch and, when ready, cue back to a march. Note that you may continue step touching for as many counts as you like, starting the anticipatory cue "4, 3, 2, _____" when you are ready to change (see figure 4.6). Be sure to say "4" when your lead foot (e.g., right foot) is striking the floor and stepping right. You should always be mindful of your lead foot.

When you return to the march, your right foot is still leading, and the foot strike occurs on the downbeat or the actual first count of the 8-count phrase (which, as explained, is counted backward in 4s to make it easier for your participants). Be aware that to finish the 8 counts of the step touch, your right foot performs a tap or touch (the last movement of the 8-count step touch) immediately before leading right in the march. This is called *finishing the movement phrase* and is a key component in staying on the downbeat. If you forget to perform this tap or last touch, you will no longer be moving with the music and your participants will eventually become confused. Finishing the phrase is much simpler than it sounds; performing these moves to music will feel quite natural. You don't even need to mention this final tap or touch to your students; they'll do it unconsciously as long as you're moving with the downbeats.

Before trying this drill with music, go back and forth between marching and step touching, continuing each move as long as necessary for you to collect your thoughts and cue properly. Practice leading with your left foot, as well. Another basic pattern to practice is to go from a march to a wide march and then back again to the march, cueing "4, 3, march it wide" and "4, 3, march it back in." Experiment with speaking in rhythm. You want to hear the ticktock of the constant rhythmic beat at all times in your head while teaching. Eventually you can expand this drill to include a wide variety of 2-count moves (see the sample list of moves on page 57).

Practice these drills with a friend who will pretend to be your student. Your friend's responses can give you instant feedback about the timeliness and effectiveness of your cues. Then, repeat the entire drill with music. Pick popular music (preferably commercially-mixed group exercise music) with a strong, easy-to-hear beat. At first, these drills and speaking in rhythm may have a slightly robotic feel. This is appropriate in the early stages of learning to cue, when hearing and moving on the downbeat may not yet be habitual and spontaneous for you.

■ **Technique and Safety Check**

When cueing, be sure to

- hear the downbeat and the 8-count phrase,
- initiate new moves at the top of the 8-count phrase on the downbeat,
- initiate new moves with your lead foot,
- finish all moves (e.g. the last tap or touch),
- cue backward starting with "4,"
- speak in rhythm (at least initially), and
- cue the next move while you're still performing the current move.

Cueing 4-Count Moves Learning to cue 4-count moves is similar to learning to cue 2-count moves; however, instead of counting on every other beat, you count on every 4th beat. For example, perform grapevines, first to the right and then to the left continuously, leading with the right foot. When you are ready to change to the next move, such as a march, begin counting backward, starting with 4 when the right (lead) foot initiates a grapevine to the right. This time, however, count each individual grapevine, or every 4th count, as shown in figure 4.7.

Finish by marching right, which should be your lead foot. Notice again the final tap of the right foot just before the march; this tap finishes the last grapevine and is essential to keeping you moving with the music. When marching, return to the 2-count cueing you have already learned, saying, "4, 3, 2, grapevine" to cue the grapevine, at which point you'll again switch to the 4-count cueing (see figure 4.7). Practice moving back and forth between 2- and 4-count moves until the anticipatory cueing feels comfortable. A grapevine is a perfect move to practice visual cueing simultaneously, which we'll discuss shortly. Participants will be grateful if you point in the direction of the initial grapevine (to help them get started) and if you hold up fingers (4, 3, 2, 1) to let them know when the next change will occur.

 See the DVD for a practice drill on cueing 2-count and 4-count moves.

Another drill that entails switching from 2-count to 4-count anticipatory cueing involves moving from singles to doubles and back to singles again. Several moves work well for this drill, including knee lifts, hamstring curls, lunges, and step touches. Start with single hamstring curls, for instance, and cue on every 2 counts: "4, 3, 2, now doubles." Once you are doing doubles, each hamstring curl requires 4 counts. When you are ready to return to singles, cue on every 4 counts: "4, 3, 2, 1, now single."

Movement Cues

A movement cue verbalizes what is seemingly obvious. Many participants need this verbal reinforcement to enhance their confidence and

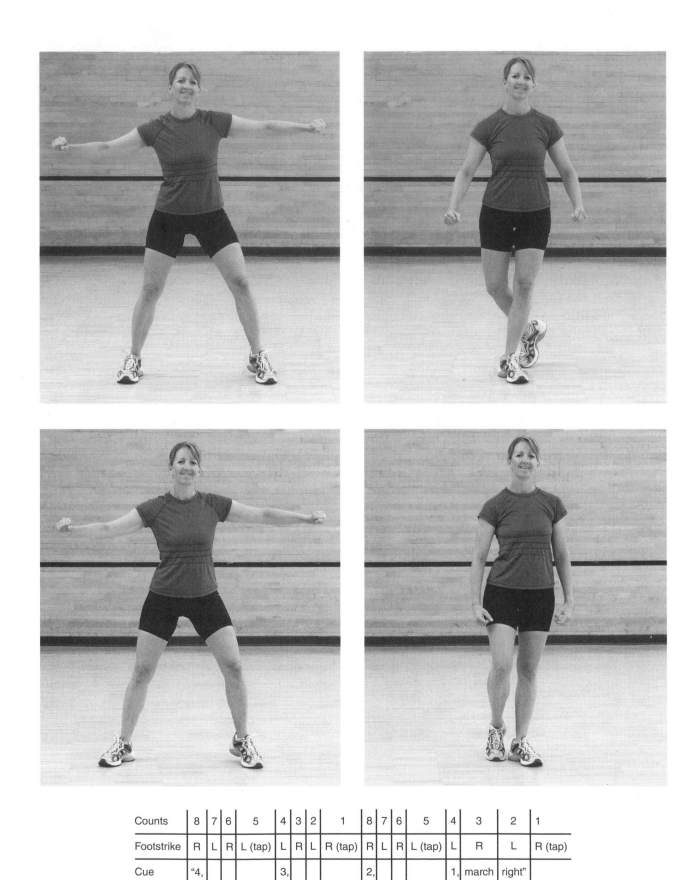

Counts	8	7	6	5	4	3	2	1	8	7	6	5	4	3	2	1
Footstrike	R	L	R	L (tap)	L	R	L	R (tap)	R	L	R	L (tap)	L	R	L	R (tap)
Cue	"4,				3,				2,				1,	march	right"	

▶ **Figure 4.7** Practice changing from a grapevine to a march while cueing.

success. A movement cue can point out foot-work, either with rhythmic counts, as in a cha-cha ("the feet go 1, 2, 1, 2, 3—1, 2, 1, 2, 3"), or with rights and lefts, as when lunging ("right foot back, left foot back, right foot back, left foot back"). It can also provide basic directions, as in a double lunge ("feet go down, up, down, switch—down, up, down, switch"). Such cues may be repeated over and over with appropriate rhythmic emphasis until participants perform the pattern correctly. Movement cues also include naming the move (e.g., "pivot turn" or "twist") and stating an actual direction, as in "grapevine right." We recommend always accompanying the words *right* and *left* with the visual cue of point-ing. Some participants experience confusion and anxiety when suddenly asked to move right or left, but these feelings can be eased or eliminated with pointing, which is a visual cue.

Motivational Cues

Motivational cue increases your participants' self-confidence and enjoyment and encourages a sense of play! Your speech should be liberally sprinkled with encouraging words and phrases: "Great," "Super," "Well done," "Fantastic job," "You people look terrific," "Outstanding." Some instructors give motivational cues every 8 to 16 counts—no wonder their classes are so popular! Additionally, many instructors cut loose with whoops, trills, yahoos, hup hup, and other noises just for fun. If you have a good time in class, the chances are good that your students will too!

Educational Cues

An educational cue delivers relevant information about the workout or about other topics related to fitness and wellness. Reviewing the benefits of aerobic training while leading simple freestyle moves is an excellent way to incorporate educa-tion into your teaching. And, of course, it's essen-tial to give intensity recommendations throughout your class. Identifying muscle groups ("These are your hamstrings.") and hydration information are other examples of educational cueing.

Alignment and Safety Cues

Skilled instructors constantly deliver pointers on alignment and safety. Common misalign-ments observed during cardiorespiratory train-ing include a forward head (chin jut), rounded and hunched shoulders, shoulders that elevate when reaching overhead, hyperextended elbows and knees, and a lack of spinal and pelvic stability (particularly during knee lifts and kicks). When participants perform lunges or repeaters, their hips, knees, and toes all need to point in the same direction. Safety cues include reminding participants to bring their heels down when jumping, to avoid excessive momentum, to stay in control, to keep their fists relaxed, to listen to their bodies, to work at their own pace, and to stay hydrated. It's nearly impossible to give too many of these types of cues! See the technique and safety section on page 69 for more ideas.

Visual Cues

Do everything possible to ensure your par-ticipants' success. If the majority of your class members consistently have trouble following or grasping new moves, their difficulty prob-ably has more to do with you than with them. Such problems can be traced to the instruc-tor's moves, transitions, sequencing, ability to work with music, and ability to cue correctly. Thus, you will want to work hard to make your cueing crystal clear. One major way to help participants move with you at all times is to use visual cueing in conjunction with verbal cueing. Adding visual cues is essential when you work with large groups or without a microphone, and in addition it can save your voice. A number of visual cues have been developed and are used commonly by cardio instructors (Webb 1989). These include hand signals for counting, show-ing direction, turning, holding a move, tapping the thigh of the lead leg, calling for everyone's attention ("Watch me!"), and pointing to various parts of your own body to indicate proper align-ment (see figure 4.8).

Most people are visual learners. Without really thinking about it, they tend to copy your body language, including your alignment, physi-cal energy, and movement style. This is good if you have excellent alignment and physical energy; however, it can be problematic if you use incorrect alignment or technique.

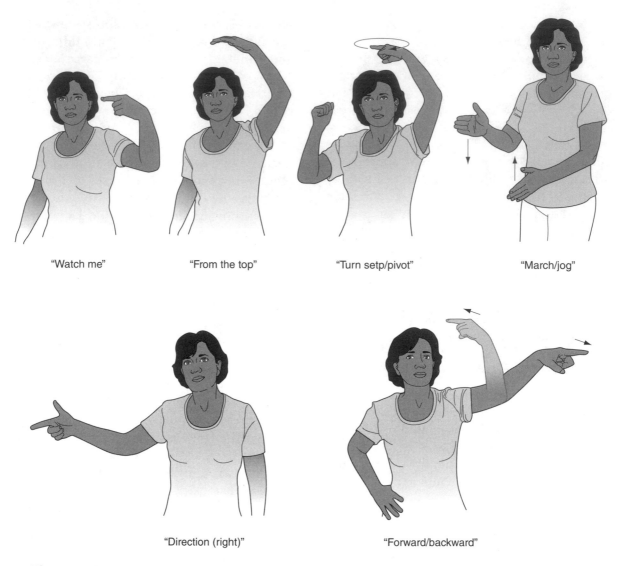

"Watch me" "From the top" "Turn setp/pivot" "March/jog"

"Direction (right)" "Forward/backward"

▶ **Figure 4.8** Visual cues.

When you face your class while moving, you are using the technique of mirror imaging. Mirror imaging is another valuable group leadership skill that takes practice. The advantages of mirror imaging include more personal and direct eye contact with your students, better vocal projection, and less temptation to become mesmerized by your own image in the mirror. Facing your class shows that you are a student-centered instructor and makes your job seem less like a performance. We recommend facing your class as much as possible, especially during the warm-up, during times you are leading freestyle choreography, and during the muscle conditioning and flexibility portions of your class. The major disadvantage of facing your class is that if your combinations are relatively complex, they'll be more difficult for your class to follow. In other words, your participants are more likely to be successful if you face away from them during intricate choreography.

Mirroring takes practice. When you want your class to move right, you have to point left with your left hand, even as you are saying "right." If you want your participants to march forward, you'll need to move backward as you motion them to come toward you. Your directional cues will be reversed for you but not for your class.

■ Practice Drill

Play your favorite music—pick something with a strong beat. Face a partner and begin a familiar move (such as a walk or step touch). Your partner should follow along, according to your visual cues. Continue the move for 4 to 16 counts, and then transition through several different moves (this works best if your transitions are smooth and natural and you use the elements of variation). Try not to speak at all; use only visual cueing to communicate with your partner. This includes having an animated face and conveying lots of enthusiasm! Note how well your partner follows your visual cues. Is there any way you could improve your visual cueing to enhance your partner's success?

For practice, repeat all the drills described in this chapter while facing a partner.

Movement Previews

When you are teaching more complex choreography, sometimes a movement preview is useful. While having your participants continue with a familiar move, you can demonstrate (preview) the new move or the more complex variation for them so that they can see it before they do it. For example, while your participants perform grapevines, you can preview the next, more complex layer by demonstrating grapevines with a turn.

Constructive Corrections

We must not underestimate the participant's overall experience in a group exercise class. How participants are treated and whether they are comfortable can make or break their attendance in your class. Bain and colleagues (1989) compared the dropout rate of group exercise participants who were overweight with the rate of those who were at their recommended weight and found that the dropout rate of the overweight participants was higher. They dropped out not because they did not like the music or the routine but because they were concerned about being embarrassed and judged by others. Wininger (2002) found that

an instructor's ability to communicate is an important aspect of the participant's overall enjoyment. Therefore, how you give your participants feedback is important. Once you have observed improper technique in your group exercise classes, take action but make sure you are kind. Some instructors find this the most challenging part of teaching because it's often hard to be a strong motivator yet also a soft encourager when a participant needs correction. See the section titled "Effective Communication When Giving Corrections" on page 75 for a few suggestions on how to cue the participant on correct position or technique without being threatening or critical. Figure 4.9 provides a cueing example.

Find ways to make your class a positive experience for all. Correcting and recommending alignment changes in a polite and nonthreatening way makes the exercise experience more comfortable for participants. If they are comfortable, they will be more likely to come back. If students are ill at ease, they may miss some of the wonderful therapeutic benefits that come from group exercise (Choi et al. 1993; Estivill 1995), such as a positive mood and increased self-esteem. These mental and emotional benefits that are derived from the group exercise experience can be just as beneficial as the physical gains.

 See the DVD for a practice drill on correcting alignment for a stationary lunge.

■ Comprehension Check

Here are the key points for cueing:

- As much as possible, cue both verbally and visually.
- Use a microphone whenever possible.
- Avoid endless counting. Instead, use your time whenever possible to deliver other types of cues (e.g., alignment, motivational).
- Always count down instead of up.
- Keep cues relatively short and to the point.
- Initiate cues on the downbeat and time them so that new moves are also on the downbeat.

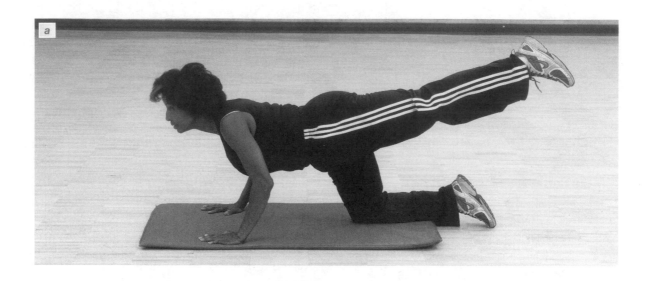

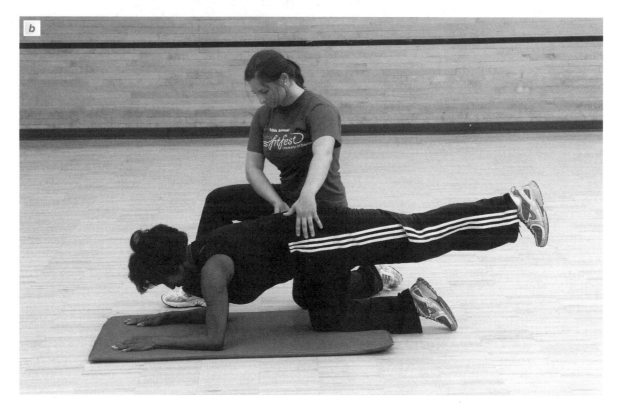

▶ **Figure 4.9** Cueing example: *(a)* poor technique and *(b)* instructor correction. You may imagine that the instructor is telling the participant, "Please bring your elbows a little closer to your knees so that your hip is directly over your support knee. Also, please keep your gaze down so that your head is in line with your spine."

Effective Communication When Giving Corrections

1. Deliver General Statements to the Whole Group

"Stop for just a moment—look at your back foot to see if your toe is facing straight ahead. The toe must be straight ahead to stretch effectively." Or, "I see people having difficulty—let me demonstrate what I want you to do."

2. Make Corrections by Moving the Person Into the Proper Position

During a wall stretch for the calves, give the following instruction to people experiencing difficulty: "I would like to turn your foot so it is straight. Is that OK? Can you feel a difference in the stretch?" Always ask permission before touching a student.

3. Exercise Next to the Participant

Stand beside the person having trouble and demonstrate what you want him to do. Perhaps he cannot quite see or hear you well enough to comply. If the person you are correcting is down on the floor, get down next to him to demonstrate. A person on the floor is more vulnerable than the person standing, so you must get down on the same level to instruct in a nonthreatening way.

4. Move Around the Room

If you stay at the front of the class, only the people in the front row will be able to observe your technique. If you are teaching step, put several benches around the room so you can move around during the cardio segment. Try teaching in the middle of the class instead of the front or regularly move from the front to the back to the side of the room.

5. Catch People Doing It Right

Most people respond much better to positive rather than negative reinforcement. If a participant is having difficulty with a movement or series of movements, point out someone performing well in class for her to watch or pair them together. Always demonstrate and instruct good alignment to keep a focus on correct technique.

6. Always Appeal to a Person's Need for Safety and Give Your Rationale

Compare "You must have your foot in this position" with "Place your foot in this position because it will prevent you from falling forward and will make this exercise easier." Or, "Don't bounce while stretching; that's the wrong technique" versus "If you bounce while stretching you might pull or tear a muscle—I don't want you to get hurt. Try holding the stretch instead." Which statement would you rather hear? Both statements tell the participant how to correct their actions; however, the second statements include a rationale and helpful alternatives.

7. Use Positive Descriptions Rather Than Labels

Words such as *good, bad, right,* and *wrong* are emotionally loaded and judgmental. Instead of saying, "Joe, you are doing this movement wrong," try, "Joe, you seem to be having trouble with this movement. Let's try this . . . I think it will help."

CHAPTER WRAP-UP

Our goal as group instructors is to make exercise fun to enhance the health and well-being of our participants. On way to do this is by using quality music played on good sound systems. This chapter covered music fundamentals as well as practical techniques for leading a high-low cardio group exercise class. Most of the topics and techniques described in this chapter also apply to other types of group exercise, such as step, slide, NIA, and kickboxing.

When developing your cardiorespiratory segment, check yourself against the group exercise class evaluation form to be sure you've met the basic criteria for leading cardio segments. To become proficient at leading group exercise, you must practice, experiment, and keep challenging yourself. The rewards are worth it; you will soon lead a class that your participants will want to take again and again!

▶ **Assignment**

Attend a group exercise class and observe an instructor getting ready to teach a class. Write down all the steps she or he takes to set up the music and microphone and how equipment is set up. Research the Web or contact one vendor from the music resource list and create a price list of a complete sound system for use in a group exercise setting. Write a one-page summary of your findings.

Class activity: In a group of 4-5 participants prepare a 2 minute high/low cardio routine to present. Use at least two 32-count blocks of simple choreography. Incorporate anticipatory cueing (on the downbeat), visual cueing, and at least one other cueing technique.

PART II

Primary Components of Group Exercise

Warm-Up and Stretching Principles

By the end of this chapter, you will

- be able to integrate the components of health into group exercise class design,
- be able to prepare a warm-up segment,
- know how to create rehearsal moves for a warm-up, and
- understand how stretching fits into the warm-up segment.

A warm-up begins by setting the atmosphere with engaging music and energy. If you are using music, the first song sets the tone for your class and gets people ready to begin moving. During the first portion of the warm-up, movements should be dynamic, using large muscle groups. The second portion should build on the first and combine warming up and stretching if appropriate. A class tends to flow better if the second portion is more upbeat and if stretching (if used) is performed in a standing position so that you can move right into the cardiorespiratory segment. We begin this chapter by reviewing the warm-up component of the group exercise class evaluation form (found in appendix A).

DYNAMIC MOVEMENT

Energetic music is one of the keys to a successful and fun dynamic segment of the warm-up. Utilizing music with a tempo of 120 to 136 beats per minute and positive lyrics is the first practical consideration of the warm-up of any group exercise class. Songs that motivate and inspire, such as the theme to *Rocky* or the songs played when introducing players at a basketball game, bring energy to the room and create a dynamic interactive aspect of a group exercise class. In essence the music selection sets the stage as much as the movement selection does. For specific ideas on music selection, see chapter 4.

Group Exercise Class Evaluation Warm-Up Essentials

- Includes appropriate amount of dynamic movement
- Provides rehearsal moves
- Stretches major muscle groups in a biomechanically sound manner with appropriate instructions
- Gives clear cues and verbal directions
- Uses an appropriate music tempo (120-136 beats per minute) or motivating music that inspires movement

---

The warm-up prepares the body for the more rigorous demands of the cardiorespiratory and muscular strength and conditioning segments; one way it does this is by raising the body's internal temperature. For each degree of temperature elevation, the metabolic rate of cells increases about 13% (Astrand and Rodahl 1977). In addition, at higher body temperatures, blood flow to the working muscles increases, as does the release of oxygen to the muscles. Because these effects allow more efficient energy production to fuel muscle contraction, the goal of an effective warm-up should be to elevate internal temperatures by 1 or 2 degrees Fahrenheit (0.5-1 C). You may notice that sweating results. Increasing body temperature has other effects that are beneficial for exercisers; see the section, "Physiological Benefits of Warming Up", on page 81. Many of these physiological effects may reduce the risk of injury because they have the potential to increase neuromuscular coordination, delay fatigue, and make the tissues less susceptible to damage (Alter 2004).

DYNAMIC MOVEMENT VERSUS STRETCHING

There is much confusion in the stretching literature due to a misinterpretation of research on warming up. Herbert and de Noronha (2007) found that warming up by itself has no effect on ROM but that when warming up is followed by stretching, ROM increases. Many people interpreted this finding to mean that stretching before exercise prevents injuries, even though the clinical research suggests otherwise. A better interpretation is that warming up prevents injury, whereas stretching has no effect on injury. Therefore, the focus during the warm-up should be on dynamic movements that increase core body temperature (see figure 5.1). Most warm-up segments of group exercise classes last 5 to 8 minutes. The sport literature recommends that the majority of this time be spent on warming up rather than stretching. However, sports are very different from the group exercise experience, which focuses more on enhancing healthy lifestyles than on improving performance. Until stretching for group exercise is researched, we will continue to suggest that incorporating brief stretches into the warm-up is acceptable.

Remember that the diaphragm, the major muscle involved in breathing, is like any other muscle group and needs time to shift gears. A rapid increase in breathing that doesn't give the diaphragm enough time to warm up properly can result in side aches and hyperventilation (rapid, shallow breathing). Sudden increases in breathing mean that the transition into the cardiorespiratory segment was not gradual enough. Incorporating a few deep breaths into the dynamic warm-up will assist in warming up the diaphragm.

REHEARSAL MOVES

Rehearsal moves make up the majority of the warm-up, preparing participants for the challenges of the workout to come (Anderson 2000). Blahnik and Anderson (1996) defined rehearsal moves as "movements that are identical to, but less intense than, the movements your students will execute during the workout phase" (50). Examples of rehearsal moves for various group exercise formats can be found on page 82. Appel (2007) feels that the right rehearsal move warms up participants mentally as well as physically. She encourages instructors to focus on dynamic flexibility rather than static stretching and to focus on exercises that improve balance, coordination, postural control, and joint stability.

Physiological Benefits of Warming Up

The physiological benefits of warming up are as follows:

- Increased metabolic rate
- Higher rate of oxygen exchange between blood and muscles
- More oxygen released within muscles
- Faster nerve impulse transmission
- Gradual redistribution of blood flow to working muscles
- Decreased muscle relaxation time following contraction
- Increased speed and force of muscle contraction
- Increased muscle elasticity
- Increased flexibility of tendons and ligaments
- Gradual increase in energy production, which limits lactic acid buildup
- Reduced risk of abnormal electrocardiogram
- Joint lubrication

The concept of using rehearsal moves in the warm-up relates to the principle of specificity of training. This principle states that the body

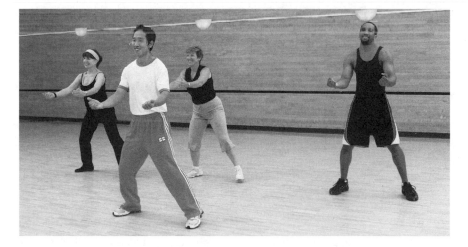

▶ **Figure 5.1** According to research, the warm-up segment should focus on dynamic movements that increase core body temperature.

adapts specifically to whatever demands are placed on it. Some researchers believe that specificity applies not only to energy systems and muscle groups but also to movement patterns (American College of Sports Medicine 1998). Because the motor units used during training demonstrate the majority of physiological alterations, movement patterns must be specifically trained. In a group exercise class, one of the main reasons participants become frustrated is that they are not able to perform the movements effectively. Introducing movement patterns in the warm-up helps wake up associated motor units and ensure that participants perform those patterns with success later on in the workout.

Using rehearsal moves in the warm-up not only specifically prepares the body for the movement ahead but also sets down neuromuscular patterns by introducing new skills. For example,

in a high-low impact class using a grapevine (R, L, R, tap; L, R, L, tap), the warm-up can be used to break down the move, identify the directional landmarks in the room, and name the specific move. If this groundwork is laid during the warm-up, when a grapevine is referred to in the cardiorespiratory segment, the class participants will know what to do. The same idea applies to complex choreography movements in a step class. You can practice the movement combination slowly in the warm-up, when maintaining a higher level of intensity is not the focus. When this movement comes up in the routine later on, it will have been rehearsed, and this will make it easier for participants to maintain their cardiorespiratory intensity level. Rehearsal moves, therefore, should make up a large part of the warm-up.

 See the DVD for a sample step warm-up. Note that this warm-up is also outlined in appendix F.

Rehearsal Move Suggestions for Various Group Exercise Formats

These suggested movements preview actions that will be used in the cardio segment following the warm-up

- Step: Use the bench during the warm-up.
- Indoor cycling: Teach participants how to climb a hill properly.
- Water exercise: Practice an interval segment (30 s rest, 30 s work) using a cross-country skier movement.
- Muscle conditioning: Use muscle-specific movements in the warm-up, such as biceps curls, triceps kickbacks, and squats.
- Kickboxing: Use shuffles, kicks, and punches.
- High-low impact class: Review a 32-count series.
- Sport conditioning: Use the ladders and walk through the movement.

STRETCHING MAJOR MUSCLE GROUPS

Whether to stretch during the warm-up is a debated issue, one on which the literature has not yet agreed. Taylor and colleagues (1990) found that flexibility gains were most significant when a stretch was held for 12 to 18 seconds and repeated four times per muscle group. Another study (Walter et al. 1995) found that stretching the hamstrings for 30 seconds produced significantly greater flexibility than stretching for 10 seconds produced. If these two studies were the complete story, we would probably recommend not stretching in a group exercise warm-up, because it is impossible to stretch a muscle group four times and hold each stretch for 30 seconds and still accomplish the goals of increasing the heart rate and core temperature. Another study (Girouard and Hurley 1995) of strength and flexibility training in older adults found that stretching before and after training did not increase flexibility. Convincing research on runners (Lally 1994; Shrier 1999; Van Mechelen et al. 1993) demonstrated that static stretches performed during the warm-up did not prevent injury. These studies encourage injury prevention through dynamic warm-up rather than stretching.

The 2006 ACSM position stand on exercise addresses flexibility, recommending that we stretch 2 to 3 days per week (the ideal is 5-7 days per week), that we hold stretches 15 to 30 seconds, and that we perform each stretch per major muscle group 2 to 4 times (American College of Sports Medicine 2006). The ACSM position stand was based on a review of many different research studies on stretching. Shrier and Gossal (2000) reviewed the stretching literature and found that one static stretch of 15 to 30 seconds per day was sufficient to enhance flexibility. It is generally agreed that flexibility exercises are beneficial, but questions remain about where to put them in the class format for group exercise. New research suggests that stretching doesn't prevent muscle soreness after exercise. In a recent systemic review and meta-analysis of 10 previously published studies on stretching, Herbert and de Noronha (2007) concluded that stretching before exercise doesn't prevent postexercise muscle soreness. They found little support for the theory that stretching immediately before exercise can prevent either overuse or acute injuries.

Most prominent exercise physiology textbooks (Baechle and Earle 2003; McArdle et al. 2006; Howley and Powers 2006; Howley and Franks 2007; Wilmore and Costill 2004) and stretching books (Alter 2004) recommend an active warm-up that includes rehearsal moves followed by brief stretching; these books recommend that the majority of flexibility work be done during the cool-down of the workout. However, these books are written with the individual and, often, the athlete in mind, and they are not necessarily specific to working with a group. Generally, they also include some stretching within the warm-up, and they all advocate that a warm-up precede any stretching. According to Neiman (2003), a warm-up will enhance the activity of enzymes in the working muscle, reduce the viscosity of muscle, improve the mechanical efficiency and power of the moving muscles, facilitate the transmission speed of nervous impulses augmenting coordination, increase muscle blood flow and thus improve delivery of necessary fuel substrates, increase the level of free fatty acids in the blood, help prevent injuries to the muscles and various supporting connective tissues, and allow the heart muscle to adequately prepare itself for aerobic exercise. Thacker and colleagues (2004) determined that there is not sufficient evidence to endorse or discontinue routine stretching before or after exercise to prevent injury among competitive or recreational athletes. Further research, especially well-conducted randomized controlled trials, is needed to determine the proper role of stretching in group exercise activities. Given that there is no conclusive evidence showing any inherent benefit to stretching during the warm-up and that there are a few studies suggesting that it might be dangerous, the warm-up should contain mostly dynamic movements with some static stretches held briefly (5-10 seconds) if this is the only place flexibility is included in the format. Many participants avoid stretching, so including it in the warm-up is a good strategy to ensure that all components of fitness are addressed.

Studies do support the finding that ROM can be increased by a single 15- to 30-second stretch for each muscle group per day. However, some people require a longer duration or more repetitions to increase their flexibility. Research also supports the idea that the optimal duration and frequency for stretching may vary by muscle group (Witvrouw et al. 2004). The long-term effects of stretching on ROM show that after 6 weeks, people who stretched for 30 seconds per muscle each day increased their ROM much more than those who stretched for 15 seconds per muscle each day. No additional increase was seen in the group that stretched for 60 seconds per muscle per day (Shrier and Gossal 2000). Overall, studies support the use of 30-second stretches as part of general conditioning to improve ROM (Andersen 2005). See chapter 7 for specific stretching movements for all the major muscle groups.

In general, proprioceptive neuromuscular facilitation (PNF) stretching creates greater increases in ROM compared with static or ballistic stretching, though some results demonstrating this finding have not been statistically significant. However, PNF stretching is not appropriate for a group exercise setting. PNF stretching is better in a one-on-one setting where there is thorough understanding of which muscle is contracting and which one is relaxing.

Static stretches are a bit easier to perform than PNF stretches and appear to have good results. However, using seated static stretches where a stretch is held for 30 seconds or more in the warm-up is not recommended, as doing so disrupts the flow of the group exercise class. We recommend brief lengthening of the muscles in the warm up by holding stretches for 5 to 10 seconds to increase range of motion for the activity to come. Studies indicate that continuous stretching without rest may be better than cyclic stretching (applying a stretch, relaxing, and reapplying the stretch); however, other studies show no difference.

Most experts believe that ballistic stretching, or bouncing while stretching, is dangerous because the muscle may reflexively contract if restretched quickly following a short relaxation period. Such eccentric contractions are believed to increase the risk of injury.

In addition to improving ROM, stretching is extremely relaxing. Most athletes also use stretching exercises to maintain a balance in body mechanics. One of the biggest benefits of stretching may be something that research just can't quantify: It feels good.

 See the DVD for an example warm-up for a high-low impact group exercise class.

The warm-up for a sports conditioning class, much like that of any other group exercise format, should involve activities that will be used in the cardiorespiratory segment. A typical sports conditioning class uses a different style than most high-low, step, or kickboxing classes use. Its warm-up is much like what you would do if you were warming up to play tennis, soccer, volleyball, and so on. It includes general calisthenics performed at a less intense effort than in the cardio segment. This warm-up can be performed in an open or circle format much like what you experienced in your physical education classes. A sports conditioning warm-up segment might involve the following movements:

- Walking in a circle on your toes to warm up your calves

- High knee walks to warm up your quadriceps and hip flexors
- High knee walks with hip rotation to warm up your abductor and adductor muscles
- Heel kicks to the seat to warm up the hamstrings while walking or jogging
- Large shoulder circles while walking to warm up the shoulder joint
- Lateral movements like a grapevine or karaoke movement to warm up the core and lower back muscles
- Rehearsal moves such as a brief walk or jog around cones to increase lateral movement and balance, which will both be used at a higher intensity during the cardio segment

 See DVD for an example of a warm-up for a sport conditioning class.

When you are designing the warm-up segment for your group exercise class, it's best to focus on rehearsal movements. If you are including static stretches, try to focus on active movement as well as stretching. For example, while performing a standing calf or hamstring stretch, keep the arms moving up and down to stay warm (see figure 5.2). Likewise, when you are designing a warm-up for a cycling class, keep the legs pedaling while performing upper-body stretches.

If you are teaching a 30-minute class, it might be better to save the stretching for the end, when it will be most beneficial in enhancing flexibility. In a short class, it might not be appropriate to do static stretching in the beginning at all. On the other hand, when you are teaching a group of seniors, you might find that they prefer performing several minutes of static stretching at the end of their warm-up. After they have warmed up, they can hold a stretch for increased flexibility and balance. By the end of the class, fatigue may prevent them from performing static stretches appropriately.

Only instructors who know their participants well will know what warm-up format fits them best. How to go about warming up and stretching is an individual decision. While there is controversy over what is the most effective for the warm-up segment, all group exercise classes ought to include this segment. We know

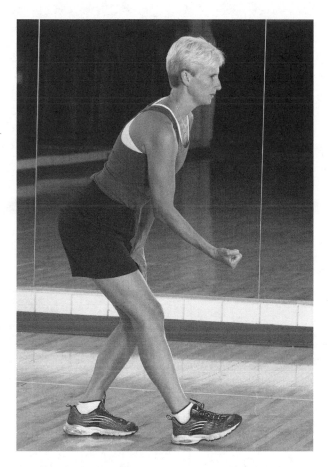

▶ **Figure 5.2** You can combine a static stretch with an active movement by performing a standing hamstring stretch with deltoid movement to keep the upper body warm. This movement may be performed with one arm while the opposite hand rests on the thigh to provide support for the low back.

that flexibility is a health-related component of fitness and should be included in the overall workout and that warming up and performing rehearsal moves before any static stretching are important no matter what group exercise format is being taught. We also know that flexibility is enhanced best at the end of any class format. Therefore save the stretching for the end of the overall workout for optimum health benefits to your participants.

CHAPTER WRAP-UP

This chapter outlined the variables that are common to the warm-up segment of most group exercise classes; these variables are listed on the evaluation form in appendix A. Whether you are teaching a cycling, sport conditioning, step, or kickboxing class, you should include an appropriate amount of dynamic movement, provide rehearsal moves, stretch major muscle groups in a biomechanically sound manner (hold briefly 5 to 10 seconds), give clear cues and verbal directions, and use music that motivates and inspires.

▶ **Assignment**

Attend the beginning of a group exercise class and notice how the instructor sets the atmosphere for the class. Using the group exercise class evaluation form, write down everything the instructor does during the warm-up. Create a 4-minute group warm-up segment (for 4-5 individuals) integrating the concepts discussed in this chapter. Prepare to practice your warm-up segment during class.

Cardiorespiratory Training

CHAPTER OBJECTIVES

By the end of this chapter, you will

- explain the importance of selecting an appropriate beginning intensity,
- understand the principles of muscle balance in cardiorespiratory programming,
- be able to give movement options and verbal cues for the cardiorespiratory segment,
- understand the importance of participant interaction,
- explain the importance of the postcardio cool-down,
- demonstrate two methods for monitoring intensity during the cardio segment, and
- review the importance of having an automated external defibrillator (AED) on site.

A few common principles apply to the cardiorespiratory segment of group exercise classes. These principles are listed under the cardiorespiratory training segment on the group exercise class evaluation form (appendix A) and repeated here on this page. During the cardiorespiratory segment of a group exercise class, it is also critical that you monitor exercise intensity. Important details for learning and teaching these techniques are discussed later in this chapter.

BEGINNING INTENSITY

Even though the human body adapts to exercise very efficiently, gradually increasing intensity is necessary for many reasons:

- Blood flow is redistributed from internal organs to the working muscles.
- The heart muscle gradually adapts to the change from a resting level to a working level.
- The respiratory rate gradually increases.

The most dangerous times for changes in the heart's rhythm are in the transitions from resting to high-intensity work and from high-intensity activity back to resting. At rest, the cardiorespiratory system circulates about 1.3 gallons (5 L)

of blood per minute. Imagine the contents of 2.5 2-liter soda pop bottles circulating through your body every minute. At maximal strenuous exercise, as much as 6.6 gallons (25 L) per minute must circulate to accommodate working muscles in a very fit person—that's 12.5 soda pop bottles per minute! Going from rest to strenuous exercise takes time and requires a gradual increase in intensity during the cardio segment. If your participants are out of breath in the first few minutes of the cardio session, you have not allowed enough time for the redistribution of blood flow to occur. Use verbal cues such as, "Keep your arms low!" You can also begin with, "We are just starting out, so let's give our bodies time to adapt to this new level of intensity."

To gradually increase intensity within a group exercise setting, start with moves that use little ROM, a short lever length, and limited traveling. In a step class, keep moves less intense by not using propulsion moves at the beginning of class. In a water exercise class, use moves that have a smaller ROM or shorter lever length. Finally, in an indoor cycling class, keep the flywheel tension set at a lower resistance for the first few minutes of cardio training.

 See the DVD for an example of proper intensity and good verbal cueing.

Group Exercise Class Evaluation Form Essentials

- Gradually increases intensity
- Uses a variety of muscle groups (especially hamstrings and abductors)
- Minimizes repetitive movements
- Promotes participant interaction and encourages fun
- Demonstrates movement options and gives clear verbal cues
- Gradually decreases impact and intensity during cool-down following the cardiorespiratory session
- Uses music volume and tempo appropriate for biomechanical movement

---

MOVEMENT OPTIONS AND VERBAL CUES FOR INTENSITY

Whether you are leading a high-low impact, treadmill, circuit, or indoor cycling class, it is impossible to be everywhere at once or help everyone simultaneously. Each participant is working at a different fitness level and has different goals. Ideally, all classes would be organized according to a given intensity and duration. The reality is that many participants come to a class because the time is convenient and not necessarily because the class length or intensity level is suitable. If participants try to exercise at the instructor's level or at another participant's level, they may work too hard and sustain an injury or they may work too little and not meet their goals. A few ways to promote self-responsibility are to encourage participants to work at their own pace, demonstrate heart rate (HR) monitoring or rating of perceived exertion (RPE) checks, and use common examples to inform participants how they should feel. For example, during the peak portion of the cardiorespiratory segment, tell participants that they should feel out of breath but still be able to talk. During the postcardio cool-down, tell them that they should feel their HR slowing down. Be as descriptive as possible concerning perceived exertion. Demonstrate high-, medium-, and low-intensity and impact options in order to reach participants at various levels. Pointing out participants who work at higher or lower levels can also help.

Help participants achieve the level of effort they need to reach, and continually remind them that reaching this point is their responsibility. It is not your job to be responsible for participants' exercise intensity, but it is your job to separate your ego from your role as an instructor. Instructing a class at your level will not allow for different intensity options. We recommend you maintain a medium intensity most of the time and present other options and intensities as the need arises. A practical example of this is demonstrating a side tap while encouraging those who want more intensity to perform a power squat

and those who want even more intensity and impact to perform a regular jumping jack (see figure 6.1). Teaching to different levels and abilities is the true art of group exercise instruction and the reason why group exercise can be more difficult to teach than one-on-one instruction.

MONITORING EXERCISE INTENSITY

Understanding HR, RPE, and the talk test is the first step in monitoring exercise intensity. One method of monitoring is not advocated over another, because all have applications depending on the type of activities the participants are performing. There is no one test that works for all group exercise participants (see "Intensity Monitoring in the Group Exercise Setting" on page 93). Many group exercise instructors have stopped using manual HR monitoring because it disrupts the flow of the class, although using a HR monitor is always an option. There are no hard and fast rules for monitoring intensity other than it must be done. See the section on intensity monitoring research for specific studies on monitoring during group exercise. Monitoring intensity or using gauges that constantly monitor

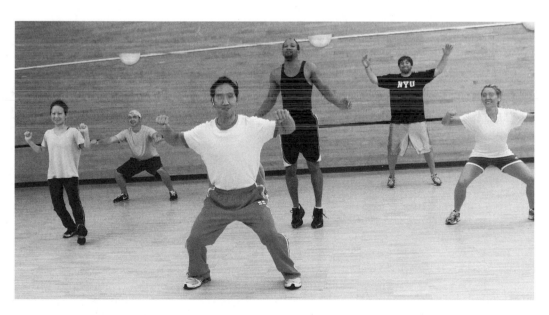

▶ **Figure 6.1** For cardiorespiratory training, you should demonstrate the low- and high-intensity options but continue moving at the middle option. In this example, the instructor performs a power squat while participants are demonstrating the step tap (lower intensity) or jumping jack (higher intensity).

intensity shows empathy for the participants. A summary of how to use target HR, RPE, and the talk test is given next.

Measuring Heart Rate

Exercise intensity within the cardiorespiratory segment must be monitored. Participants need to know the purpose of monitoring HR during exercise and how to obtain a pulse rate. Proper instruction on how to measure HR is the first step to monitoring intensity effectively.

There are many sites on the body to monitor heart rate. The potential sites that are the easiest to use for measuring heart rate are outlined in Figure 6.2.

- Carotid pulse site. This pulse site is on the carotid artery, just to the side of the larynx. Use light pressure from the fingertips of the first two fingers, not the thumb, to take your pulse. Never palpate both carotid arteries at the same time, and always press lightly.

- Radial pulse site. This pulse site is on the radial artery at the wrist, in line with the thumb. Use the fingertips of your first two or three fingers to take your pulse. Keep your hand below your heart. Many people

find a pulse in this location right where they wear their watchbands.

- The temporal site is just to side of the eye right above the ear. This site can often be felt without palpating a pulse. Marching lightly and paying attention to this area can result in feeling your pulse rate.

- The brachial site is on the inside of the arm where one would measure a blood pressure. This is a difficult one to palpate and is often the least used in a group exercise setting.

Be very careful when using the carotid site for checking your pulse. Near the carotid site are baroreceptors that are very sensitive to pressure. When you press on the carotid artery, these baroreceptors send a message to the brain to decrease HR and increase blood pressure to allow the brain better access to oxygen. If you press too firmly and cut off the oxygen going to your brain, you will find yourself horizontal on the ground very quickly. Instruct participants to press lightly whenever they use the carotid artery site. Also discourage the use of this site with older adults, as they may have plaque buildup in these arteries. If participants insist

Intensity Monitoring Research

Parker and colleagues (1989) performed a research study on intensity monitoring in group exercise, in which they determined that HRs taken during high-low impact group exercise reflect a lower relative exercise intensity ($\dot{V}O_2$max) than HRs taken during running. Other research (Roach et al. 1994) on different forms of group exercise (step, interval high-low impact, and progressive treadmill training) concluded that HR may not be an appropriate predictor of exercise intensity and that RPE is the preferred method of monitoring intensity. Grant and coworkers (2002) compared RPE and physiological responses for two modes of aerobic exercise (walking and aerobic dance) in men and women aged 50 years and older. They found that aerobic dance was a bit more intense than walking was for this age group. However, both modes of exercise met the ACSM requirements for exercise intensity. Finally, research by Frangolias and Rhodes (1995) suggests that using land HRs when the chest is submerged in water during water exercise is not appropriate. Janot (2005) suggests that it is best to combine methods of intensity monitoring in order to maximize effectiveness in a group exercise setting. Many research studies on HR were performed on runners and cyclists, not participants in group exercise. Therefore, in a treadmill class or an indoor cycling class, HR monitors can be effective, while in a kickboxing class in which the arms are moving in many different directions, RPE might be a better choice.

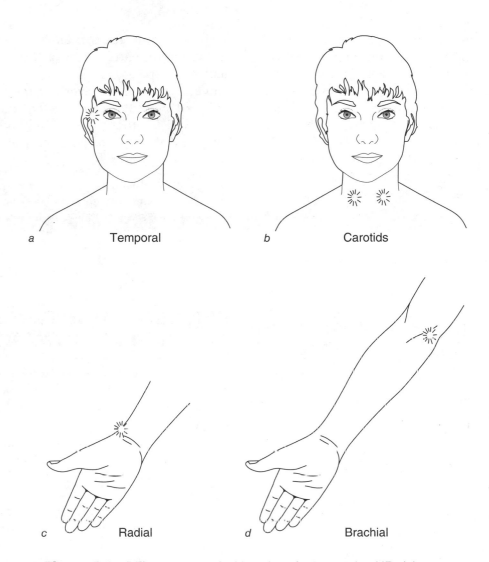

a Temporal   *b* Carotids

c Radial   *d* Brachial

▶ **Figure 6.2** Different anatomical locations for measuring HR: *(a)* temporal, *(b)* carotid, *(c)* radial, and *(d)* brachial.

on using this site they can obtain an incorrect reading and also decrease blood flow to the brain.

Heart Rate Reserve and Target Heart Rate

A method for determining target HR is the HR reserve method, commonly known as the *Karvonen formula* (see the section titled "Using HR Reserve to Determine Target HR" on page 93). The recommended intensities when monitoring with the HR reserve method (50%-85%) correspond to similar recommended percentages of maximal oxygen uptake. The HR reserve method takes into account resting HR when determining

target HR. It is estimated that a participant's maximal heart rate (HRmax) equals 220 beats per minute minus the participant's age. Currently, there are many equations for predicting HRmax that take into account variables other than age, but these may contain large standard errors of estimate, which may result in inaccuracy when applied to general populations (Robergs and Landwehr 2002). There are also population-specific prediction equations (i.e., equations designed for people who smoke, who are obese, who are elderly, and so on) that may provide more accurate estimates of HRmax (Miller et al. 1993; Whaley et al. 1992). Keep in mind that 220 minus age is only an estimate of

HRmax. It is based on a regression equation, which means that 220 minus age will not be appropriate for everyone. Participants taking prescribed medications that alter HR who want to use the HR reserve method to calculate target HR should use an HRmax measured during a stress test. The key to the HR reserve method is to take a percentage of the difference between HRmax and resting HR and then add that percentage to the resting HR to identify the target HR. See page 93 for a sample calculation of target HR using the HRR method.

Rating of Perceived Exertion

Rating of perceived exertion (RPE) is another common method of determining exercise intensity. Participants use their subjective perceptions of intensity to rate their level of steady-state work on the 6 to 20 RPE scale or the 0 to 10 RPE scale developed by Borg (1982). Interestingly, RPE is both valid and reliable (Dunbar et al. 1992; Robertson et al. 1990) and is closely associated with increases in most cardiorespiratory parameters, including work, maximal oxygen uptake, and HR. In a group exercise setting, RPE can be used with or without HR to monitor the relative exercise intensity of most participants. Participants taking medication that alters HR can use RPE to monitor their relative exercise intensity. The verbal description of each level of the RPE scale is important when using RPE. The descriptions must give participants a clear idea of the intensity that each level represents. For example, a rating of 6 to 7 could be described as the intensity of standing still, 11 could be walking to the store, 13 could be breathing hard during an activity, and 15 could be chasing the dog down the street. Relating real-life tasks to RPE helps participants understand how they should feel.

Talk Test

The talk test is another subjective method of gauging exercise intensity and can be used as an adjunct to HR and RPE. When participants exercise, their breathing should be rhythmic and comfortable. Particularly for newer clients, talking while exercising can indicate whether they are achieving an appropriate intensity. As the intensity increases, their breathing rate will become faster and shallower. If the participant needs to gasp for breath between words when conversing, then the exercise intensity is too high and should be reduced. The talk test may work well for those possessing higher fitness levels but it does not work as well for beginners.

 Watch the DVD to see how the instructor puts the concepts of monitoring exercise intensity into practice. Notice how the participants are kept moving, the instructor suggests modifications, and the HR and RPE are used to help the participants check their exercise intensity in two ways.

PARTICIPANT INTERACTION AND ENJOYMENT

One reason people like to exercise in a group is because they enjoy interacting with others. Promote participant interaction in your classes so that participants will get to know each other and reap the social benefits of exercise. Keep in mind the research on group cohesion that was presented in chapter 1—people who adhered to a program experienced higher levels of group cohesiveness. Many participants derive a great deal of satisfaction and a feeling of belonging from interacting with other class members. This increase in self-esteem, through exercise and social contact, is as important as the physical changes that take place. In fact, Ornish (1998) believes that interpersonal interaction might be the single most important concept that breeds a loving and accepting environment in your program. This interaction may be extremely important to the whole exercise experience in terms of making a difference in participants' health. Group cohesiveness does not just happen, however—it needs to be fostered with your leadership skills. See the highlighted section on promoting participant interaction for suggestions on how to increase interaction in your classes.

Involving your participants in interpersonal interaction lets them feel good about exercise and your class in general. This camaraderie makes up for the hard work of exercise. Although techniques like these are challenging

Using HR Reserve to Determine Target HR

A 40-year-old participant with a resting HR of 60 beats per minute wants to exercise at 50% to 70% of her HR reserve. What is the range of her target HR?

Step 1: Estimate HRmax.

- Estimated HRmax = 220 – age.
- Estimated HRmax = 220 – 40.
- Estimated HRmax = 180 beats per minute.

Step 2: Find HR reserve.

- HR reserve = estimated HRmax – resting HR.
- HR reserve = 180 – 60.
- HR reserve = 120 beats per minute.

Step 3: Find 50% to 70% of the HR reserve.

- 50% of HR reserve = HR reserve × 0.50.
- 50% of HR reserve = 120 × 0.50.
- 50% of HR reserve = 60 beats per minute.
- 70% of HR reserve = 120 × 0.70.
- 70% of HR reserve = 84 beats per minute.

Step 4: Find target HR range (50%-70%).

- Target HR range = % of HR reserve + resting HR.
- 50% target HR = 60 + 60 = 120 beats per minute.
- 70% target HR = 84 + 60 = 144 beats per minute.
- Target HR range = 120 to 144 beats per minute.

Intensity Monitoring in the Group Exercise Setting

Whether you are using target HR, RPE, or the talk test to monitor exercise intensity, there are a few practical application points to remember and share with the group. Several of these points are listed on the group exercise class evaluation form in appendix A.

- When measuring HR, turn off the music so the beats do not influence the counting of the pulse rate.
- Encourage use of the radial pulse rather than the carotid pulse; if you are using the carotid pulse, remind participants to press lightly to avoid reducing blood flow to the brain.
- Check intensity toward the middle of the workout so it can be modified if necessary.
- Keep participants moving while checking intensity to prevent blood from pooling in the lower extremities.
- Use a 10-second pulse count if using target HRs and start counting with 1. Count each beat and multiply this number by 6 to get beats per minute. Many group exercise facilities have charts that do this multiplication in the group exercise area.
- Give modifications based on HR or RPE results and encourage participants to work at their own levels.

POSTCARDIORESPIRATORY COOL-DOWN

The last few minutes of any group cardio session should be less intense to allow the cardiorespiratory system to recover. Lack of a postcardio cool-down is correlated with an increased risk of heart arrhythmias (American Council on Exercise 2000). Because metabolic waste products can get trapped inside the muscle cells if the intensity is not decreased gradually, many

and require motivation on your part, they can make you an extraordinary instructor and can keep your people coming back. If you believe in yourself and the power of exercise, it will be very easy for you to project fun and enthusiasm to all who attend your class.

people experience increased cramping and stiffness if they do not cool down. A proper cool-down enables waste products to disperse and the body to return to resting levels without injury. The cool-down also prevents blood from pooling in the lower extremities and allows the cardiovascular system to make the transition to more gradual workloads. This is especially important if muscle work will follow the cardiorespiratory segment. During the cool-down, encourage participants to relax, slow down, keep their arms below the level of the heart, and put less effort into their movements. Use calmer music, change your tone of voice, and verbalize the transition to the participants to help create this atmosphere.

 See the DVD for a demonstration of a post-cardiorespiratory cool-down.

Promoting Participant Interaction

- Talk to people and call them by name.
- Introduce new people to other members of the class.
- Post your name where it's visible.
- Have people choose partners and perform hand-slap activities while moving or have people introduce themselves to one another.
- Play musical themes and schedule special activities on holidays.
- Hold social gatherings before or after class.
- Keep records of birthdays. Have participants sprint on the bike for 1 second for each year of their age.
- Use partner exercises in muscular conditioning.
- Devise circuit classes where participants work together in small groups.
- Form circles and have participants demonstrate or lead their favorite move.

Automated External Defibrillators

It seems fitting to include a discussion of automated external defibrillators (AEDs) within the cardiorespiratory section of this book. An AED is a computerized medical device that can check a person's heart rhythm, recognize a rhythm that requires a shock, and advise the rescuer to deliver that shock. Fitness facilities in several U.S. states are required by law to provide AEDs, and most CPR classes now include AED training. It is important to determine if your facility is in a state that requires an AED to be present for the safety of the participant. According to Larkin (2007), IHRSA has found that there is no legal standard of care requiring that AEDs be placed in all fitness centers. However, the association does encourage health club operators to consider the advantages of installing AEDs in their facilities. A study of U.S. demographics demonstrates that the number of health club members aged 35 years and older is steadily increasing. In fact, this population currently accounts for more than 55% of club memberships. The number of members with some form of cardiorespiratory disease is also on the rise (American Heart Association 2002). Having an AED on site definitely shows that your primary concern is for the safety of your participants. This is the most important reason to consider keeping one on site. If you are going to work so hard to make sure your participants are fit and healthy, then you should also work hard to be able to help their cardiovascular system in an emergency. We suggest all facilities have an AED on site and believe that eventually the AED will be a required piece of equipment in all workout areas.

CHAPTER WRAP-UP

This chapter outlined the variables that are common to cardiorespiratory segments of most group exercise classes. Whether you are teaching a cycling, water, step, or sports conditioning class, you should increase intensity gradually, vary muscle groups used, give movement options, interact with participants, monitor intensity, and lead a postcardio cool-down. Later chapters on various group exercise classes (the chapters of part III) will refer you back to these principles.

▶ **Assignment**

Attend (and participate in) a group exercise class that contains a cardiorespiratory segment. Observe how the instructor monitors intensity. Monitor your intensity every 5 minutes, switching between HR and RPE. Be sure to record your values. Describe in a one-page paper which method worked better for you and why. Also reflect on how well the instructor led the class in monitoring exercise intensity.

Muscular Conditioning and Flexibility Training

CHAPTER OBJECTIVES

By the end of this chapter, you will

- understand basic muscle anatomy, joint actions, and kinesiological terms;
- be able to show exercise progressions and multiple muscle group modifications;
- know a variety of muscular conditioning and core stability exercises appropriate for the group setting;
- be familiar with equipment used in group muscular conditioning;
- understand basic safety issues in muscular conditioning;
- be able to demonstrate exercises with proper form and alignment;
- be able to cue muscular conditioning exercises using a variety of cues;
- be familiar with basic safety issues in flexibility training;
- know a variety of flexibility exercises appropriate for the group setting;
- be able to demonstrate and cue flexibility exercises with proper form and alignment;
- know how to use music appropriately for flexibility training; and
- understand relaxation, visualization, and deep-breathing techniques.

The development of muscle strength, endurance, and flexibility is essential for overall fitness and is an integral part of any group fitness program (see the special sections titled "Benefits of Resistance Training" on page 99 and "Benefits of Flexibility Training" on page 100). To be a competent group instructor in muscular (muscle) conditioning and flexibility, you must understand basic anatomy, kinesiology (joint actions), safety and equipment issues, and appropriate cueing. You also need to know a large variety of exercises and stretches. A few common principles guide the muscle conditioning and flexibility segments of most group exercise classes. In this chapter, we discuss muscular conditioning first and then cover flexibility and cooling down. After that, we provide detailed descriptions and photographs of exercises and stretches; these make up the majority of this chapter. The descriptions begin with the upper-body muscles, move through the torso muscles, and conclude with the lower-body muscles. The main points on the group exercise class evaluation form (found in appendix A) that apply to muscular conditioning and flexibility training are listed on this page.

GIVING POSTURE AND ALIGNMENT CUES

Because 8 of 10 Americans will experience back problems during their lifetime (Frymoyer and Cats-Baril 1991), it is essential to give verbal cues on posture and spinal alignment in each segment of the class; giving appropriate postural and alignment cues is especially critical during the muscular conditioning and stretching segments. Following are points to remember when teaching correct posture in the standing position (the numbers listed here correspond to those in figure 7.1.

1. Keep the head suspended (not pushed back or dropped forward), the ears in line with the shoulders, the shoulders over the hips, the hips over the backs of the knees, and the knees over the ankles.

2. Allow the arms to relax and hang from the shoulders. Let the palms of the hands face the sides of the body. Circle the shoulders back and down. The shoulder blades should be in a neutral position (depressed, slightly retracted).

3. Maintain the four natural curves of the spine. A decrease or increase in the low-back curvature changes the compression forces on the spine.

4. Lightly compress the abdominal muscles to help support the spinal column, especially when lifting. Abdominal compression helps distribute weight over the entire torso so that it is not concentrated on the low back. Extreme abdominal compression, however, restricts breathing.

5. Hold the pelvis in its neutral position (not tilted anteriorly or posteriorly). Individuals with swayback, pregnant women, and par-

---

Group Exercise Class Evaluation Form Essentials

Muscular Conditioning

- Gives verbal cues on posture and alignment
- Encourages and demonstrates good body mechanics
- Observes participants' form and suggests modifications for participants with injuries or special needs as well as progressions for advanced participants
- Gives clear verbal directions and uses appropriate music volume
- Uses appropriate music tempo for biomechanical movement

Flexibility Training

- Chooses appropriate music
- Includes static stretching
- Appropriately emphasizes relaxation and visualization

Benefits of Resistance Training

- Easier performance of daily activities
- Increased lean body (muscle) mass
- Increased metabolism due to increased lean body mass
- Stronger muscles, tendons, and ligaments
- Stronger bones
- Decreased risk of injury
- Decreased risk of low-back pain
- Enhanced feelings of well-being and self-confidence

ticipants with a large protruding abdomen may tuck the pelvis slightly.

6. Keep the knees unlocked or soft. Hyperextended knees shift the pelvis anteriorly, increasing the low-back curve and contributing to back strain. Hyperextended knees can also gradually overstretch the knee ligaments, leading to knee joint instability and potential injury.

7. Make sure feet are shoulder-width apart and body weight is evenly distributed. Participants who roll their feet to the inner or outer edges need to concentrate on keeping their weight over the entire bottom surface of each foot.

8. Drop an imaginary plumb line from the head to the floor. This line should pass through the cervical and lumbar vertebrae, hips, backs of knees, and ankles.

When giving alignment cues, focus on joints of the neck, spine, pelvis, scapulae, shoulders, wrists, elbows, hips, knees, and ankles. As a general rule, most conditioning exercises engage the stabilizer muscles. Give several posture cues *before* providing instruction on the specific muscle groups to be worked or stretched. For example, when leading the class in a latissimus dorsi strengthening exercise using elastic tubing, cue the participants to soften the knees, get a good base of support with the feet apart comfortably, and contract the abdominals while keeping the spine in a neutral position. In other

words, clearly cue the exercise setup. After that, you may cue the movement itself, in this case a standing lat pull-down for the latissimus dorsi.

Encouraging and Demonstrating Good Body Mechanics

You must perform exercises and stretches correctly when giving verbal cues. If you say to keep a leg movement at a 45° ROM but at the same time lift your leg higher than that, you will confuse the participants. Whatever instructions you give need to be duplicated in your demonstration of the movement. Most participants are visual learners and will copy what they see you doing. Practice is the key to becoming an effective visual demonstrator. Work constantly on your own form and alignment so that you can inspire your class and enhance safety and effectiveness by becoming a superior role model.

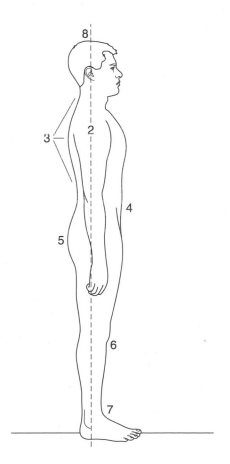

▶ **Figure 7.1** Proper posture and alignment in the standing position.

Benefits of Flexibility Training

- Enhanced performance of daily activities
- Decreased low-back pain
- Increased motor performance
- Decreased risk of injury
- Reduced muscle tension
- Increased relaxation
- Increased ROM
- Decreased muscle soreness
- Decreased stress and tension
- Increased mind–body connection
- Improved posture

Observing Form and Suggesting Modifications for Special Needs

A big difference between the teacher-centered instructor and the student-centered instructor is that the student-centered instructor helps individual participants make their exercise safer and less painful or problematic. To help your participants, you must observe them and understand their problems and limitations.

In addition to knowing the basic exercises, skilled instructors are familiar with a wide variety of modifications that they can use to suggest appropriate exercises for every person in their class. If a participant complains that his knee, shoulder, back, or any other body part hurts in an exercise, you need to modify the exercise to make it more comfortable for him or give him a completely different exercise that works the same muscle group. For example, imagine that a student tells you her wrists hurt when she does push-ups. You can suggest that she try the push-up on her fists or on her fingers or that she curl her hands around sturdy dumbbells; all of these modifications help keep the wrists in a straight line during the push-up movement and may alleviate the problem. Or you might suggest that she try push-ups on the wall, where she has to lift less of her body weight. If none of these options relieves the pain, you can suggest an alternative exercise that still targets the chest muscles, such as a bench press. If her wrists still hurt, you can recommend that she see her physician if she hasn't already done so.

The functional training continuum (discussed in chapter 3 and later in this chapter) ranks the exercises for a particular muscle group according to their difficulty level. As a participant gradually improves his strength and endurance, he will be able to perform harder and harder exercises and will be able to move up the continuum. Conversely, a participant who is having trouble performing an exercise from the more difficult end of the continuum can move back down to a modification or a different exercise that she can do safely with good form. The ACSM (2002) recommends that novice exercisers start with simple exercises and progress to complex exercises as they become more advanced.

All group exercise instructors should get out on the floor to observe and assist their participants. You should demonstrate the exercise, perform a few repetitions, and then begin to move around the room watching the participants. When you stay in one place, you give your participants only one frame of reference. Plus, coaching participants is a large part of the group exercise experience, and when you are nearby and observing, participants will listen and perform more effectively. When you move around the room, you allow participants to see that you have empathy as well as the knowledge to modify exercises that are problematic for them.

RECOMMENDATIONS AND GUIDELINES FOR MUSCULAR CONDITIONING

Most group exercise instructors include some form of muscle strength and endurance training in their classes. To promote total fitness, you must include exercises for maintaining muscular strength, endurance, and tone as well as exercises for promoting flexibility and cardiorespiratory fitness. The ACSM (2006) has published the following guidelines regarding resistance training for the average healthy adult:

- Perform a minimum of 8 to 10 separate exercises that train the major muscles of the hips, thighs, legs, back, chest, shoulders, arms, and abdomen.

- Perform one set of each exercise to the point of volitional fatigue for healthy individuals, while maintaining good form.
- Perform 8 to 12 repetitions to achieve an appropriate repetition range, although if desired, anywhere between 3 and 20 repetitions can be performed. Spend about 3 seconds on the concentric phase and about 3 seconds on the eccentric phase.
- Exercise each muscle group 2 to 3 nonconsecutive days per week, and if possible, perform a different exercise for each muscle group every 2 to 3 sessions.
- Maintain a normal breathing pattern; breath holding can cause increases in blood pressure.

According to Feigenbaum and Pollock (1999), single-set programs performed a minimum of two times per week are recommended over multiple-set programs because they are less time consuming, are more cost efficient, and still produce most of the health and fitness benefits of resistance training. Other studies, however, report that multiple-set programs provide superior results, especially for intermediate and advanced exercisers (Wolfe et al. 2004). The NSCA adds that training should occur at least 3 days per week and that there should be a minimum of 24 hours of rest between training sessions (Pearson et al. 2000). The bottom line is that strength training is an important health-related fitness component that needs to be included in group exercise instruction. Teaching resistance training is not always easy to do in the group setting, because you may not have access to heavier weights.

Group exercise class participants often ask the following question: "How many sit-ups (curl-ups, leg lifts, and so on) should I do?" The answer is, "It depends." Participants should do as many as they can while maintaining good form and alignment and should stop when they reach the point of fatigue (not total muscle failure). The optimal number of repetitions varies from exercise to exercise and from person to person. Also, the more challenging the exercise, and the harder you push yourself during the exercise, the more quickly you'll reach the point of fatigue.

For example, you will find that you are able to do more abdominal curl-ups when you hold your arms at your sides rather than overhead (holding them overhead creates a longer lever and thus is more biomechanically challenging). Participants who are performing more difficult variations may do fewer repetitions than participants who are performing an easier modification or participants who are not pushing themselves.

How do you increase intensity when instructing muscular conditioning in the group exercise setting? There are at least three ways to increase intensity:

1. Have your students focus on consciously contracting the muscle with each repetition. Conscious muscle contractions create tension similar to that experienced during isometric muscle actions. Most people can squeeze their biceps while holding their elbow at a fixed angle. Continuing that squeeze while moving the elbow through its full ROM is what we mean by conscious muscle contraction, and it's a great technique to teach your students. In addition to increasing the exercise intensity, conscious muscle contractions promote increased body awareness and better alignment.

2. Use various resistance devices to increase intensity and provide overload. Commonly used devices include dumbbells, Body Bars, barbells, Kettlebells, medicine balls, elastic tubing, and elastic bands. Steps can be inclined or declined to increase the resistance depending on the exercise. You can also use stability balls, BOSU balance trainers, foam rollers, and core boards to increase the potential for overload in a wide variety of exercises. Resistance in water exercise can be increased with aquatic gloves, dumbbells, barbells, paddles, fins, elastic bands and tubes, and buoyancy boots. Because it is impractical to supply a wide range of dumbbells or weight plates in the group setting, most facilities stop stocking large quantities of dumbbells at 8 or 10 pounds (3.6-4.5 kg). This means that you must be more creative in order to provide sufficient overload for more advanced participants.

3. Another important option for overload is to change the exercise mode (Yoke and Kennedy 2004). In group resistance training, this means using the functional training continuum (see figure 3.4, page 38) to progress from easier to more difficult (compound) exercises. To do this you need a comprehensive knowledge of a wide variety of exercise choices for all major muscle groups and the ability to evaluate which exercises are appropriate for which participants. As a general rule, the more advanced a student becomes, the more she needs to emphasize multimuscle, multijoint exercises (Sorace and LaFontaine 2005). Many exercises have several variations that can move them along the functional training continuum. For example, push-up modifications from easiest to hardest include: wall push-up, hands and knees (tabletop) push-up, knee push-up with hands on step, knee push-up with hands on floor, knee push-up with knees elevated on step, full-body push-up with hands on step, full-body push-up with hands on floor, full-body push-up with feet on step, full-body push-up with feet on stability ball, and full-body one-arm push-up. A competent instructor will be familiar with these modifications and be able to help participants determine which one is right for them.

Another technique that instructors commonly use to increase exercise difficulty is to increase the duration of the strength training or to encourage more repetitions. Although this method may be appropriate in some classes, you must be cautious with this approach. It's hard to challenge 8 to 10 major muscle groups in a 1-hour class that also includes a cardio component if you are prescribing large numbers of repetitions for each exercise.

When it comes to monitoring intensity, you should not use heart rate due to the fact that oxygen consumption does not increase proportionately to heart rate during muscular conditioning. A higher heart rate during a strength and endurance session is caused by sympathetic nervous system activation and doesn't necessarily mean you're getting a great workout (Beckham and Earnest 2000). Heart rate may be used as an intensity indicator during cardio activities such as step, high-low, and stationary indoor cycling—all activities that repeatedly engage large muscle groups for a prolonged duration.

 See the DVD for muscular conditioning progression options and instructor cueing for the following exercises: squat, bent-over row, push-up; and abdominal exercises performed on a stability ball and a BOSU balance trainer.

RECOMMENDATIONS AND GUIDELINES FOR FLEXIBILITY TRAINING

Stretching a muscle group immediately after strengthening it promotes relative balance between flexibility and strength for that group. Note that, contrary to popular misconceptions, resistance training alone does not improve flexibility (Nobrega et al. 2005). Coupling a strengthening exercise with a stretching exercise ensures that you have included both aspects in your class format and optimizes the benefits of each.

Flexibility training is an integral part of any exercise session; it helps release tight muscles and can reduce the risk of injury by correcting muscle imbalances (see "Benefits of Flexibility Training" on page 100). There are several points during a group exercise class when stretching is appropriate. These include the warm-up, the postcardio cool-down, the end of a resistance training exercise for a specific muscle or muscle group, and the end of class. Alternatively, learning to teach an entire class devoted to flexibility and relaxation can expand your opportunities as a group leader. If you teach your class how to release and relax each muscle as well as how to breathe deeply and slowly to release excess tension, you'll have many grateful students!

Remember to focus on stretching the muscle groups that are relied on the most in the class you teach. For instance, after teaching an indoor cycling class, stretching the quadriceps, calves, and hamstrings makes sense because they are the major muscles used for cycling. After a kickboxing class, lead the participants in stretching the muscles that surround the hip and are used in kicking; it is also important to work on stretching the anterior chest muscles, which are used in punching.

Following are the ACSM (2006) guidelines for flexibility:

- Precede stretching with a warm-up to elevate muscle temperature.
- Do a static stretching routine that focuses on muscle groups (joints) that have reduced ROM.

- Stretch a minimum of 2 to 3 days per week; ideally, you should stretch 5 to 7 days per week.
- Stretch to the end of your ROM without inducing discomfort.
- Hold each stretch for 15 to 30 seconds.
- Repeat each stretch 2 to 4 times.

Other stretching recommendations include the following:

- Encourage your participants to tune in and listen to their bodies. Stretching should feel good!
- Encourage muscle balance (see chapter 3).
- Encourage participants with extreme flexibility around a joint to focus on strengthening the muscles around the joint instead of working toward more mobility. Flexibility without strength can lead to injury.

The guidelines above are for the improvement of flexibility. Note that stretches do not need to be held as long during the warm-up segment; the goal of the warm up is not to make flexibility gains but to move joints and muscles through their full ROM prior to vigorous activity.

Stretching should be comfortable. Encourage proper form by giving cues such as, "Move to the position where you can feel the muscle stretch slightly, and then hold that position. You should feel the sensation of stretch, but no pain. If you are shaking, reduce the intensity of your stretch." A student-centered teacher will provide options for stretching and will model average flexibility so that participants do not imitate a form they cannot safely match. As with any other fitness activity, it is important to move participants ahead appropriately and progressively. Yoga (see chapter 13) has long been touted as an activity that enhances flexibility. Be careful, however, when incorporating challenging yoga postures into your general fitness classes; these postures are meant to be practiced by advanced yoga students in a mindful setting such as an actual yoga class.

When you are stretching, reminding participants of proper alignment promotes overall body awareness and enhances the effectiveness of the stretching experience. You should give at least 2 to 3 verbal cues for every stretch to make sure body positioning is effective. For example, when you are leading a class in a standing hamstring stretch (see figure 7.2), you should cue the participants to tilt the pelvis anteriorly to lengthen the hamstring muscle. Sullivan and colleagues (1992) studied anterior and posterior pelvic tilt using two types of stretching techniques and found that the anterior pelvic position was the most important variable for enhancing hamstring flexibility.

The final flexibility segment of a class is the time when stretching for long-term improvement is optimal. Students are warm and psychologically ready to relax and hold a given stretch. During this segment, the focus is on providing a variety of stretches held for long durations (15-30 seconds each). Studies show that flexibility improvement

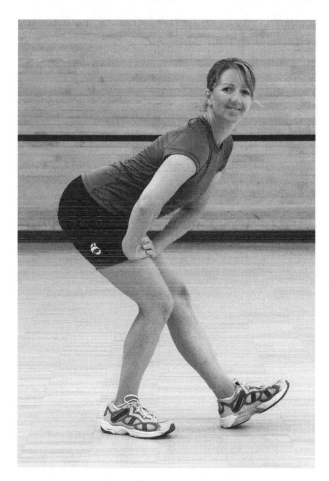

▶ **Figure 7.2** Standing hamstring stretch with anterior pelvic tilt. Instructors must always keep in mind the tenets of good alignment and use injury prevention strategies to protect the major joints.

relates to both the frequency and duration of a stretch (Bandy and Irion 1994; Feland 2000). We have found that one of the best techniques for promoting comfortable stretching that helps to reduce stress is to have your students count their breaths while holding a position; have them count 3 to 5 deep, slow breaths per stretch. Suggest that they imagine that all their stress and tension (both muscular and otherwise) is draining out of their bodies with each prolonged exhalation, leaving them more and more relaxed and refreshed.

Figuring out how to stretch a muscle is easy if you know your kinesiology (joint actions). To stretch a muscle, simply move it into the opposite position of its concentric joint action. For example, if you have just led your class members in shoulder abduction exercises such as lateral raises and overhead presses for the deltoids, you can now lead them in a stretch involving shoulder adduction, which is the opposite position from the concentric muscle shortening action of the deltoid exercises. Once you understand this principle, you can come up with your own stretches for any muscle group (just make certain that you also abide by safety guidelines). Later in this chapter you will see standing stretches (appropriate for both the warm-up and the final flexibility segment of class) and floor stretches (generally not used during the warm-up) for each major muscle group.

 See the DVD for an example of a flexibility segment that covers the inner and outer thigh, low back, hamstrings, abdominals, quadriceps, hip flexors, upper back, neck, deltoids, triceps, and pectorals as well as breathing, relaxation, and visualization.

SAFETY

Safety is a major concern when you are leading a group fitness class. In general, group exercise instructors need to be more cautious and conservative than personal trainers when designing a muscular strength and conditioning program. Responsible personal trainers take thorough health histories on all their clients, require physicians' clearances when appropriate, and create individualized programs that account for each client's unique musculoskeletal needs Group leaders usually don't have the luxury of individually assessing

each participant in their class or tailoring their program to a specific participant. Ideally, each exercise that is given in a class is safe for everyone in that class, including beginners or deconditioned members. You may show progressions for students who are in better shape, although after demonstrating an advanced move, you should return to demonstrating the variation that best fits the majority of your participants. The reason for this is that most students will try to copy whatever the instructor is demonstrating, even though that particular variation may be inappropriate for them. (Participants will also unconsciously copy your form and alignment, so always demonstrate all exercises with excellent alignment.)

The major cause of exercise-related injury is doing too much, too soon. Students must progress gradually to harder, more intense exercises and longer duration. Your exercise choices must be appropriate for the students in your class, This means that you must be prepared to alter your class plan on a moment's notice, depending on the fitness levels and skills of the participants who have shown up for the session. Experienced instructors have a large repertoire of exercises and exercise modifications that they can use to reformat or even individualize a class on the spot.

When teaching your class, follow the tenets of good technique and correct alignment. Avoid the following:

- Hyperextended knees or elbows
- Excessive momentum
- Inappropriate torque (a rotational twisting force applied to a joint, as in the hurdler's stretch)
- Hyperflexed knees (knees bent past 90°) in a weight-bearing position such as a squat or lunge

Avoid risky moves and follow industry guidelines on high-risk exercises to protect your students and yourself. Moves that are considered higher risk include

- ballistic stretches,
- deep squats (in which the hips drop below the knees),
- extreme or ballistic lumbar hyperextension,
- cervical spinal hyperextension,

Key Definitions

Stress Adaptation

Increasing the intensity of the workout by increasing the number of repetitions or the amount of resistance should be gradual and progressive. Sudden increases in intensity, such as abruptly doubling the repetitions or the resistance, can result in muscle damage. On the other hand, staying at the same intensity will not allow musculoskeletal stress adaptation to occur. Instruct your participants to add 1 to 2 pounds (0.5-1 kg) or to go to the next thickness of rubber band if they can perform 15 or more repetitions at their current level. The ACSM recommends that resistance be increased by 2% to 10%, depending on the muscle groups used, when the participant can complete 1 to 2 repetitions beyond the desired number and has done so for at least two consecutive sessions (American College of Sports Medicine 2002).

Rebuilding Time

When a muscle is stressed beyond its normal limitations, it needs time for repair, recovery, and positive physiological change. This time is known as *rebuilding time*. Generally, muscles require 1 to 2 days (24-48 hours) to rebuild, so resistance training should be performed every other day. If you are strength training daily, you should emphasize different muscle groups on each day, especially if your intensity is high.

Controlled Movement

Slow, smooth, and controlled movement speed ensures consistent application of force throughout the entire ROM. Keep in mind that music tempos of 130 beats per minute or faster increase momentum and the risk of injury. Slower music tempos (~116 beats per minute) demand control and strength. If you want to progress a class, use slower music tempos as the class session proceeds.

Full Range of Motion

Use the full ROM of the muscle and joint structure to help preserve flexibility. Training the muscles and tendons through a greater ROM enables more muscle fibers to perform work. Pulsing (or performing a limited ROM) is discouraged unless limited ROM is your goal, as it is in some abdominal work. Using limited ROM may be appropriate for rehabilitation or for injury avoidance. For example, performing partial ROM exercises during weight training can help an injured rotator cuff to heal.

Training Specificity

The principle of specificity states that specific adaptations occur in response to specific exercises, activities, or stretches. This means that the results of exercise training are specific to the part of the body being trained; for example, training the upper body has very little effect on the lower body, and vice versa.

- unsupported forward flexion of the lumbar spine (avoid toe touches without back support; place hands on a block, the floor, ankles, shins, or thighs),
- unsupported forward flexion with rotation (e.g., windmills),
- unsupported lateral spinal flexion,
- hurdler's stretch,

- full sit-ups,
- full straight-leg sit-ups,
- double straight-leg raises,
- deadlifts,
- good mornings,
- plow (yoga),
- full cobra (yoga), and
- V-sits (Yoke 2006).

For the average class participant interested in health-related fitness, the risks of performing these exercises outweigh any potential benefits. Always consider the risk-to-benefit ratio and the issue of appropriateness when choosing exercises and stretches for your class. For example, the hurdler's stretch is appropriate for hurdlers who are training to run hurdles in competition, but for all other groups, the benefits of the hurdler's stretch are outweighed by the risk to the medial collateral ligaments of the knee (overstretching these ligaments can lead to knee instability, which can lead to serious knee injury). Instead of using the hurdler's stretch, teach a modified version (much safer for the knees) or present a completely different hamstring stretch (see figure 7.3).

Encourage your participants to listen to their bodies and note twinges or slight annoyances, which can be warning signals of future injury. Most participants have heard the saying, "No pain, no gain," and think that if they don't hurt after an exercise session, it wasn't a good workout. No pain, no gain may be appropriate for competing athletes but is completely inappropriate in a group health and fitness setting.

Educate your students about the difference between muscle soreness and joint pain. Muscle soreness usually disappears after 24 to 48 hours and may be acceptable for students who want to challenge themselves. Joint pain, however, is never OK and is a sign that something is wrong. Teach your students to distinguish between the two and stop whatever activity is causing joint pain. Remember, if there is pain, there is little gain!

Additionally, participants must take precautions when stretching. Ballistic (bouncing) stretching and passive overstretching can be dangerous. Researchers have shown that the risk of injury from ballistic stretching is greater than any potential benefit, at least for most exercisers (Knudson 1995). Both passive overstretching and ballistic stretching can initiate the stretch reflex. Whenever you suddenly stretch or put excessive tension on your muscle, special receptors (Golgi tendon organs and muscle spindles) within the muscle fiber detect the action (American College of Sports Medicine 2005). There is a complicated and continual interplay between opposing muscle groups that leads to precise, controlled, and coordinated movement, and if a muscle is

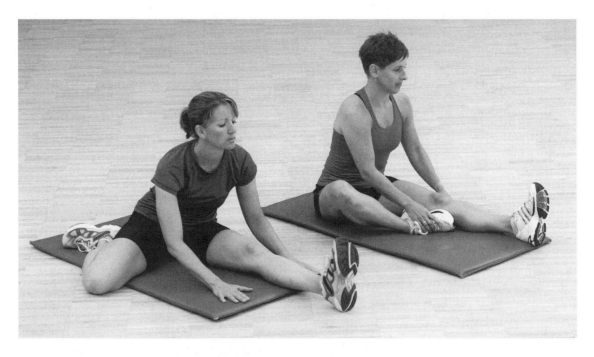

▶ **Figure 7.3** Avoid the hurdler's stretch (left) due to increased risk of knee injury. Instead, perform the modified version (right) that is shown here.

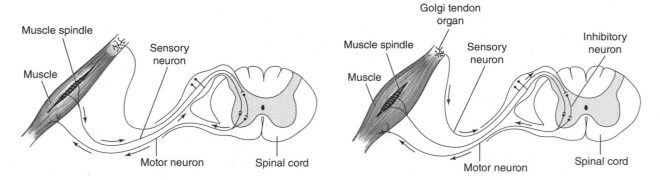

▶ **Figure 7.4** Special receptors are active during a strong contraction or stretch. They inhibit or facilitate contraction in order to protect the muscle.

activated by a sudden stretch or is continually overstretched, then the system stimulates the muscle to contract rather than lengthen and maintains the contraction to oppose the excessive lengthening force. Simply put, if you overstretch or bounce and stretch, then the muscle shortens to protect itself. Keep pulling on a shortened muscle and it will either cramp up or tear—but it will not lengthen. This process is often referred to as the *myotatic stretch reflex* (figure 7.4). It is an involuntary reflex that happens at the spinal cord level; we cannot mentally override it no matter how hard we try.

 See the DVD for an example of destabilizing exercises for the biceps, triceps, and hamstrings.

MUSCULAR CONDITIONING AND FLEXIBILITY EXERCISES

In this section we examine the major muscles, joint by joint. For each major muscle, we show anatomical illustrations, list joint actions, and include appropriate strengthening and then stretching exercises—both with corresponding verbal cues.

Shoulder Joint and Shoulder Girdle

Figures 7.5 and 7.6 illustrate the major muscles of the shoulder joint and shoulder girdle. Tables 7.1 and 7.2 list common activities using these muscles as well as basic strengthening exercises appropriate for the group setting. Tables 7.3 and 7.4 list the shoulder joint and shoulder girdle muscles and their joint actions. Table 7.5 gives the ROM of select shoulder joint actions. Photos on pages 112 through 126 demonstrate muscular conditioning exercises and stretches for the shoulder joint and shoulder girdle. Remember that keeping the shoulder girdle (scapular) muscles strong is very important for good posture and injury-free shoulders.

SHOULDER JOINT AND SHOULDER GIRDLE

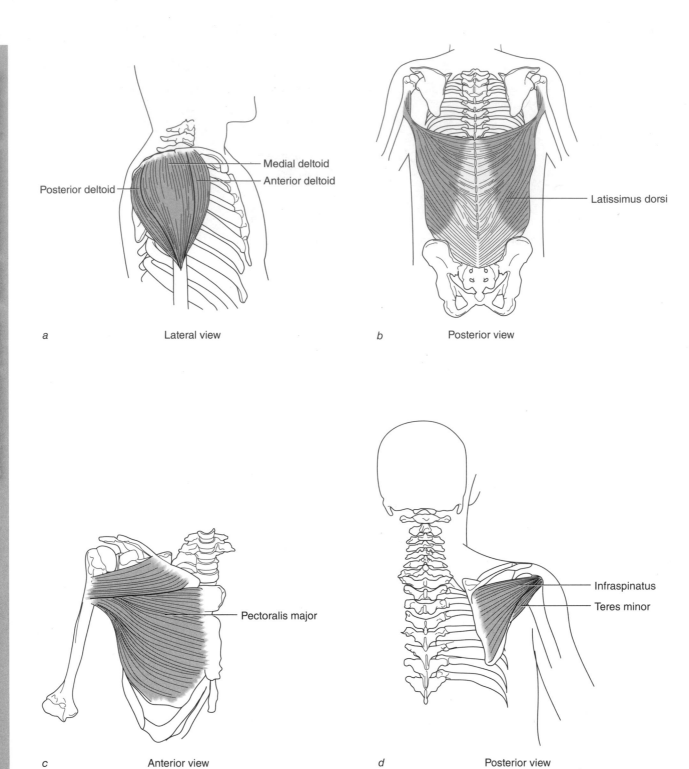

a   Lateral view

Medial deltoid
Anterior deltoid
Posterior deltoid

b   Posterior view

Latissimus dorsi

c   Anterior view

Pectoralis major

d   Posterior view

Infraspinatus
Teres minor

▶ **Figure 7.5** Shoulder joint muscles: *(a)* anterior, medial, and posterior deltoids; *(b)* latissimus dorsi; *(c)* pectoralis major; and *(d)* external rotator cuff (infraspinatus and teres minor).

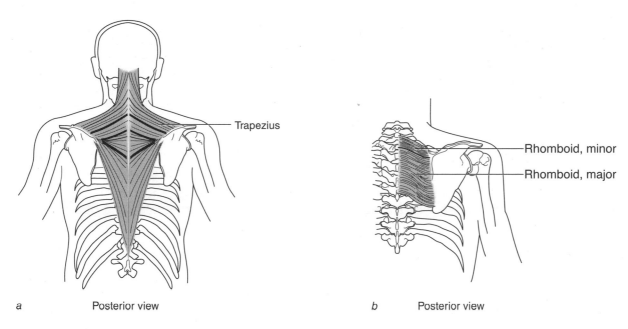

a   Posterior view   *b*   Posterior view

▶ **Figure 7.6**   Important shoulder girdle muscles: *(a)* posterior view including trapezius I, II, III, and IV and *(b)* rhomboids.

Table 7.1   Shoulder Joint Muscles

Muscle	Daily activities	Exercises for groups
Anterior and medial deltoid	Lifting and carrying, pushing items up overhead	Front raise, lateral raise, overhead press, upright row
Latissimus dorsi	Pulling items toward the body, lifting	Bent-over low row, bent-over shoulder extension, seated low row, unilateral adduction with tube
Pectoralis major	Pushing items in front of the body, lifting, throwing	Push-up, bench press, dumbbell fly, standing chest press with tube
Posterior deltoid (works with scapular retractors)	Pulling items toward the body, lifting	Bent-over high row, reverse fly, prone dorsal lift, seated high row
Rotator cuff muscles (supraspinatus, subscapularis, infraspinatus, teres minor)	Opening and closing doors, stabilizing the shoulder joint	Side-lying external shoulder rotation, supine internal rotation, standing rotation with tube

SHOULDER JOINT AND SHOULDER GIRDLE

Table 7.3 Shoulder Joint Muscles and Their Actions

Muscle	Flexion	Extension	Abduction	Adduction	Internal rotation	External rotation	Horizontal adduction	Horizontal abduction
Anterior deltoid	PM		Asst		Asst		PM	
Medial deltoid			PM					PM
Posterior deltoid		Asst				Asst		PM
Latissimus dorsi		PM		PM	Asst			Asst
Teres major		PM		PM	PM			Asst
Pectoralis major, clavicular	PM		Asst		Asst		PM	
Pectoralis major, sternal		PM		PM	Asst		PM	
Supraspinatus			PM					
Subscapularis	Asst		Asst	Asst	PM		Asst	
Infraspinatus						PM		PM
Teres minor						PM		PM
Biceps, long head			Asst					
Biceps, short head	Asst			Asst	Asst		Asst	
Triceps, long head		Asst		Asst				

PM = prime mover; Asst = assistant mover.

Adapted, by permission, from P.J. Rasch, 1989, *Kinesiology and applied anatomy*, 7th edition (Philadelphia, PA: Lippincott, Williams and Wilkins), 172.

Table 7.2 Shoulder Girdle (Scapulothoracic) Joint Muscles

Muscle	Daily activities	Exercises
Trapezius I and II	Holding phone to ear	Shrug
Trapezius III and rhomboids	Posture stabilizer	High row, reverse fly, prone dorsal lift, seated high row
Trapezius IV	Stabilizer when pushing out of a chair	Resisted depression in a dip position

Table 7.4 Shoulder Girdle (Scapulothoracic) Muscles and Their Actions

Muscle	Elevation	Depression	Protraction	Retraction	Upward rotation	Downward rotation
Trapezius I	PM					
Trapezius II	PM			Asst	PM	
Trapezius III				PM		
Trapezius IV		PM		Asst	PM	
Rhomboid	PM			PM		PM
Levator scapula	PM					
Pectoralis minor		PM	PM			PM
Serratus anterior			PM		PM	

PM = prime mover; Asst = assistant mover.

Adapted, by permission, from P.J. Rasch, 1989, *Kinesiology and applied anatomy*, 7th edition (Philadelphia, PA: Lippincott, Williams and Wilkins), 158.

Table 7.5 ROM of Select Shoulder Joint Movements

Joint movement	ROM
Flexion	90°-120°
Extension	20°-60°
Abduction	80°-100°
Horizontal abduction	30°-45°
Horizontal adduction	90°-135°
Internal rotation	70°-90°
External rotation	70°-90°

Muscular Conditioning Exercises for the Deltoids

FRONT RAISE

Anterior deltoid, clavicular pectoralis major (shoulder flexion)

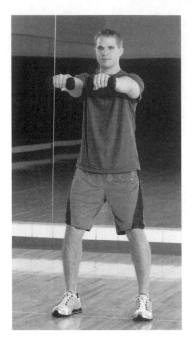

Cues: Stand (or sit on a step or stability ball) with feet shoulder-width apart, knees slightly bent, and neck, spine, and pelvis in neutral. Elbows are straight but not hyperextended. Shoulder blades are down and slightly retracted (neutral position). Wrists are straight throughout. Palms are down (pronated). Keep torso stable while flexing shoulders to about shoulder height (90°). Avoid momentum.

FYI: Consider limiting the use of this exercise when leading a group. The reason is that everyday activities (and high-low and step classes) challenge the anterior muscles much more frequently than they challenge the posterior muscles. Dumbbells, barbell, or tubing may be used for resistance. This exercise may be performed bilaterally or unilaterally; the unilateral version is safer for the back.

LATERAL RAISE

Medial deltoid, supraspinatus (shoulder abduction)

Cues: Stand (or sit on a step or stability ball) with the feet shoulder-width apart and the knees slightly flexed. Maintain the neck, spine, and pelvis in neutral. In addition, keep the scapulae neutral (down and slightly retracted). Wrists should also be neutral (neither flexed nor extended). Elbows may be bent at 90° for a short-lever variation or flexed at about 15° (so that arms are nearly straight) for the more traditional long-lever version (using the long lever is more difficult). Palms face the sides (midpronated position) at the start of the exercise and maintain this position throughout, thumbs facing straight ahead. As the shoulders abduct, they stay in partial internal rotation, lifting to no more than 90°. At the end of the movement, the shoulders are slightly higher than the elbows, which are slightly higher than the wrists.

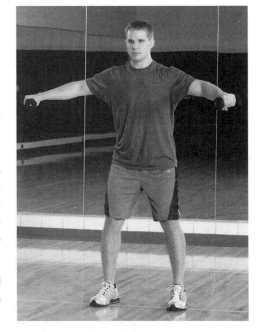

FYI: During this exercise it is particularly important to avoid momentum and to avoid bringing the arms higher than the shoulders (they should not abduct any higher than 90°). Both of these actions can cause shoulder impingement.

Lateral raises can be performed with dumbbells or tubing for added resistance.

OVERHEAD PRESS

Medial and anterior deltoids, supraspinatus, triceps (shoulder abduction, elbow extension)

Cues: Stand (or sit on bench or stability ball) with feet shoulder-width apart for stability. Knees are soft, and spine, neck, and pelvis are in neutral. The shoulder girdle is down and slightly retracted (neutral). Start in the down position, with the palms facing forward (pronated) and the hands slightly wider than the shoulders. When pressing up, straighten but do not lock (hyperextend) the elbows. Keep the chest lifted and avoid leaning backward.

FYI: This exercise can be performed with dumbbells, barbell, or tubing for added resistance. The press should be performed in front of the head to minimize injury to the shoulder joint; the behind-the-neck press has become controversial because of the vulnerable shoulder position and the increased risk of injury of external rotation behind the frontal plane. This exercise may be performed unilaterally or bilaterally.

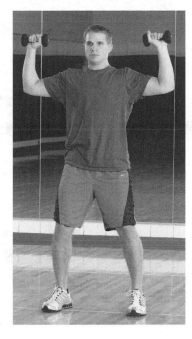

UPRIGHT ROW

Medial and anterior deltoids, supraspinatus, biceps brachii (shoulder abduction, elbow flexion)

Optional: upper trapezius, rhomboids, and levator scapulae (scapular elevation)

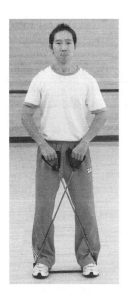 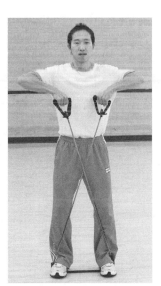

Cues: Stand with feet shoulder-width apart, knees flexed, and spine, neck, and pelvis in neutral. Hands are pronated (overhand grip) and 6 to 8 inches (15-20 cm) apart. Lead with the elbows (not the wrists), and do not lift the elbows above the shoulders. Keep wrists as neutral as possible (watch for the tendency to flex the wrists, which increases the risk of wrist and elbow injuries). Avoid momentum.

FYI: The upright row has become somewhat controversial due to concerns about shoulder joint injury. Because the exercise is performed while the shoulders are internally rotated, it is very important that the elbows do not come higher than the shoulders (no more than 90° of abduction) because of the risk of shoulder joint impingement. Even though the traditional variation of the upright row includes shoulder girdle elevation, we do not recommend this for the general public or for group exercise. From a functional training perspective, most fitness and health exercisers need to strengthen the muscles required to keep the scapulae down, not up. Therefore, scapular elevation can be considered an optional movement in an upright row. This exercise may be performed with dumbbells, barbell, or tubing for added resistance.

DELTOID STRETCHES

Anterior, medial, and posterior deltoids

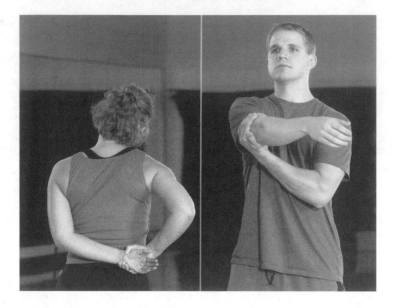

Cues: *(left)* To stretch the medial and anterior deltoids, stand in ideal standing alignment and bend one elbow behind the body. Gently press the arm across and toward the back of the body. Try tilting your head to the opposite side for a great stretch of the side of the neck (upper trapezius). *(right)* To stretch the medial and posterior deltoids, stand with the feet shoulder-width apart, knees slightly flexed, and pelvis, spine, and neck in neutral. Keep the shoulder blades down and maintain a large space between shoulders and ears. Gently press your arm across the body and in toward the torso.

FYI: These stretches may also be performed in a seated position.

Muscular Conditioning Exercises for the Latissimus Dorsi

BENT-OVER ROW

Latissimus dorsi, teres major, posterior deltoid, biceps brachii
(shoulder extension, elbow flexion)

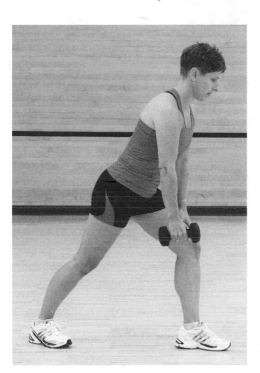
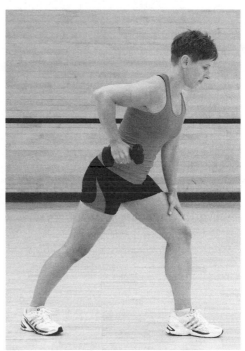

Note: The middle trapezius and rhomboids are strong stabilizers because of their antigravity position. If the exercise is performed bilaterally, the erector spinae and abdominals are also very important stabilizers of the spine.

Cues: Stand with the feet staggered and the nonworking hand placed on the front thigh (front knee bent) for support. All joints face the same direction, with the hips and shoulders evenly squared and level. Ideally, one long line is created from the back heel to the top of the head. The spine is in neutral, with no rounding or hunching of the upper back. The neck continues the line of the spine with no ducking toward the weight. Keep scapulae stabilized in neutral; do not protract or retract with the exercise. The only moving joints are the working-side shoulder and elbow; all else is kept still. The moving arm brushes against the rib cage. Avoid rotating the spine when lifting the weight. Keep shoulders level throughout.

FYI: This exercise is one of the best choices for working the latissimus dorsi in group exercise; we recommend performing it unilaterally when in a group. Although the bilateral version is excellent, it is quite unlikely that every student in a group class will be able to correctly stabilize the spine and maintain proper alignment for the bilateral version. This exercise may be performed with dumbbells or tubing or, for advanced participants, both. Another variation is long-lever shoulder extension with the elbow held straight.

SEATED LOW ROW

Latissimus dorsi, teres major, sternal pectoralis major, posterior deltoid, biceps brachii (shoulder extension, elbow flexion)

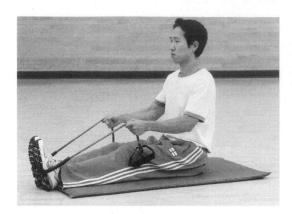 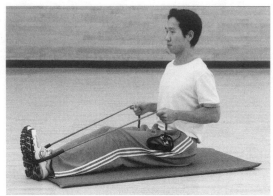

Cues: Sit on the floor (or step) and bend knees slightly to ensure that the pelvis and spine are aligned directly over the sitting bones (ischial tuberosities). Hold the spine erect and tall, maintaining neutral alignment throughout. Keep the neck in line with the spine and the scapulae down and away from the ears. Move the arms through the sagittal plane, keeping the upper arms close to the rib cage. Hold the handles of the tubing in a midpronated position (palms face each other). Move only the shoulders and elbows; keep the lower back still.

UNILATERAL LAT PULL-DOWN

Latissimus dorsi, teres major, sternal pectoralis major, biceps brachii (shoulder adduction, elbow flexion)

Cues: Stand with feet shoulder-width apart for stability. Spine, neck, and pelvis are in neutral. Grasp the elastic tubing or band with one hand, keeping it anchored overhead. Perform the pull-down with the other hand, keeping the shoulder blades down and the head high. Release the tubing or band upward slowly, with control.

FYI: Without a high pulley (found in most weight rooms), the only way to make this exercise effective in the group setting is to use elastic resistance. Although some instructors try to duplicate the pull-down exercise with dumbbells, the muscles actually resisting gravity's pull when holding free weights are the deltoids, not the latissimi dorsi.

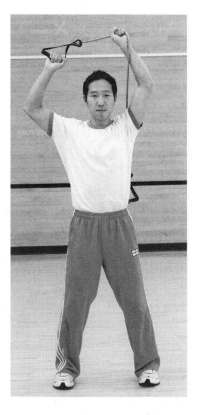 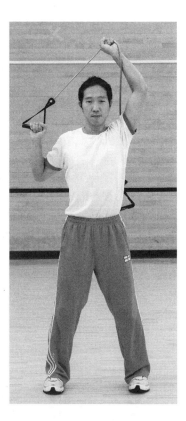

LATISSIMUS DORSI STRETCHES

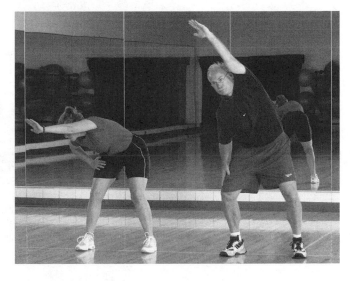

Cues: *(left)* Stand with feet shoulder-width apart, knees bent, and pelvis tucked under (posterior pelvic tilt). Curve (flex) the spine, pull the abdominals in, and reach one arm up and out in front, allowing the upper back to round and curve slightly to one side to increase the lengthened feeling through the latissimus dorsi. Keep the opposite hand on the thigh to support the low back. *(right)* Stand with feet shoulder-width apart, knees slightly bent, and pelvis, spine, and neck in neutral. Place one hand on outer thigh and reach the other hand overhead. Lengthen along your side as you lift up your hand, separating the ribs from the hip; perform a comfortable, gradual side bend, allowing the neck to continue the line of the spine. Leave the opposite hand on the thigh to help support the low back.

FYI: These stretches may be performed in a seated position.

Muscular Conditioning Exercises for the Pectoralis Major

CHEST FLY

Pectoralis major, anterior deltoid (shoulder horizontal adduction)

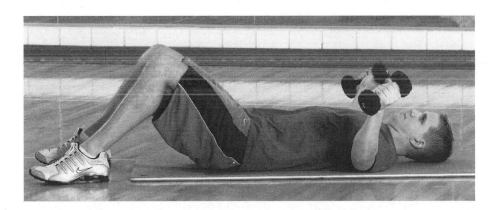

Cues: Lie supine, with the feet flat on the floor or bench and the knees bent. Keep the neck, spine, and pelvis in neutral alignment. Start in the up position, with the elbows just slightly flexed. Palms can be pronated or midpronated (facing each other). Moving only the shoulder joints, stabilize the elbows, wrists, scapulae, spine, and pelvis. Lower the arms out to the sides until the upper arms are parallel with the chest, being especially careful not to exceed the appropriate end ROM, which can lead to shoulder injury.

FYI: This exercise is performed with dumbbells and can be inclined or declined on a step. Another variation is the short-lever fly, or pec dec, in which the elbows are flexed at a 90° angle.

BENCH OR CHEST PRESS

Pectoralis major, anterior deltoid, triceps (shoulder horizontal adduction, elbow extension)

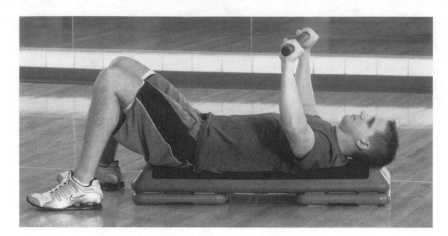

Cues: Lie supine on the floor or bench with the knees bent and the feet on the floor. Keep the spine, neck, and pelvis in neutral and the abdominals engaged. Use a wide, pronated grip. Stabilize all joints, including the scapulae, wrists, and spine, while the shoulders and elbows move. Angle the upper arm 80° to 90° out from the torso; forearms are perpendicular to the floor. Keep the movement slow and controlled, avoiding a sudden descent. If on a step, avoid letting the elbows drop too far below the bench, as doing so increases the shoulder joint stress. Avoid rolling the wrist, arching the back, and hyperextending the elbows.

FYI: The narrower the grip, the more the triceps are involved and the less the chest is involved. This exercise can be performed with dumbbells or a bar and may be inclined or declined on a step. Performing this exercise while lying supine on the floor hinders the ROM—the floor gets in the way of the movement.

PUSH-UP

Pectoralis major, anterior deltoid, triceps (shoulder horizontal adduction, elbow extension)

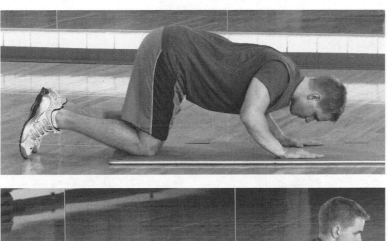

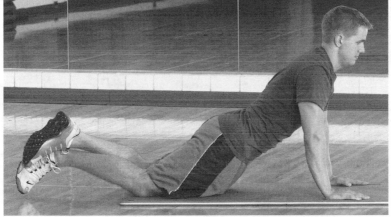

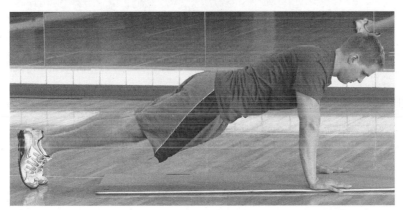

Note: There are several important stabilizers used for this exercise—the abdominals, erector spinae, gluteus maximus, trapezius, rhomboids, serratus anterior, and pectoralis minor.

Cues: Keep the head, neck, spine, and pelvis in neutral. The head and neck continue the line of the spine. In all positions except tabletop, the hips are in neutral as well (in the tabletop position, the hips are flexed at 90°). The fingers point straight ahead to minimize wrist stress; the hands are slightly wider than the shoulders and the upper arms are perpendicular to the torso (in the horizontal plane). The only moving joints are the shoulders and elbows; all other joints are stabilized. This is very important for injury prevention. Avoid sagging through the back, hyperextending the elbows, or hyperextending the cervical vertebrae. Exhale on the way up.

FYI: Push-ups are a good option for chest work in the group setting. Always show at least three variations to accommodate varying ability levels. Here are a few variations, listed from easiest to hardest: wall push-up, tabletop push-up *(top)*, knee (intermediate) push-up with hands on step, knee push-up with hands on floor *(middle),* knee push-up with knees on step and hands on floor (decline), full-body push-up with hands on step, full-body push-up with hands on floor *(bottom),* full-body push-up with feet on step, and full-body push-up on one leg. The closer the elbows are to the ribs, the more the exercise becomes a triceps push-up and the less it challenges the chest muscles.

STANDING CHEST PRESS

Pectoralis major, anterior deltoid, triceps (shoulder horizontal adduction, elbow extension)

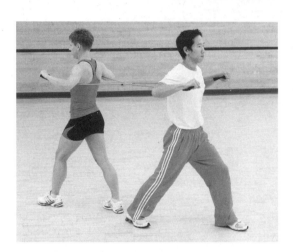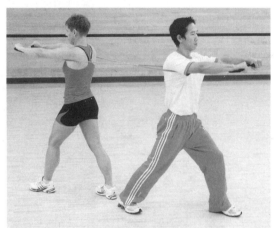

Cues: Stand with feet parallel and shoulder-width apart or staggered and hip-width apart. Loop elastic tube or band around a ballet barre or hook and face away from the barre, grasping the ends of the tube or band in the hands with the elastic under the arms. Place spine, neck, pelvis, scapulae, and wrists in neutral; contract abdominals. Moving only the shoulders and elbows, exhale and press directly away from the anchor point of the tubing. Stabilize the entire torso throughout the movement.

FYI: For an ideal line of pull and optimal muscle recruitment, the tube or band must be anchored on a stationary object behind the body; wrapping the elastic behind the back instead of anchoring it reduces the exercise effectiveness. (Alternatively, loop two bands around each other as in the partner exercise shown above.) Traditional standing chest exercises with dumbbells are not an effective choice because gravity does not directly oppose the muscle action. The muscles holding the arms up against gravity are the deltoids; the chest muscles actually do very little work.

PECTORALIS MAJOR STRETCHES

Cues: *(left)* Stand with the feet hip-width or shoulder-width apart, knees soft, and pelvis, spine, and neck in neutral. Bring your arms behind your body, clasping the hands together if possible (although this is not essential). Keep the shoulders down and abdominals contracted; avoid arching the lower back. Hold a towel or strap if desired to help increase the stretch. *(right)* Stand with the feet shoulder-width apart, knees soft, and pelvis, spine, and neck in neutral alignment. Place the hands behind the ears with the elbows high and shoulders down, and gently open the elbows toward the back while lifting and opening the chest. Feel the shoulder blades scrunch together in the back as the chest muscles stretch.

FYI: These stretches may be performed in the seated position.

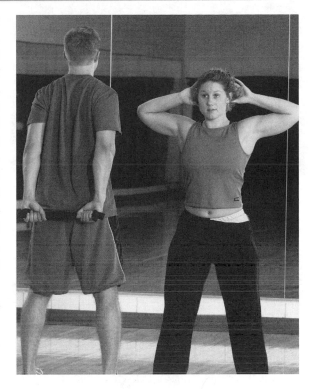

Muscular Conditioning Exercises for the Middle Trapezius and Rhomboids

PRONE SCAPULAR RETRACTION (PRONE DORSAL LIFT)

**Middle trapezius, rhomboids, posterior deltoids
(scapular retraction, shoulder horizontal abduction)**

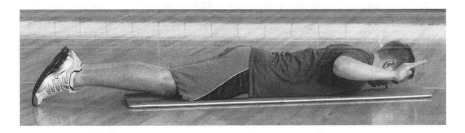

Cues: Lie prone on the floor (or on a step) with the forehead down and the neck in line with the spine. Place arms on the floor with the upper arms at a 90° angle to the torso and the elbows flexed at 90°. Place palms down on the floor. Retract the scapulae, pulling the shoulder blades toward each other. Keep your forehead on the floor and your neck and spine in neutral. Be sure to lift the elbows up toward the ceiling, not back toward the hips.

FYI: This exercise requires no equipment other than a mat and can make a great superset when alternated with sets of push-ups. Most participants will have a small ROM in this position and will be unable to lift much more than the weight of their arms. Even so, prone scapular retraction is an excellent exercise for posture correction and education.

SEATED HIGH (HORIZONTAL) ROW

Middle trapezius, rhomboids, posterior deltoids, biceps brachii (scapular retraction, shoulder horizontal abduction, elbow flexion)

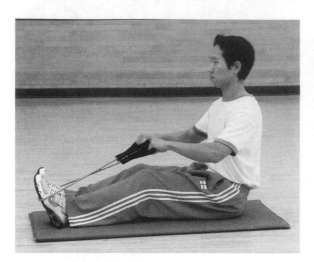 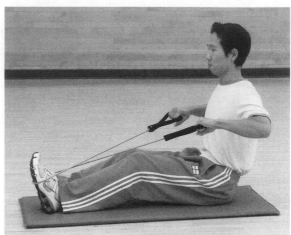

Cues: Sit on the floor with the hips flexed at 90° and the spine and neck in neutral. Keep the knees slightly bent to help keep the torso aligned over the sitting bones. Wrap the elastic tubing around the feet and grasp the handles with your palms down (pronated). Start with the elbows extended and the arms in the horizontal plane in front of the chest. Row the elbows back (keeping them in the horizontal plane, parallel to the floor) and consciously retract the shoulder blades. Keep the wrists straight and avoid rocking the lower spine.

FYI: Do not confuse this exercise with a low row, which targets the latissimus dorsi. In a high row, the arms are held up in the horizontal plane just slightly below the shoulders. Perform a standard row, or, for variety, try a 4-count row: pull back on 1, retract the shoulder blades on 2, release the shoulder blades on 3, and release the row on 4.

REVERSE FLY

**Middle trapezius, rhomboids, posterior deltoid
(scapular retraction, shoulder horizontal abduction)**

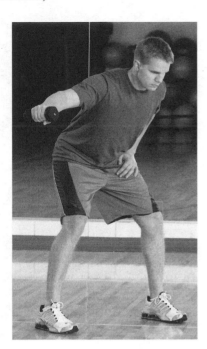

Cues: Choose whichever standing bent-over position feels the most comfortable: feet shoulder-width apart and parallel with one hand on thigh or feet staggered with one hand on the front thigh. Square the hips and shoulders and place the spine and neck in neutral alignment. Press the shoulders and shoulder girdle down, away from the ears. With the working arm perpendicular to the torso, lift the arm backward toward the ceiling, finishing the move with the scapula moving toward the spine (retraction). Only the scapula and shoulder joint move; the spine, neck, hips, elbow, and wrist remain perfectly still. Consciously contract the rear deltoid, middle trapezius, and rhomboids.

FYI: This exercise may be performed with dumbbells, band, or tube for resistance. Bilateral bent-over reverse flys are not recommended for most group exercise classes. Most participants are unable to properly stabilize the torso and maintain strongly contracted abdominal and erector spinae muscles when working bilaterally. Bent-over movements performed unilaterally with one hand on the thigh to support the spine are much less risky. This exercise may also be performed in the half-kneeling position or prone on a step.

SHOULDER JOINT AND SHOULDER GIRDLE

BENT-OVER HIGH ROW

**Middle trapezius, rhomboids, posterior deltoid, biceps brachii
(scapular retraction, shoulder horizontal abduction, elbow flexion)**

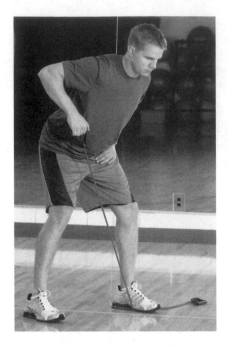

Cues: Choose whichever standing bent-over position feels the most comfortable: feet shoulder-width apart and parallel with one hand on thigh or feet staggered with one hand on the front thigh. Square the hips and shoulders and place the spine and neck in neutral alignment. Press the shoulders and shoulder girdle down, away from the ears. With the working arm perpendicular to the torso, lift the elbow backward toward ceiling, finishing the move with the scapula moving toward the spine (retraction). Only the scapula, shoulder joint, and elbow move; the spine, neck, hips, and wrist remain perfectly still. Consciously contract the rear deltoid, middle trapezius, and rhomboids.

FYI: This exercise may be performed with dumbbells, barbell, band, or tubing for resistance. Do not confuse this exercise with a low row, which targets the latissimus dorsi. In a high row, the arms are held in the horizontal plane just slightly below the shoulders. For variety, try a 4-count row: Pull back on 1, retract the shoulder blade on 2, release the shoulder blade on 3, and release the row and return to start on 4. Again, be very cautious with bilateral bent-over high rows in the group setting; most participants have difficulty stabilizing the torso when moving bilaterally in the bent-over position.

TRAPEZIUS STRETCHES

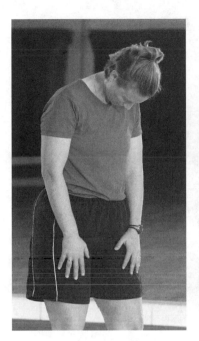 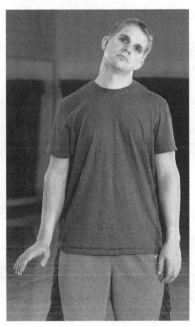 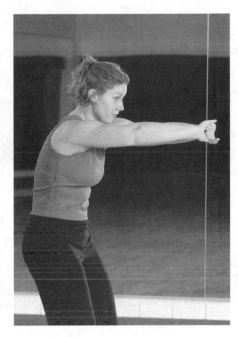

Cues: *(left)* To stretch the upper trapezius, stand in ideal standing alignment and gently tip the head forward (cervical spinal flexion), moving the chin toward the chest. Do not allow the upper back to round forward; this stretch is only for the neck. If desired, the hands can rest lightly on the top of the head; do not pull. Experiment with slightly and carefully tipping your head diagonally (in the direction of your left little toe and then your right little toe) to release neck and shoulder tension. *(middle)* To stretch the upper trapezius, stand with feet shoulder-width apart, knees soft, and pelvis and spine in neutral. Consciously press the shoulder blades down. Tilt the head sideways (lateral flexion) to the left and feel a comfortable stretch on the right side of your neck. If you like, gently rest your left hand on your head to increase the stretch sensation (do not pull). Repeat on the other side. *(right)* To stretch the middle trapezius and rhomboids, stand with the knees flexed, pelvis slightly tucked under (posterior pelvic tilt), back rounded and flexed, and hands clasped together directly in front of your chest. Allow your shoulder blades to come apart as far as possible. Contract the abdominals, bringing navel to spine, and allow your head to gently continue the line of the spine. Maintain your upper body over your hips (avoid unsupported forward spinal flexion).

Muscular Conditioning Exercises for the External Rotators

STANDING SHOULDER EXTERNAL ROTATION

Infraspinatus, teres minor (shoulder external rotation)

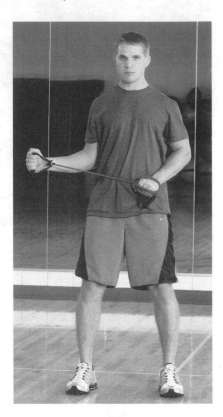

Cues: Stand with the feet shoulder-width apart and the spine, neck, and pelvis in neutral. Keep the shoulder blades down and slightly retracted (neutral scapulae). Anchor the tube by holding it on the opposite hip with the nonworking hand. On the working side, flex the elbow to 90° and grasp the tube or band. Hold the upper arm close to the side of the body and move the forearm to the side, externally rotating the shoulder joint (as if you were opening a door). Keep your forearm parallel to the floor and maintain a neutral wrist. Move slowly and with control.

FYI: Strengthening the external rotator cuff is important to counteract the large forces generated by the powerful internal rotator muscles of the shoulder. These muscles include the subscapularis, teres major, pectoralis major, anterior deltoids, latissimus dorsi, and biceps brachii. Strong external rotator muscles help to maintain proper function of the shoulder joint and decrease the risk of injury. We recommend occasionally incorporating this exercise into your class.

Elbow Joint

The major muscles of the elbow joint are illustrated in figure 7.7. Table 7.6 lists the common activities that use these muscles as well as basic strengthening exercises for these muscles. Table 7.7 lists the elbow and radioulnar joint muscles and their joint actions. Table 7.8 lists the ROM of the elbow and radioulnar joints. Photos on pages 129 through 133 demonstrate exercises and stretches for the elbow joint.

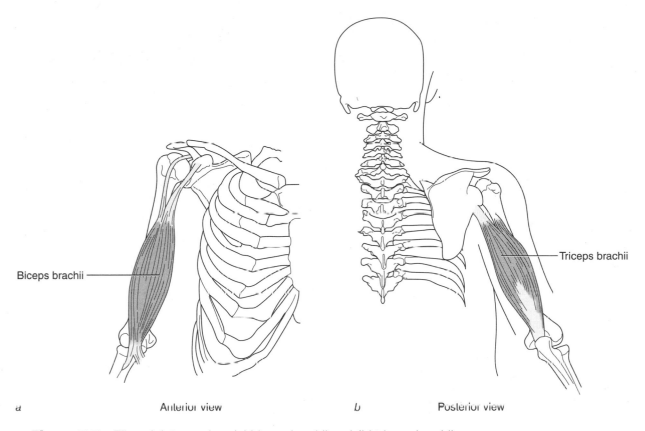

Biceps brachii

Triceps brachii

a Anterior view b Posterior view

▶ **Figure 7.7** Elbow joint muscles: *(a)* biceps brachii and *(b)* triceps brachii.

Table 7.6 Elbow Joint Muscles

Muscle	Daily activities	Exercises
Biceps brachii, brachialis, brachioradialis	Carrying, lifting	Biceps curl, concentration curl, hammer curl, reverse curl
Triceps brachii	Getting in and out of chairs, throwing balls	Dip, kickback, press-down with tube, supine elbow extension

ELBOW JOINT

Table 7.7 Elbow and Radioulnar Joint Muscles and Their Actions

Muscle	Flexion	Extension	Pronation	Supination
Biceps brachii	PM			Asst
Brachialis	PM			
Brachioradialis	PM		Asst	Asst
Pronator teres	Asst		Asst	
Pronator quadratus			PM	
Triceps brachii		PM		
Anconeus		Asst		
Supinator				PM
Flexor carpi radialis	Asst		Asst	
Flexor carpi ulnaris	Asst			
Extensor carpi radialis longus		Asst		Asst
Extensor carpi ulnaris		Asst		

PM = prime mover; Asst = assistant mover.

Adapted, by permission, from P.J. Rasch, 1989, *Kinesiology and applied anatomy,* 7th edition (Philadelphia, PA: Lippincott, Williams and Wilkins), 190.

Table 7.8 ROM of Elbow and Radioulnar Joint Movements

Joint movement	ROM
Flexion	135°-160°
Supination	75°-90°
Pronation	75°-90°

Muscular Conditioning Exercises for the Biceps Brachii

ALTERNATE DUMBBELL BICEPS CURL

**Biceps brachii, brachialis, brachioradialis, optional supinator
(elbow flexion optional radioulnar joint supination)**

Cues: Stand with the feet shoulder-width apart, the knees flexed, and the spine, neck, and pelvis in neutral. Press the shoulders down and slightly back (neutral scapulae). Hold the upper arms close to the ribs (shoulder joints are neutral), palms facing the outer thighs. Curl one arm and then the other, smoothly supinating the palms (turning the palms faceup) at the end ROM. Keep hands as relaxed as possible, maintaining tension in the biceps. Wrists stay completely neutral (no active wrist flexion or extension). Control the movement on the way down, avoiding elbow hyperextension. Return the palms to the midpronated position (facing the thighs) on the way down.

FYI: This exercise may be performed while standing or while seated on a step. Barbell, dumbbells, or tubing may be used for resistance. Supinating the wrist (turning the palms faceup) at the end of the lift is optional. Other variations include maintaining supination throughout and performing the exercise bilaterally, without alternation. The hammer curl (palms stay in midpronated position throughout the movement) and reverse curl (palms are pronated and facing down throughout the movement) are additional exercises that challenge the biceps, brachialis, and brachioradialis.

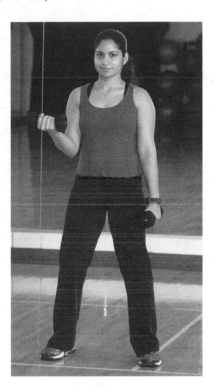

CONCENTRATION CURL

Biceps brachii, brachialis, brachioradialis (elbow flexion)

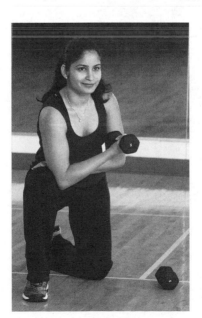

Cues: Kneel, placing one knee on the floor. Rest the opposite foot on the floor so that the opposite knee is bent at 90°. Place the elbow of the working arm slightly inside the thigh of the bent leg and place the opposite hand behind the elbow for support. Hinge forward from the hips, maintaining a neutral spine and neck and keeping the shoulders down. Flex the elbow, lifting the weight diagonally across the body; keep the wrist neutral. Slowly return to the starting position, keeping the elbow from locking (hyperextending).

FYI: This exercise may also be performed while seated on a step.

BICEPS STRETCHES

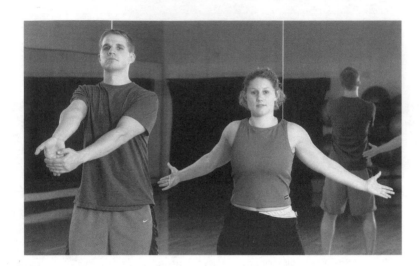

Cues: *(left)* Stand with the feet shoulder-width apart, the knees soft, and the pelvis, spine, neck, and scapulae in neutral. Hold one arm out in front of your body (shoulder flexion), elbow straight, and use your other hand to gently support the wrist, extending your wrist if desired. *(right)* Stand in the same alignment; reach your arms behind your body with your elbows extended and shoulders externally rotated; your palms should face forward and up (thumbs up). Allow the biceps muscles to lengthen.

Muscular Conditioning Exercises for the Triceps Brachii

SUPINE TRICEPS EXTENSION

Triceps brachii (elbow extension)

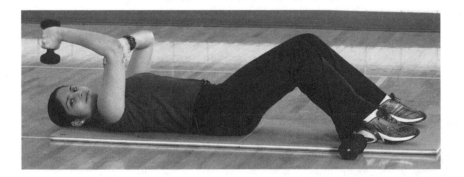

Cues: Lie supine on the floor or on a step. Keep the knees bent with the spine and neck in neutral and the abdominals contracted. Flexing the shoulder of the working arm, point the elbow straight up toward the ceiling; your hand should be near the side of your head. Smoothly extend the elbow to lift the dumbbell, contracting the triceps. Without flaring the elbow, carefully lower the dumbbell back to the starting position. Keep the upper arm still throughout the movement.

FYI: This exercise may be performed unilaterally, which is the easiest variation. It may also be performed bilaterally by holding a dumbbell in each hand, by holding a single dumbbell in both hands, or by holding a barbell (this last variation is the most challenging).

TRICEPS PRESS-DOWN WITH TUBE

Triceps brachii (elbow extension)

Cues: Stand with the feet shoulder-width apart and the spine, pelvis, and neck in neutral. Contract the abdominals and press the shoulders down. Holding one end of the tube or band in the working-side hand, use the other hand to anchor the tube or band to the working-side shoulder. Extend the elbow so that the working arm presses straight down. Straighten the elbow without hyperextending it, and keep the wrists as neutral as possible. Control the motion on the way up (eccentric phase), maintaining a conscious muscle contraction.

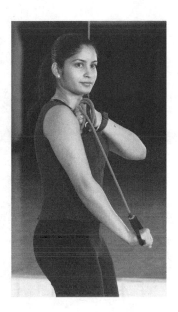

TRICEPS KICKBACK

Triceps brachii (elbow extension)

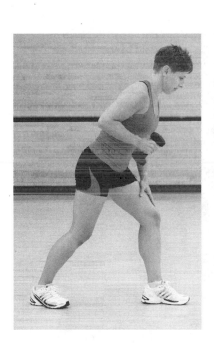
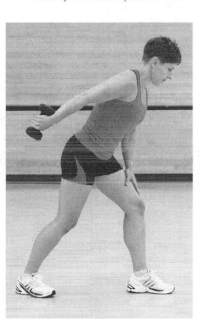

Cues: Stand in a bent-over position with the feet staggered and all joints pointing in the same direction; keep the hips and shoulders squared. Place the nonworking hand on the same-side thigh for low-back support. Place the spine and neck in neutral and pull the abdominals in; be sure the shoulders are pressed down and the scapulae are neutral. Bring the working arm up so that the upper arm is parallel to the floor (shoulder stays down). With control and conscious muscle contraction, straighten the elbow without hyperextending it. Maintain a neutral wrist.

FYI: Although this exercise may be performed bilaterally, we don't recommend doing so in the average group fitness class. Most students are unable to assume the proper bent-over position with a neutral spine and correct alignment; in addition, sufficient core stability is critical for low-back protection. Performing the exercise unilaterally is a fine modification for almost everyone. Kickbacks can also be performed in the half-kneeling position. Common mistakes when performing the kickback include rotating the spine, hunching the shoulders, locking the elbow, and using momentum.

FRENCH PRESS (OVERHEAD PRESS FOR TRICEPS)

Triceps brachii (elbow extension)

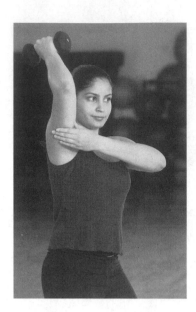

Cues: Stand (or sit on a step) with the knees soft; the pelvis, spine, and neck in neutral; and the abdominals contracted. Point the working elbow straight up to the ceiling; the working forearm should be behind the head. Support the upper arm with the opposite hand. Smoothly, maintaining careful control, move the weight straight up toward the ceiling and carefully lower it back behind the head. Hold your head high and maintain a perfectly neutral neck throughout the exercise, keeping your elbow next to your head.

FYI: This exercise is difficult for participants with tight shoulder muscles or kyphosis. If proper alignment is difficult or impossible, suggest a different triceps exercise (such as a press-down or kickback) that participants can more safely perform. The French press may be performed bilaterally, but doing so is especially inappropriate for those with poor upper-body flexibility.

TRICEPS DIP

Triceps brachii (elbow extension)

Cues: Place your hands on the floor or step with the fingers pointing forward. Suspend your buttocks off the floor or step, supporting your body weight on your hands. Press the shoulder blades down and away from the ears, lengthening the neck. Stabilize the lower body, and avoid moving the legs and hips. The elbow joint should be the only moving joint. Straighten and flex the elbows, keeping them close to the sides of the body. Avoid hyperextending the elbows as you straighten them.

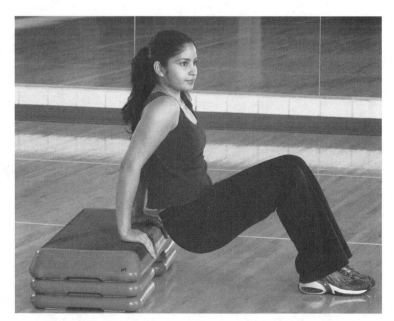

FYI: This is an advanced exercise. Even the beginner version (seated with the hands behind the buttocks) demands heightened body awareness. Avoid flexing the elbows more than 90° and extending the shoulder joints too far back (avoid dips that are too deep), as doing so increases the risk of shoulder joint injury. A dip progression, listed from easiest to hardest , is as follows: dip while seated on the floor, dip on floor with buttocks lifted, dip with hands on step, dip with hands on step and feet on another step, and dip with hands on a stability ball.

TRICEPS STRETCHES

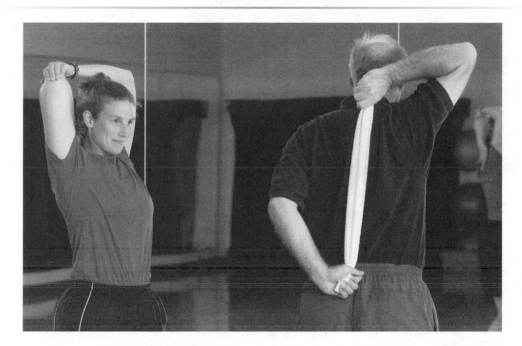

ELBOW JOINT

Cues: *(left)* Stand with feet shoulder-width apart, knees flexed, tailbone pointing straight down, abdominals in, and spine in neutral. Point one elbow toward the ceiling and reach your hand down your back. Gently support the stretch by placing your other hand on either your upper arm or elbow. Keep the head and neck in alignment; avoid hunching the shoulders or hanging the head forward. Keep the shoulders down and away from the ears. *(right)* For a more intense triceps stretch that also stretches the anterior deltoids and the external rotators on the opposite side, stand in the same ideal alignment, again pointing one elbow toward the ceiling so that the hand reaches down the back. Reach the opposite hand behind the back, bringing it up along the spine so that it is reaching toward the other hand. Use a towel or strap to help move the hands toward each other and deepen the stretch.

FYI: This stretch can identify dramatic muscle imbalances between the right and the left sides. Many people will have one side that is noticeably tighter than the other—keep stretching! Try not to force this stretch, particularly on the side with the elbow pointing down toward the floor; the weaker external rotator cuff muscles are already in a strong stretch on this side, and injuries may easily occur when trying to force the stretch deeper. Release from the stretch gradually.

Spinal Joints and Torso Muscles

The major muscles of the torso are illustrated in figure 7.8. Table 7.9 lists muscles of the spinal joints, activities that use these muscles, and basic strengthening exercises for these muscles. Table 7.10 lists the spinal joint muscles and their joint actions. Table 7.11 gives the ROM of various spinal movements. Photos on pages 137 through 142 show muscular conditioning exercises and stretches for the spinal joint muscles.

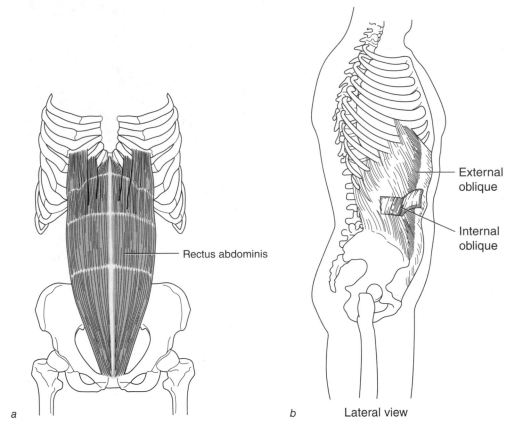

a

Rectus abdominis

External oblique

Internal oblique

b   Lateral view

▶ **Figure 7.8** Spinal muscles: *(a)* rectus abdominis, *(b)* internal and external obliques, *(c)* transverse abdominis, and *(d)* erector spinae.

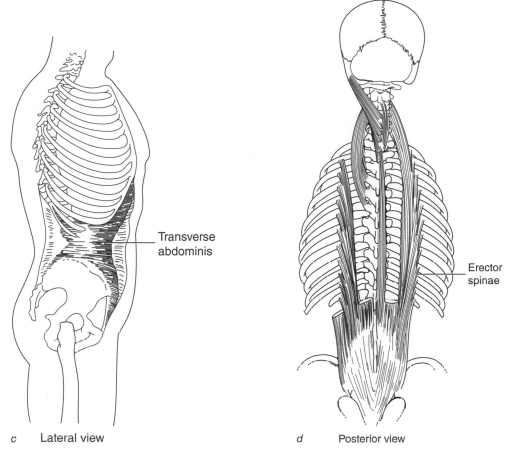

c   Lateral view   d   Posterior view

▶ **Figure 7.8**   (continued)

Table 7.9   Spinal Joint Muscles

Muscle	Daily activities	Exercises
Rectus abdominis	Getting out of bed, posture maintenance	Crunch, pelvic tilt, hip lift
Internal and external obliques	Bending sideways to pick something up, maintaining posture	Diagonal twist crunch
Transverse abdominis	Laughing, coughing, maintaining posture	Hollowing in plank, crunch, Pilates exercises, quadruped
Erector spinae	Bending forward to pick something up, maintaining posture	Prone extension, quadruped

SPINAL JOINTS AND TORSO MUSCLES

Table 7.10 Spinal Joint Muscles and Their Actions

Muscle	Flexion	Extension	Lateral flexion	Rotation to same side	Rotation to opposite side
Sternocleidomastoid	PM		PM		
Erector spinae group (iliocostalis, longissimus, spinalis)		PM	PM	PM	
Multifidus		PM	PM		PM
Rectus abdominis	PM		Asst		
Internal obliques	PM		PM	PM	
External obliques	PM		PM		PM
Quadratus lumborum			PM		

PM = prime mover; Asst = assistant mover. Transverse abdominis performs no joint actions but is responsible for abdominal compression, vigorous exhalation, and expulsion.

Table 7.11 Spinal ROM

Spinal movement	ROM
Flexion	30°-45°
Extension	20°-45°
Lateral flexion	10°-35°
Rotation	20°-45°

Muscular Conditioning Exercises for the Abdominals

PELVIC TILT FOR ABDOMINALS

**Rectus abdominis, transverse abdominis
(spinal flexion and posterior pelvic tilt, abdominal compression)**

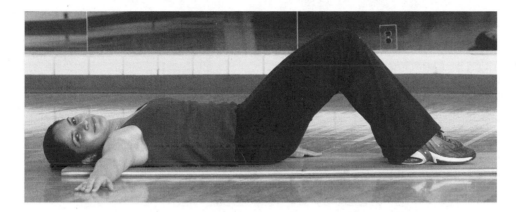

Cues: Lie supine with the knees bent, the upper body relaxed on the floor, and the spine in neutral. Using a diaphragmatic or abdominal breath, exhale and firmly contract the abdominals, allowing them to tilt the pelvis posteriorly. Because this exercise is focusing on the abdominals, avoid allowing the buttocks muscles to participate. Work to isolate the abdominals, feeling a tug on the pubic bone attachment. Keep the movement small; more is not better. Avoid arching the lower back on the return; simply go back to the neutral spine.

FYI: This is an excellent exercise to teach abdominal awareness and proper diaphragmatic breathing. Here is a progression for the pelvic tilt (modifications are listed in order from easiest to hardest): feet flat on floor with knees bent, legs somewhat straight with heels on floor, supine on a slanted bench with pelvis below head, and pelvis hanging off a stability ball. In all variations, try to perform lumbar spinal flexion and posterior pelvic tilt by using the abdominals but not the buttocks.

BASIC CURL-UP (CRUNCH)

Rectus abdominis (spinal flexion and posterior pelvic tilt)

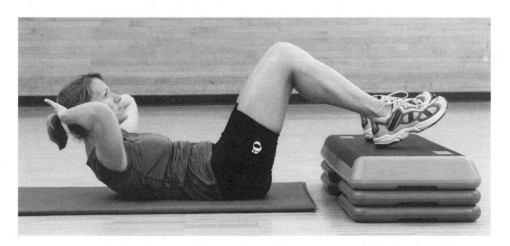

Cues: Lie supine with the knees bent and the spine and neck in neutral. Perform a diaphragmatic breath, exhale, and flex the spine, pulling the ribs toward the hips. Keep the neck in neutral; it has no independent movement of its own (it just goes along for the ride). Avoid performing neck-ups or hyperextending the neck. Bring the shoulder blades up off the floor, and avoid arching the low back on the descent, returning only to neutral.

FYI: There are many variations of this exercise. Arm variations (listed from easiest to hardest) include arms at sides, arms crossed on chest, hands behind ears, hands on forehead, arms crossed behind head, and arms extended overhead. Lower-body variations (again listed from easiest to hardest) include feet supported on a wall or bench (great for participants with low-back problems), lying supine on an inclined step (hips below head) with knees bent, supine with feet on floor and knees bent, supine with legs elevated and knees bent, supine with legs elevated and knees straight, lying supine on declined step (head below hips), lying supine on a stability ball (may be inclined, flat, or declined), and lying supine with a medicine ball toss. For variety and increased difficulty, combine the upper-body curl-up with a hip lift and pelvic tilt.

ABDOMINAL HIP LIFT

Rectus abdominis (spinal flexion and posterior pelvic tilt)

Cues: Lie supine and elevate the legs with the knees slightly bent. Stabilize the knees and the hips at one joint angle. Keep this angle (or position) constant, exhale, and contract the abdominals firmly, posteriorly tilting the pelvis. The movement will be small. Avoid active hip flexion or swinging and rocking the legs.

FYI: This exercise is the more difficult version of the pelvic tilt described earlier. Before progressing to the hip lift, make certain your participants can perform a correct pelvic tilt with coordinated abdominal breathing. The knees may be bent or straight during the hip lift, depending on hamstring flexibility and low-back status. Using an inclined step with the hips below the head increases the difficulty, as does adding an upper-body crunch (full spinal flexion). For variety, try this 4-count variation: Tilt the pelvis (legs are in the air) on 1, curl the upper body up on 2, curl the upper body down on 3, and lower the pelvis on 4.

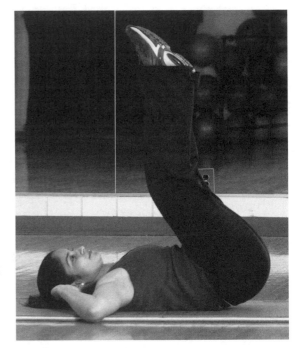

RECTUS ABDOMINIS STRETCHES

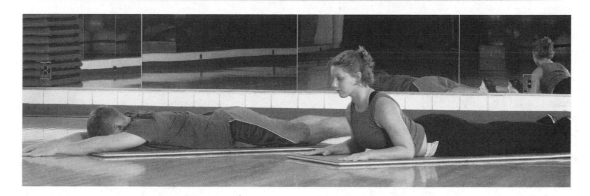

Cues: Lie prone and prop yourself up onto your elbows, stretching the spine up and away from your hips. Lengthen the neck and allow it to continue as a natural extension of the spine (avoid cervical spinal hyperextension). Press down against the floor with your forearms to lower the shoulders away from the ears; slide your shoulder blades down your back. If this position is uncomfortable, modify it by reaching your arms out in front and lifting your upper torso just slightly off the floor, lengthening the abdominals. Keep the neck in alignment.

FYI: The full cobra pose, used in yoga, is an advanced version of this stretch. Since the cobra pose has a greater tendency to overstretch the long ligaments of the spine, we do not recommend including it in a group exercise class.

Muscular Conditioning Exercises for the Obliques

DIAGONAL TWIST CRUNCH

External and internal obliques (spinal flexion and rotation)

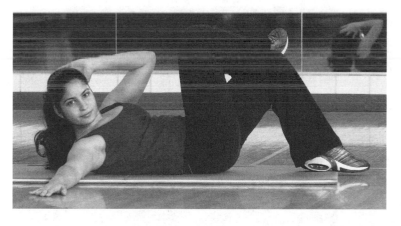

Cues: Lie supine with one knee bent, foot on the floor. Place your other foot on the thigh of your bent leg. Place one hand on the floor and the other hand behind your head. Exhaling, crunch diagonally, moving the ribs toward the opposite hip. Keep your neck in neutral (apple-sized space between chin and chest) and bring the shoulder blade off the floor. Keep the movement slow and controlled, avoiding momentum. Change legs and repeat the set on the opposite side.

FYI: Many variations exist for this exercise. Upper-body variations may be performed unilaterally and bilaterally and include, from easiest to hardest, arms at sides, arms crossed on chest, hands behind ears, arms crossed behind head, and arms stretched overhead. Lower-body variations include both feet on floor (knees bent), both legs in the air (knees bent or straight), and one foot on the floor with the other leg extended in the air. In addition, a slanted step or a stability ball may be used for additional overload.

OBLIQUE STRETCHES

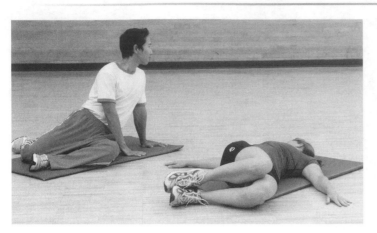

Cues: *(left)* Sit with your knees bent, one hip externally rotated (open) and the other hip internally rotated. Walk your hands around to the externally rotated side as far as is comfortable, stretching the obliques as well as the latissimus dorsi. Allow your arm to reach up and over in this position if desired. *(right)* Lie supine with both knees bent in toward the torso. Allow the knees to slowly drop toward the floor. Reach your opposite arm off and away to the other side, turning your head in that direction. Breathe deeply, relax, and enjoy this multiple-muscle stretch (the obliques, pectorals, hip abductors, erector spinae, and rectus abdominis are all being stretched).

Muscular Conditioning Exercises for Training the Core

SINGLE-LEG CIRCLE

Iliopsoas, rectus femoris, transverse abdominis (hip circumduction, abdominal compression)

Note: The purpose of this and the next exercise is to train the core muscles to stabilize the spine in neutral. The first exercise, single-leg circles, is easier since it is performed in the supine position; the quadruped that follows requires greater balance and core stability.

Cues: Lie supine with one leg extended along the floor and the other leg extended toward the ceiling, toes pointed. Firmly anchor the torso by hollowing the abdominals and pulling the navel toward the spine, all the while staying in neutral spinal alignment that maintains the four natural curves of the spine. Press both hips and shoulders evenly into the floor. Make small circles in the air with the perpendicular leg, moving first clockwise and then counterclockwise. Increase the size of the circles only as long as the pelvis can be kept level and absolutely still. Repeat on the other side.

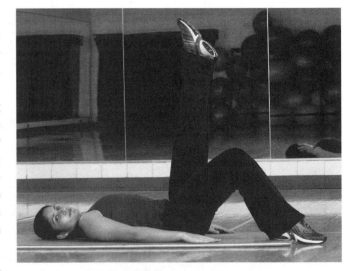

FYI: In this Pilates exercise, the hip flexors act as the prime movers; the rectus abdominis, obliques, transverse abdominis, and erector spinae muscles stabilize the spine. Adequate hamstring flexibility is required to perform the exercise as described; keeping the bottom knee bent is an acceptable modification.

QUADRUPED

Erector spinae, transverse abdominis, gluteus maximus, hamstrings, deltoids, serratus anterior (maintenance of neutral spine and scapulae, abdominal compression, hip extension, shoulder flexion)

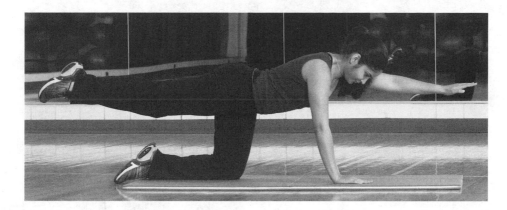

Cues: Kneel on all fours with the hands directly under the shoulders and the knees directly under the hips. Place the pelvis, spine, neck, and scapulae securely in neutral alignment. Slowly extend one arm and the opposite leg, maintaining level hips and shoulders and the neutral spine and neck. Hold. Return slowly to all fours without disturbing your alignment and repeat on the other side.

FYI: This exercise may be performed statically (holding 5-30 seconds per side) or dynamically (smoothly alternating back and forth between sides). The purpose of both variations is to promote torso stability and to challenge both the erector spinae and the abdominals as stabilizers.

Muscular Conditioning Exercises for the Erector Spinae

PRONE SPINAL EXTENSION

Erector spinae (spinal extension)

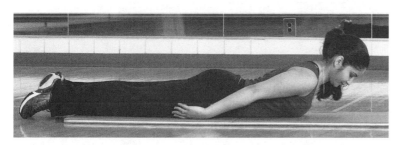

Cues: Lie prone with your forehead on the mat and your neck in neutral. Press your hips into the floor and keep your arms at your sides. Lengthening the spine, slowly lift the upper body, maintaining a neutral neck (chin will remain slightly tucked). Lower smoothly and repeat.

FYI: Active lumbar extension or hyperextension can be problematic for some participants. Always ask your participants how they feel and provide modifications when needed. Tell participants to stop if they feel any pain. The most conservative approach to strengthening the lower back is to perform isometric extension only and encourage students to work with their physicians. Other variations of this exercise, moving from easiest to hardest, include extension with arms at 90°, extension with arms overhead, extension with opposite arm and leg, and extension performed on a stability ball.

ERECTOR SPINAE STRETCHES

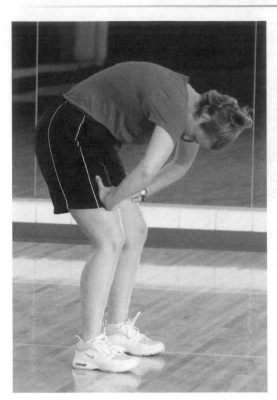 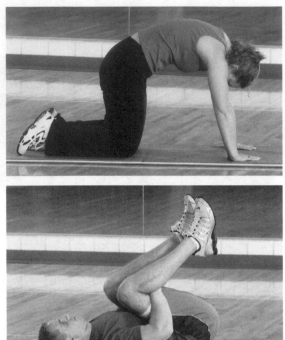

Cues: *(left)* Stand with the feet shoulder-width apart and the knees bent. Placing your hands on your thighs, tuck your pelvis (posterior pelvic tilt) and round (flex) your spine, pulling your navel in. Allow your head and neck to be a natural extension of the spine and your hands to support your back as you press your waist backward, lengthening the muscles of the lower back. *(top right)* Kneel on all fours and perform the angry cat stretch, flexing your spine upward and contracting your abdominals up and in. Keep your pelvis tucked under and tailbone pointing down. Allow your head and neck to flex gently, following the line of the spine. Press your waist back and up to increase the low-back stretch. *(bottom right)* Lie supine and hug both knees to your chest, placing your hands behind the knees. Allow your spine to flex and your tailbone to curve upward. If comfortable, gently rock side to side, back and forth, or in a circular pattern, massaging the low-back muscles. Allow the head and neck to rest in neutral alignment on the floor.

FYI: Encourage your participants to find low-back and abdominal stretches that make their backs feel good. Provide them with several options and let them discover their preference.

Hip and Knee Joints

Since so many lower-body exercises use the hip and knee joints simultaneously, we combine the information for these two joints into this section. Figures 7.9 and 7.10 show the muscles of the hip and knee joints. Tables 7.12 and 7.15 list the major muscles of each joint, activities of daily living that use each joint, and basic strengthening exercises for each joint. Tables 7.13 and 7.16 list the muscles and joint actions of the hip and knee. Tables 7.14 and 7.17 give the ROM of selected hip and knee movements. Photos on pages 148 through 157 demonstrate muscular conditioning exercises and stretches for the hip and knee joint muscles.

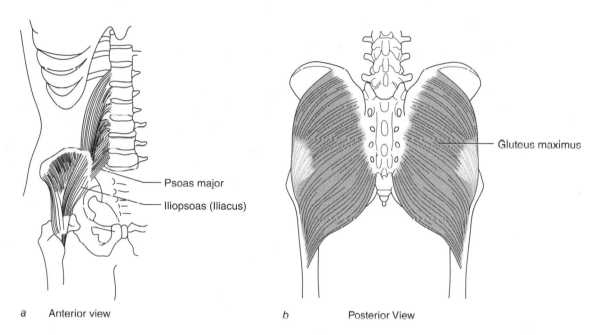

a   Anterior view

— Psoas major
— Iliopsoas (Iliacus)

— Gluteus maximus

b   Posterior View

▶ **Figure 7.9**   Hip joint muscles: *(a)* anterior view of the iliopsoas, *(b)* gluteus maximus, *(c)* posterior view of the gluteus medius, and *(d)* anterior view of the hip adductors.

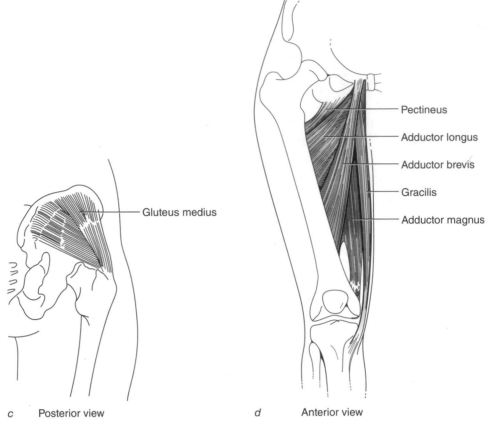

c   Posterior view   *d*   Anterior view

▶ **Figure 7.9**   *(continued)*

Table 7.12   Hip Joint Muscles

Muscle	Daily activities	Exercises
Psoas and rectus femoris	Climbing stairs, walking, getting in a car, kicking a ball	Standing and supine leg lift (hip flexion)
Gluteus maximus, hamstrings	Climbing stairs, running, walking uphill	Squat, lunge, leg lift in all-fours position, pelvic tilt
Gluteus medius	Stabilizing hip when walking, balancing	Side-lying leg lift, standing abduction
Hip adductors	Stabilizing hip when walking, horseback riding	Side-lying leg lift, supine adduction

Table 7.13 Hip Joint Muscles and Their Actions

Muscle	Flexion	Extension	Abduction	Adduction	Inward rotation	Outward rotation
Psoas	PM		Asst			Asst
Iliacus	PM		Asst			Asst
Rectus femoris	PM		Asst			
Sartorius	Asst		Asst			Asst
Gluteus maximus		PM	Asst[a]	Asst[b]		PM
Biceps femoris		PM				Asst
Semitendinosus		PM			Asst	
Semimembranosus		PM			Asst	
Gluteus medius	Asst[c]	Asst[a]	PM		Asst[c]	Asst[a]
Gluteus minimus	Asst[c]	Asst[a]	Asst		PM	Asst[a]
Tensor fasciae latae	Asst		Asst		Asst	
Pectineus	PM			PM	Asst	
Gracilis	Asst			PM	Asst	
Adductor longus	Asst			PM	Asst	
Adductor brevis	Asst			PM	Asst	
Adductor magnus	Asst[a]	Asst[b]		PM	Asst	
Six outward rotators						PM

PM = primo mover; Asst = assistant mover. The six outward rotators are the piriformis, obturator internus, obturator externus, quadratus femoris, gemellus superior, and gemellus inferior. [a]Upper fibers; [b]lower fibers; [c]anterior fibers

Adapted, by permission, from P.J. Rasch and R.K. Burke, Kinesiology and applied anatomy, 7th edition (Philadelphia, PA: Lippincott, Williams and Wilkins), 282.

Table 7.14 ROM of Select Hip Joint Movements

Joint movement	ROM
Flexion	90°-135°
Extension	10°-30°
Abduction	30°-50°
Adduction	10°-30°
Internal rotation	30°-45°
External rotation	45°-60°

HIP AND KNEE JOINTS

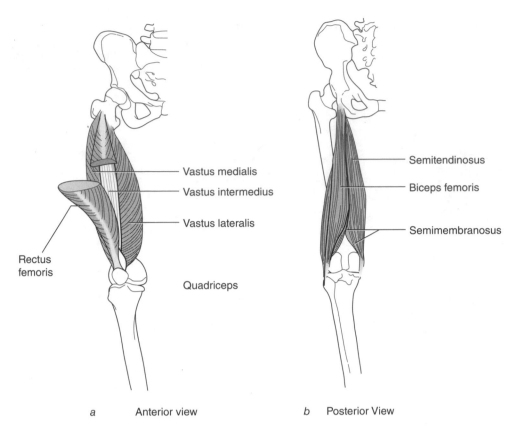

Vastus medialis

Vastus intermedius

Vastus lateralis

Rectus femoris

Quadriceps

Semitendinosus

Biceps femoris

Semimembranosus

a   Anterior view   *b*   Posterior View

▶ **Figure 7.10**   Knee joint muscles: *(a)* quadriceps and *(b)* hamstrings.

Table 7.15   Knee Joint Muscles

Muscle	Daily activities	Exercises
Quadriceps	Walking, cycling, stair-climbing, sitting down, standing up	Squat, lunge, knee extension, plié
Hamstrings	Swimming, running	Prone knee curl, knee curl on all fours

Table 7.16 Knee Joint Muscles and Their Actions

Muscle	Flexion	Extension	Inward rotation	Outward rotation
Biceps femoris	PM		PM	
Semitendinosus	PM		PM	
Semimembranosus	PM			PM
Rectus femoris		PM		
Vastus lateralis		PM		
Vastus intermedius		PM		
Vastus medialis		PM		
Sartorius	Asst		Asst	
Gracilis	Asst		Asst	
Popliteus[a]	Asst		PM	
Gastrocnemius	Asst			
Plantaris	Asst			

PM = prime mover; Asst = assistant mover. [a]Unlocks the knee at the start of knee flexion.

Adapted, by permission, from P.J. Rasch and R.K. Burke, Kinesiology and applied anatomy, 7th edition (Philadelphia, PA: Lippincott, Williams and Wilkins), 309.

Table 7.17 ROM of Knee Joint Movements

Joint movement	ROM
Flexion	130°-140°
Extension	5°-10°

Muscular Conditioning Exercises for the Quadriceps, Gluteus Maximus, and Hamstrings

SUPINE LEG LIFT AND KNEE EXTENSION

Iliopsoas, quadriceps (hip flexion, knee extension)

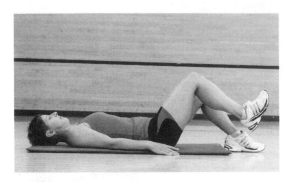

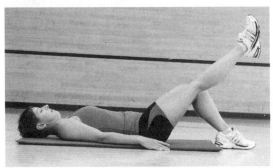

Cues: Lie supine with the spine in neutral and the abdominals firmly anchored. Place one foot on the floor with the knee bent. Straighten the other knee and raise it to a 45° angle off the floor. Using a controlled, smooth motion, bend and straighten the elevated knee; alternate with hip flexion, if desired.

FYI: Knee extension *(top)* and hip flexion *(bottom)* can be performed supine, supine propped up on elbows, or standing. Supine is the easiest position. In addition, the knee extension can include a quad set (isometric-type contraction of the quadriceps that tighten the patella) and terminal knee extensions (moving the knee joint only through the last few degrees of motion). These variations help to correct potential muscle imbalances around the knee joint. Bands or ankle weights can be added for additional overload.

SQUAT

Quadriceps, gluteus maximus, hamstrings (knee extension, hip extension)

Cues: Stand with the feet shoulder-width apart and the toes straight ahead or slightly rotated outward (in the same direction as the knees). The spine, neck, and pelvis are in neutral, and the abdominals are pulled up and in. Bending the knees, press the tailbone and the middle third of the body back. Keeping the torso erect, the chest lifted, and the head in line with the spine, lower the body until the thighs are almost parallel to the floor or until the lumbar curve becomes excessive. Do not allow your hips to drop below your knees; avoid overshooting the toes or lifting the heels off the floor. Keep the abdominals contracted and the spine stable throughout the movement. Keep one hand on your thigh for low-back safety and allow the other arm to flex forward, providing a counterbalance.

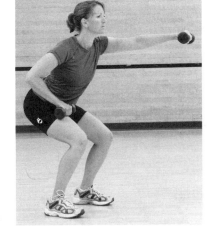

FYI: Almost everyone can benefit from learning to squat properly. This very functional exercise helps students have better mechanics in lifting, getting in and out of chairs, and other daily activities. Variations, listed in order from easiest to hardest, include a sit-back squat while holding onto a ballet barre, a squat while holding onto a Body Bar placed vertically in front of the body, a squat with hands on thighs, a squat with one hand on one thigh, a squat with dumbbells held at the sides, a back squat with a barbell, and a front squat with a barbell (the last three variations pose a greater risk for the low back).

PLIÉ

**Quadriceps, gluteus maximus, hamstrings, adductors
(knee extension, hip extension, hip adduction)**

Cues: Stand with the feet wide apart and the toes angled away from the midline of the body. Turning out from the hips, make sure that the knees are aligned in the same direction as the toes (if this isn't possible, adjust the feet so that the toes and knees are in the same line). The pelvis is in neutral with the tailbone pointing straight down, and the spine is in neutral with the shoulders level and chest lifted. Maintaining this lifted, turned-out alignment, bend the knees to no more than a 90° angle (thighs will be parallel to the floor). Straighten the knees and return to the starting position, consciously contracting the buttocks and inner thighs.

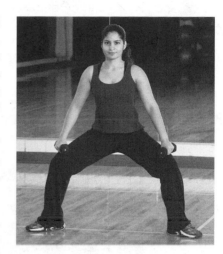

FYI: This exercise may be performed with dumbbells or a barbell for added resistance; upper-body exercises can be combined with the plié once good alignment has been mastered. A plié is really just a modified squat. Some students may find it easier than a squat because the pelvis is kept neutral and the spine is kept upright. Other students may find it more difficult because of the amount of turnout required. Although the quadriceps is the prime mover of this exercise, the gluteus maximus isometrically contracts to maintain external hip rotation, and the adductors can be recruited during the lifting phase of the movement (although there is no resistance against gravity).

LUNGE

**Quadriceps, gluteus maximus, hamstrings, hip abductors, hip adductors
(knee extension, hip extension, hip stabilization)**

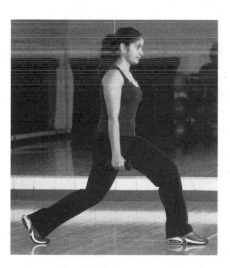

Cues: For a stationary lunge, stand with the feet staggered at least 3 feet (1 m) apart; participants with long legs should stand with their feet even farther apart. Lift up onto the ball of the back foot. Place the pelvis in neutral, the tailbone down, and the spine and neck in neutral; contract the abdominals. The hips and shoulders are level. Bending both knees, slowly lower your body. Go only low enough that the front knee bends to a right angle (90°) and the front thigh is parallel to the floor. Avoid dropping the hips below the knee or letting the back knee touch the floor. Keep the pelvis and spine upright; avoid leaning forward. Return to the starting position, keeping the back heel elevated. To perform a front lunge, start in a standing position with the feet shoulder-width apart and the spine, pelvis, and neck in neutral. Step forward and land on the heel, ball, and then toe. Slowly lower the body and bend the front knee to no more than 90°. Keep the front knee behind the toes (avoid overshooting). The torso remains completely upright (requiring hip flexor flexibility), and the heel of the back foot is off the floor. Push off with the front foot and return to standing. When performing a long lunge with the back leg straight, it may be necessary to stutter step back with the front foot—this more advanced move uses two or three smaller steps.

FYI: In general, lunges are a more advanced exercise. To perform a proper lunge, students need lower-body strength, flexible hip flexors, stable torsos, balance, and coordination. There are many variations of the lunge, including the front, back, side, and crane lunges. All of these can be performed with stationary, dynamic, or traveling variations. Front, back, and crane lunges can be performed with the back leg bent or straight (using the straight leg is more difficult and requires much more flexibility). The lunge can be an excellent lower-body strengthener, but care must be taken to maintain strict form (especially with regard to the knees) to avoid injury.

ALL-FOURS BUTTOCKS AND HAMSTRINGS EXERCISE

Gluteus maximus, hamstrings (hip extension, knee flexion)

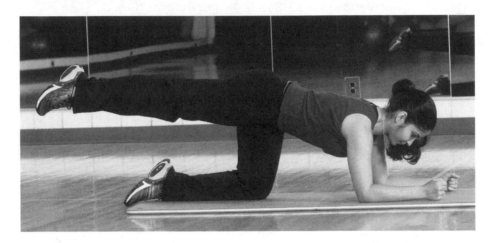

Cues: Assume the all-fours position; place the hands directly under the shoulders and the knees directly under the hips, forming a tabletop with the spine, neck, and head. Lift the abdominals, placing the spine in neutral with the head and making the neck a natural extension of the spine. The hips and shoulders are level. Keeping the torso absolutely still, slowly raise one leg on 1, flex the knee on 2, straighten the knee on 3, and lower the leg on 4. Consciously squeeze the buttocks and hamstring muscles as you perform this exercise.

FYI: The hip extension and knee curl can be performed prone, on all fours, or even standing. Hip extension can be performed alone and knee flexion can be performed alone, or the two moves can be combined, as described previously. The prone position is the most stable and appropriate for beginners, although ROM at the hip joint is small. Both the all-fours and standing positions are more difficult to stabilize, and both challenge the abdominal and low-back muscles isometrically. Avoid momentum in this position, because performing the movements too quickly can lead to back hyperextension and potential injury. Performing the exercise on elbows and knees is an excellent alternative to hands and knees; ROM may be increased without as much risk of back hyperextension.

ILIOPSOAS (HIP FLEXOR) STRETCHES

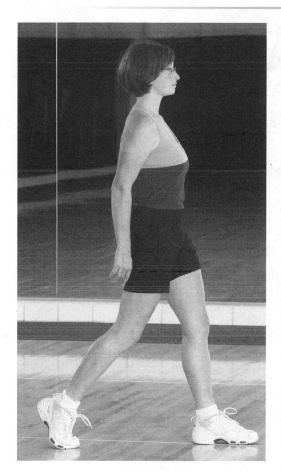

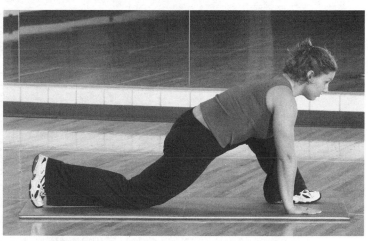

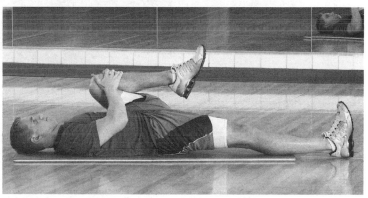

Cues: *(top left)* Stand with the feet staggered, as pictured. Your feet should be far enough apart to prevent your front knee from bending excessively (the front knee should be directly over the heel, with the lower leg perpendicular to floor). Turn all the joints in the same direction: The toes, knees, hips, and shoulders should all face the same way. Firmly squeeze the buttocks and press the pelvis into a posterior pelvic tilt (tailbone tips slightly forward and under). Hold the abdominals securely in and the torso upright with neutral spine, scapulae, and neck. Feel the hip flexor muscles lengthen and stretch across the front of the right hip. If necessary, stand by a wall for balance. *(top right)* For a more intense version of this stretch, move into a runner's lunge, bringing the back foot even farther back. The front knee will now make a right angle; the shin will be perpendicular and the thigh will be parallel to the floor. Keep the torso as upright as possible, place your hands on the floor or balance them on your thighs. The back knee may be placed on the floor, if desired (although avoid placing it directly on a wood floor—use a mat for cushioning). If you choose to show the runner's lunge first, always show the easier version as well, as many participants will be uncomfortable in the runner's lunge. Pay special attention to the front (bent) knee, as overbending is a common mistake and can lead to knee problems. The rectus femoris is also stretched in these first two stretching examples. *(bottom)* Lie supine on the floor with one knee pulled into the chest (hands behind the thigh) and the other leg stretched out straight on the floor. Lie with the spine and neck in neutral and the abdominals contracted. Gently attempt to press the back of the straight knee toward the floor while maintaining the bent knee pressed into the chest. Feel the hip flexor stretch on the top of the extended hip.

QUADRICEPS STRETCHES

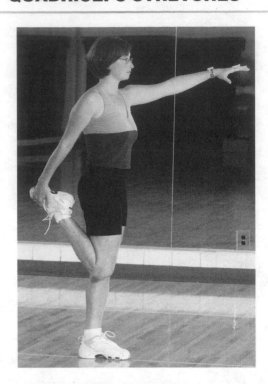

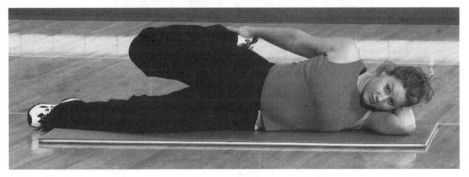

Cues: *(top)* Stand on one foot. and keep the knee soft, the abdominals contracted, and the pelvis, spine, neck, and scapulae in neutral. Grasp the other foot with your hand (usually the same-side hand, although either hand is acceptable as long as it feels comfortable) and gently pull the heel into your buttocks, making certain that the hip, knee, and ankle joints are all in a line (no torque) and the knee is pointing toward the floor. Check to see that your hips and shoulders are level and even. If balance is a problem, stand near the wall for support. If you cannot comfortably reach your foot or ankle, try holding onto your pants leg or sock, or place your foot on a bench or chair and then squeeze your buttocks, tucking your pelvis posteriorly. *(bottom)* Lie on your side and grasp your top foot with your top hand, flexing the knee and gently pulling it toward your buttocks. Keep your hips stacked, abdominals in, and spine and neck in neutral, with your bottom arm bent under your head (do not place your head up on your hand, because this takes your neck out of alignment).

FYI: Another excellent position for quadriceps stretching is the prone position. The participant simply places one hand under the forehead (avoiding cervical hyperextension) and reaches back with the other, grasping the same-side ankle and gently pulling it in toward the buttocks.

GLUTEUS MAXIMUS AND HAMSTRING STRETCHES

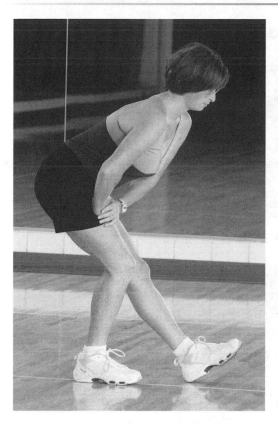
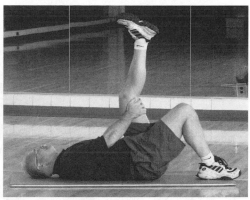
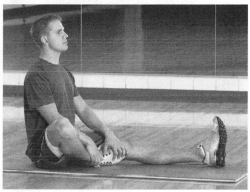

Cues: *(left)* Stand with the feet hip-width apart, with the heel of one foot in line with the toes of the other foot. Press the tailbone backward, as if preparing to sit or squat; keep the hips and shoulders square. Hinging at the hips (no spinal flexion), fold the torso forward while maintaining a long, neutral spine. Contract the abdominals and place both hands on the thigh of the bent knee (this helps protect the low back). The leg with the bent knee is the support leg, whereas the other leg is the stretching leg. The knee of the stretching leg is straight but not hyperextended. Your foot may be dorsiflexed or plantar flexed. Keep the hips square and hip hinge in the direction of the straight leg so you are stretching along the longitudinal line of the hamstring muscle. *(top right)* Lie supine with one knee bent, the foot on the floor, and the spine, neck, and scapulae in neutral. With the other knee straight (but not hyperextended), gently pull your leg in toward your torso (your foot may be pointed or flexed). *(bottom right)* Sit perfectly upright on the sitting bones (ischial tuberosities) so that your pelvis, spine, and neck are in neutral alignment. If you find it difficult to sit upright without slumping, wedge a towel slightly under the tailbone or use a stretch strap (or towel) around the foot, enabling you to pull yourself upright. (It is harmful to your spine to slouch in this position.) Extend one leg. Keeping the hips square and the opposite knee bent out to the side, hinge at the hip as much as possible in the direction of your extended leg, keeping your spine long and straight, your chest lifted, and your head and neck a natural extension of the spine.

FYI: Be familiar with the modifications for the seated hamstring stretches: Many participants won't be able to perform them with acceptable alignment and will risk hurting their backs. Have participants use props (a wedge or towel under the edge of the buttocks and a strap around the feet), place their hands behind the body for support (instead of reaching forward), or choose an alternative hamstring stretch. The seated stretch can be performed either unilaterally or bilaterally (both legs in front), although the bilateral position is potentially more stressful to the low back.

Muscular Conditioning Exercises for the Gluteus Medius

HIP ABDUCTION

Gluteus medius

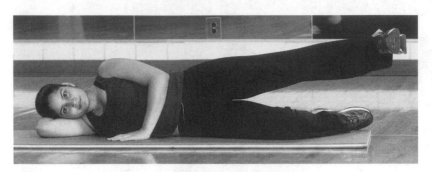

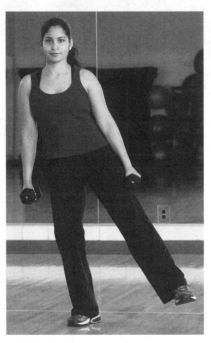

Cues: To perform side-lying hip abduction, lie on your side with your head resting on your arm. Maintain a neutral neck and spine (do not place your head on your hand, as doing so can place undue stress on the neck), and keep your hips stacked. Both kneecaps must face forward (to avoid external hip rotation and flexion and the subsequent use of muscles other than the hip abductors) if the goal is to isolate the outer thigh muscles. Consciously contract the abductors and slowly raise and lower the leg. If you are performing this exercise while standing, make certain that the standing knee is bent slightly, allowing the pelvis and spine to maintain a neutral position. Keep the hips level, keep the moving kneecap facing forward, and maintain a stable torso as the leg abducts and returns.

FYI: Effective isolation-type exercises for the abductors may be achieved in either the side-lying or the standing position. The side-lying position is the safest and arguably the most effective choice because of its stability and direct resistance against gravity. There are several variations of this exercise, including top leg straight, top leg bent, top leg in line with the body, and top leg at 45° of hip flexion. There are also numerous rhythm variations. Bands or ankle weights may be added for additional overload.

GLUTEUS MEDIUS STRETCHES

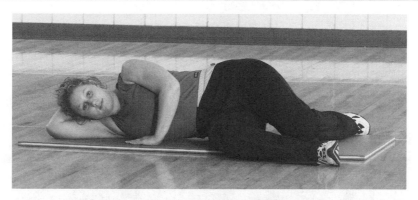

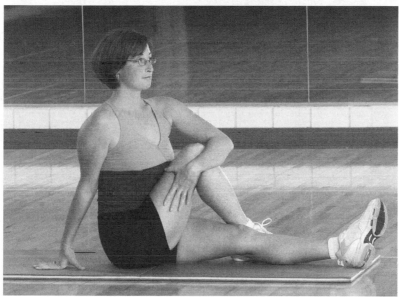

Cues: *(top)* Lie on your side with your arm comfortably under your head, your hips stacked, and your spine in neutral. Flex the bottom hip so that your bottom leg is in front of your body (knee can be bent). Place your top leg in a straight line with your torso and bend the knee. Gently lower the bent top knee toward the floor, maintaining level, stacked hips and avoiding any lateral spinal flexion. Do not let your top leg move in front of or in back of the torso; it needs to be in exactly the same plane for the most effective outer thigh stretch. *(bottom)* Sit in good alignment, up on the sitting bones, with the spine, neck, and scapulae in neutral and one leg extended out in front. Bring the opposite knee diagonally across the torso, attempting to press the knee into the opposite shoulder. Feel the stretch in the right outer thigh and buttock muscles.

Muscular Conditioning Exercises for the Hip Adductors

HIP ADDUCTION

Adductor longus, adductor brevis, adductor magnus, gracilis, pectineus

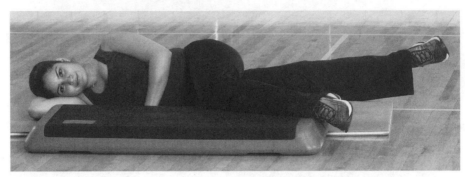

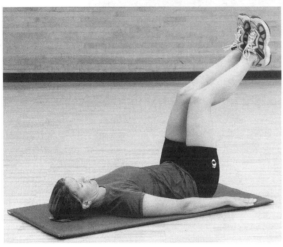 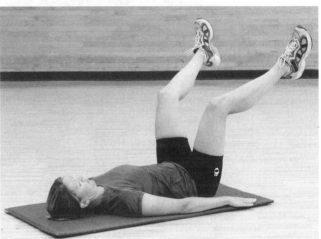

Cues: To perform hip adduction from the side-lying position, lie on your side with your head resting on your arm. Keep your hips stacked and your spine and neck in neutral (do not place your head in your hand because this takes the neck out of alignment). The bottom (moving) leg is in line with the body, and the top leg is in front of the body with the inside edge of the foot resting on the floor. Unless students have long thigh bones and narrow hips, they should hold the top knee in a slightly elevated position to ensure that the hips remain stacked—unstacking the hips leads to greater reliance on muscles other than the hip adductors and can stress the back. Consciously contract the muscles and slowly raise and lower the bottom leg. To perform hip adduction from the supine position, lie supine with the legs elevated in the air. Participants with tight hamstrings should bend their knees to ensure that the weight of the legs is over the torso and not over the floor. Anchor the abdominals to help maintain torso stability. Open and close the legs, consciously tightening the inner thigh muscles.

FYI: Isolation of the adductors can be performed in the side-lying or the supine position; the side-lying position is more effective because it optimizes resistance against gravity's pull. Hip adduction exercises may be varied by using short or long levers, adding rhythmic variations, and using bands or weights. To help maintain the slight elevation of the top knee in the side-lying position, use a step, towel, or small ball.

HIP ADDUCTOR STRETCHES

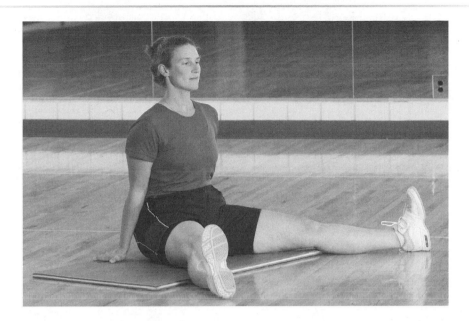

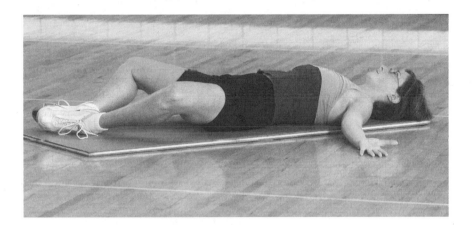

Cues: *(top)* Sit on the floor in the straddle position, legs wide apart, weight securely on sitting bones (ischial tuberosities). If necessary, place the hands on the floor behind the body to help place the pelvis, spine, scapulae, and neck in a neutral alignment directly in line with the sitting bones. Rotate the hips open so that the kneecaps face the ceiling; the feet may be pointed or flexed. Hinging at the hips, not the waist (no spinal flexion), point the tailbone backward and bring the torso forward, maintaining neutral alignment. The farther you are able to hinge at the hips and bring the torso forward, the more you'll need to place your hands in front for support. *(bottom)* Lie supine with the knees bent, the feet on the floor, and the pelvis, spine, scapulae, and neck in neutral. Allow the legs to fall open (abduct) until you feel a comfortable inner thigh stretch; keep the feet together on the floor and the knees bent.

Ankle Joint

Figure 7.11 shows the major muscles of the ankle joint. Table 7.18 lists the ankle joint muscles, activities that use these muscles, and basic strengthening exercises for these muscles. Table 7.19 lists the ankle joint muscles and their joint actions. Table 7.20 gives the ROM of ankle joint movements. Photos on pages 159 through 161 demonstrate exercises and stretches for the ankle joint muscles.

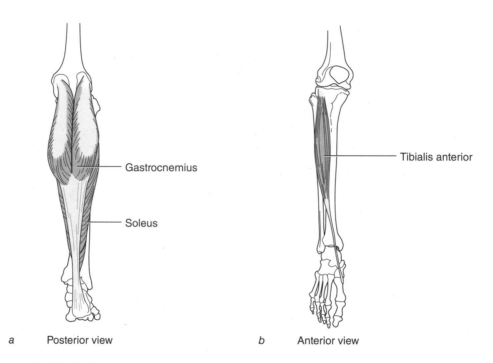

a   Posterior view   b   Anterior view

▶ **Figure 7.11**   Ankle joint muscles: *(a)* gastrocnemius and soleus and *(b)* tibialis anterior.

Table 7.18   Ankle Joint Muscles

Muscle	Daily activities	Exercises
Tibialis anterior	Walking uphill, toe tapping	Toe lift
Gastrocnemius, soleus	Walking, running, jumping	Heel raise

Table 7.19 Ankle Joint Muscles and Their Actions

Muscle	Dorsiflexion	Plantar flexion	Inversion	Eversion
Tibialis anterior	PM		PM	
Extensor digitorum longus	PM			PM
Peroneus tertius	PM			PM
Gastrocnemius		PM		
Soleus		PM		
Peroneus longus		Asst		PM
Peroneus brevis		Asst		PM
Flexor digitorum longus		Asst	Asst	
Tibialis posterior		Asst	PM	

PM – prime mover; Asst – assistant mover.

Adapted, by permission, from P.J. Rasch and R.K. Burke, Kinesiology and applied anatomy, 7th edition (Philadelphia, PA: Lippincott, Williams and Wilkins), 330.

Table 7.20 ROM of Ankle Joint Movements

Joint movement	ROM
Dorsiflexion	15°-20°
Plantar flexion	30°-50°
Inversion	10°-30°
Eversion	10°-20°

Muscular Conditioning Exercises for the Shin Muscles

SHIN EXERCISE

Anterior tibialis (ankle dorsiflexion)

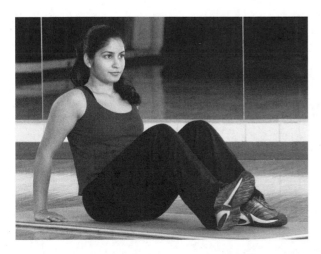

Cues: Sit in good alignment, with your weight over your sitting bones and your spine and neck in neutral alignment. Keeping the knees slightly bent, point and flex each foot one at a time. Move through the full ROM, allowing each foot to point fully and then bringing the toes as far toward the shin as possible. Consciously contract the shin muscles.

FYI: This exercise may be combined with basic abdominal crunches. As you curl up, simultaneously dorsiflex one ankle, releasing as the spine returns to neutral. Alternate ankles with each curl-up.

ANKLE JOINT

SHIN STRETCHES

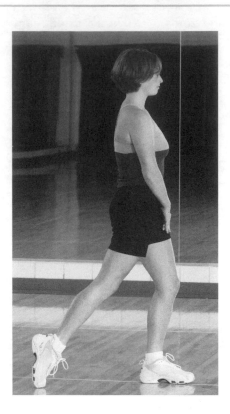

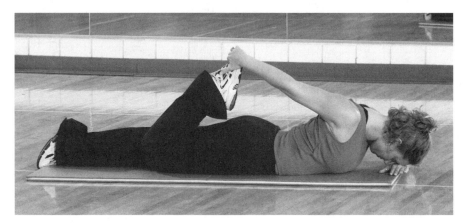

Cues: *(top)* Stand in the position for the calf stretch, feet staggered with one foot behind the body. Maintaining one long line from the back foot to the head, contract the abdominals as you balance on the front leg and point the back foot (ankle plantar flexion). Keep all joints in line and avoid letting the ankle collapse to the right or left side. Feel the stretch through the shin and along the top (front) of the foot. *(bottom)* Lie in the prone position for the quadriceps stretch, one hand under your forehead and the other hand holding your foot. Point your foot as you gently bring the heel toward the buttocks, feeling the stretch not only in the quadriceps but also in the shin (anterior tibialis) and the top (front) of the foot.

Muscular Conditioning Exercises for the Calves

CALF EXERCISE

Gastrocnemius and soleus (ankle plantar flexion)

Cues: Stand with the knees soft; the pelvis, spine, and neck in neutral; the abdominals tight; and the feet hip-width apart. Lift both heels off the floor, rising onto the balls of the feet as far as possible. Return to the floor.

FYI: To achieve full ROM for the calf muscles, stand on the edge of a step, lowering the heels as far off the step as possible and then returning to normal standing.

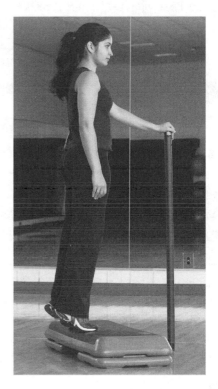

CALF STRETCHES

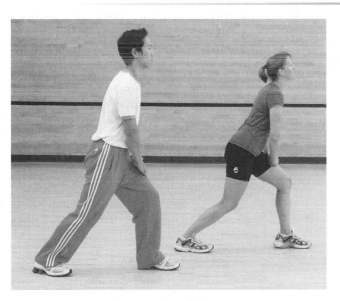

Cues: *(left)* Stand with the feet staggered, one foot behind the body. Adjust the distance between your feet so that your back heel comfortably reaches the floor yet your front knee is still directly over the heel and the front lower leg is perpendicular to floor. Turn all joints in the same direction: The toes, knees, hips, and shoulders should all face the same way. Place both hands on your front thigh and check to see that your body forms one long line from heel to head; the spine should be neutral. Contract your abdominals, keep the chest slightly lifted, and keep the shoulders back and down. This stretch may also be performed with the hands on a wall. *(right)* Stand in the position just described and let your back knee bend as far as feels comfortable; your back heel should remain down and your joints should remain in alignment—pointing in the same direction. Bending the knee provides a deeper stretch for the soleus muscle and helps lengthen the Achilles tendon (which is often too tight).

Practice Drill

Practice each of the preceding exercises and stretches with a partner, taking turns performing each movement. Study the pictures, cues, and other information and practice giving cues as your partner performs the exercise. Make sure to perform each exercise and stretch with excellent form and alignment. Write down two cues for every exercise and stretch in this chapter.

MUSCULAR CONDITIONING EQUIPMENT

A wide variety of equipment can be used in group exercise muscle conditioning. Dumbbells, elastic tubes, and resistance bands are standard in most fitness facilities, and many clubs also stock weighted bars, barbells with plates, stability balls, BOSU balance trainers, medicine balls, foam rollers, core boards, wobble boards, fitness circles, and more. The following sections discuss the use of various equipment options.

Dumbbells

Most health clubs and fitness centers supply several sets of dumbbells ranging from 1 to 10 pounds (0.5-4.5 kg) for use during group exercise class. Dumbbells provide a practical and convenient way to overload the musculoskeletal system and can be used in a wide variety of exercises. Here are recommendations for the safe and effective use of dumbbells:

1. Do not let participants use weights until they can perform muscle conditioning exercises with proper form and technique against gravity alone; this includes being able to consciously contract the targeted muscle throughout its entire ROM. The eccentric, or lengthening, phase of the muscle action (when the weight is lowered) should be performed with awareness and care. An uncontrolled eccentric action is a primary mechanism of musculoskeletal injury (see "Common Mistakes in Weight Training" on page 162).

2. Teach participants to hold the weights with a relaxed grip, as lifting with tight fists may inadvertently raise blood pressure. Many participants also hold their breath and strain when clenching their fists. This action, called the *Valsalva maneuver,* can be potentially dangerous for people with heart disease, people with high blood pressure, and women who are pregnant. The Valsalva maneuver also increases the possibility of fainting, light-headedness, and irregular heart rhythms. Consistently remind your students to breathe!

3. Make sure participants maintain a neutral wrist throughout all exercises, especially when holding hand weights, tubes, or bands. Repeatedly flexing or extending the wrists while holding weights or tubes increases the likelihood of developing carpal tunnel syndrome or tennis elbow.

4. Encourage participants to select a weight load that allows them to move with proper form yet still fatigues the targeted muscle group after several repetitions.

Use caution when adding hand weights to the cardio segment of class. Studies have shown that adding 1- to 2-pound (0.5-1 kg) weights to the cardio routine does not significantly increase the caloric expenditure or oxygen uptake (Blessing et al. 1987; Kravitz et al. 1997; Stanforth et al. 1993; Yoke et al. 1988). Although adding weight to cardio sessions may improve local muscle endurance, the risk-to-benefit ratio must be

Common Mistakes in Weight Training

- Using weights that are too heavy for maintaining good form
- Failing to stabilize the core (pelvis, spine, and scapulae)
- Holding the breath (Valsalva maneuver)
- Using excessive speed or momentum, especially during the eccentric phase
- Range of motion problems (too little or too much)

considered; rapidly moving 1- to 2-pound (0.5-1 kg) hand weights while performing complex lower-body patterns offers questionable benefit while increasing the risk of injury, especially to the vulnerable shoulder joint. Upper-body form may be compromised when the attention and focus are on footwork. We encourage you to reserve the use of weights for the time when they can provide the greatest benefit—the muscular conditioning portion of your class.

Barbells and Weighted Bars

Some facilities invest in sets of barbells and weight plates for group exercise. Barbells can provide an excellent option for participants who are more advanced. They may be troublesome in a mixed-level class that includes beginners and intermediates, however, as many of the exercises that are performed bilaterally with barbells are more challenging because of the increased need for core stabilization. Instructors must provide several modifications and be wary of continually demonstrating and exercising with barbells while in front of the group. Even when the instructor gives an easier variation, if she or he continues to demonstrate the more advanced version, participants are likely to copy whatever is being demonstrated even if it goes beyond their level. Examples of barbell exercises that are not appropriate for many group exercise participants are the weight room–style back or front squat, bent-over bilateral lat row, bent-over bilateral high (horizontal) row, upright row, and deadlift. All of these exercises require a high degree of core stability and body awareness for safe execution.

Additionally, participants need to be able to perform a proper weight room–style squat to safely pick up the barbell from the floor. We encourage you to reserve group barbell work for classes clearly labeled as advanced.

Elastic Resistance

Elastic bands and tubes are another option for overloading the muscular system. Many facilities stock tubing and bands in different strengths and thicknesses, allowing participants to progressively overload their exercises. Elastic resistance is different from most weighted exercise in that the tension is less at the starting position and the greatest at the end of the range of motion. For instance, when participants perform a biceps curl with the tubing anchored under the foot, the tension is greatest at the top of the curl—the end range of motion (Miller et al. 2001; Stoppani 2005). In contrast, when participants perform a biceps curl with a dumbbell, the tension is greatest at the sticking point, the point where the elbow is at approximately 90° of flexion and the force needed to overcome gravity is at its greatest. Providing a variety of exercises with both free weights and elastic resistance is an optimal way to provide overload and stimulate improvement throughout a muscle's entire ROM. Note that even more exercises can be created by combining elastic resistance with dumbbells or barbells.

The following are recommendations for safe and effective band and tubing use:

■ Technique and Safety Check

Teach participants how to pick up and put down their weights correctly without jeopardizing their lower backs:

- Face the dumbbells with the feet shoulder-width apart. Placing one hand on the front of the thigh for support, use the other hand to reach for a dumbbell.

- Pick up the dumbbell and transfer it to the hand that is resting on the thigh. Hold the dumbbell against the thigh, continuing to lean on the thigh for support.

- Pick up the other dumbbell with your free hand. Hold this dumbbell against your other thigh and press up to standing.

- Reverse this process to put the dumbbells back on the floor. The idea is to always keep one hand on the thigh for support and perform a one-handed lift. This is a great method for protecting the spine when picking up objects; whenever possible, use one hand to lift the object while supporting your back by keeping the other hand on the thigh.

1. Always match the line of pull with the direction of the tubing or bands. In other words, the elastic resistance must always be in the same plane as the muscle action of the exercise. In a biceps curl, for example, the tubing must fall straight down from the forearm; the anchor point should be directly below, behind, or even in front of the moving arm. If the anchor point is off to the side (not in the same plane), the exercise is both less effective and less safe; a rotary force, or torque, is applied to the moving joints and ligaments and may lead to injury (Page and Ellenbecker 2003).

2. Adjust the resistance by choosing different thicknesses of bands or tubing or by choking up on the tubing to shorten it. Multiple pieces of thin tubing may also be used to increase the resistance. This method has the advantage of allowing for multiple lines of pull within the plane of motion. For example, tubing can be anchored both anteriorly and posteriorly to the elbow joint in a standing biceps curl.

3. Make certain participants maintain a neutral wrist when holding tubes or bands. Have participants who have carpal tunnel syndrome check with a physician before using elastic resistance.

4. Remind participants to maintain a relaxed grip whenever possible so as not to elevate blood pressure. Using tubing with handles makes it easier to avoid a clenched fist and keep the hands relaxed.

5. Teach your participants to control the eccentric (negative) phase of the exercise. Avoid the rebound effect and joint stress that occur when students abruptly stop their contraction and let the elastic yank the joint back to its starting point.

6. Regularly inspect the tubing or bands for cracks and tears.

7. When placing tubing under a step, use tubing designed for that purpose (usually there is a nylon strip that prevents excessive rubbing and deterioration of the tubing as it contacts the step).

8. Place tubes and bands over clothing whenever possible to avoid pinching or rubbing the skin and pulling body hair.

9. Look away from the band (especially in upper-body resistance work) to protect the face in the event that the band might break.

Steps

Steps, or benches, can be used to increase or decrease the amount of resistance in a given exercise and to change the muscle group focus. If you place the steps on risers only at one end, participants can be inclined or declined, and the exercise can be gravity-assisted or gravity-resisted. For example, if participants are inclined (head is higher than the hips) when performing an abdominal curl-up, the exercise becomes easier than if they were lying flat (supine). The exercise is gravity assisted. If participants are declined (head is lower than the hips), the curl-up is harder than if they were supine and the gravitational resistance is greater (gravity resisted).

The muscle group focus can also be altered by inclining or declining an exercise. A classic example is the bench press, an exercise that in the supine position targets the majority of the pectoralis major muscle fibers as well as the anterior deltoid. If the bench press is performed in an inclined position, anterior deltoid and clavicular pectoral involvement increases and sternal pectoral involvement decreases. When the bench press is performed in a declined position, the reverse is true: There is increased sternal pectoral and latissimus dorsi involvement and less anterior deltoid and clavicular pectoral recruitment.

Steps are also useful props for lower-body conditioning. The lunge, squat, and one-leg step-up are all exercises that can be performed with a step. The use of steps adds variety to your muscular conditioning segment and increases your potential for individualizing your conditioning sessions and appropriately overloading your students.

Stability Balls and BOSU Balance Trainers

Large, resilient stability balls (also known as *Swiss balls*) have been used for years by physical therapists for both strength and flexibility training. The BOSU balance trainer (*BOSU* stands for *both sides up*), on the other hand, is a relatively new device for muscle training. Stability balls are an extremely effective prop for training the core muscles (abdominals and lower back) to stabilize the trunk and spine (Hahn et al. 1998; Willardson 2004). Other muscle groups can also be strengthened effectively on the stability ball and BOSU balance trainer. Studies show that core muscles are recruited to a greater extent when exercises targeting other muscle groups (e.g., the bench press for the chest and triceps) are performed on the stability ball (Marshall and Murphy 2006). In general, exercises performed using stability balls and BOSU balance trainers are more advanced than those performed without these devices because they require greater balance and thus greater recruitment of the stabilizer muscles (Cosio-Lima et al. 2001). The ball, of course, provides an unstable surface and improves balance by improving muscle reflex,

proprioception, and small muscle involvement. Depending on how the BOSU is used (dome side up or flat side up), it can also significantly challenge balance and coordination (see figure 7.12). We recommend that participants develop basic muscle strength and endurance before progressing to stability ball and BOSU exercises. Stability balls should be sized according to the participant's height or leg length and should always be inflated to the designated amount (see table 7.21). The following pages describe some of the common exercises using the stability ball.

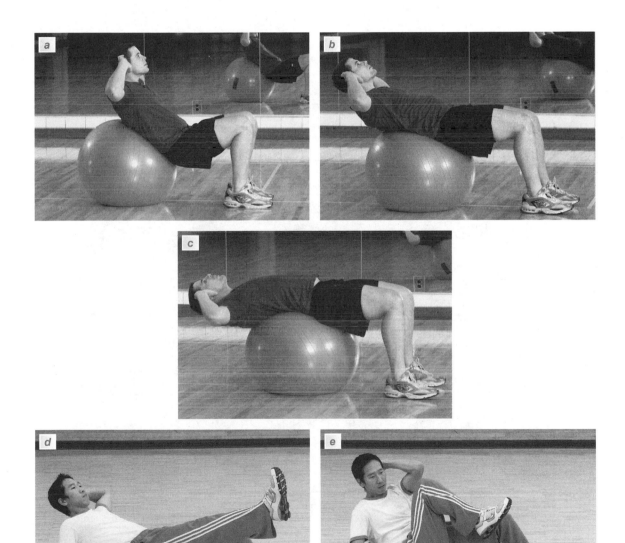

▶ **Figure 7.12** Curl-ups performed on a stability ball can be *(a)* inclined (gravity assisted), *(b)* parallel to the floor, and *(c)* declined (gravity resisted), *(d and e)* diagonal twist crunch (with added leg movement) for obliques on the BOSU.

Table 7.21 Stability Ball Size Recommendations

Participant height	Ball size
<60 in. (<152 cm)	18 in. (45 cm)
60-67 in. (152-170 cm)	22 in. (55 cm)
68-74 in. (173-188 cm)	26 in. (65 cm)
>74 in. (>188 cm)	30 in. (75 cm)

The knees and hips should both form 90° angles when the participant sits on the ball.

Muscular Conditioning Exercises Using the Stability Ball

SEATED KNEE EXTENSION WITH BAND AND SEATED OVERHEAD PRESS

Quadriceps; Deltoids and triceps

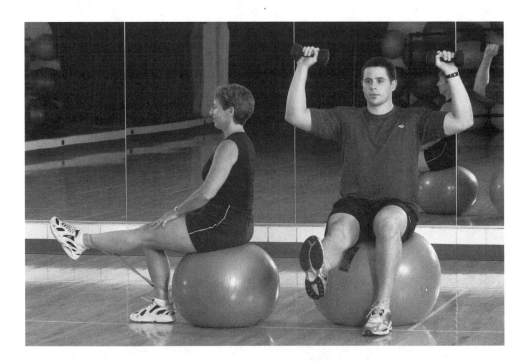

Cues: *(left)* The seated knee extension is executed by sitting with good posture on the ball, with the band around both ankles, smoothly extend one knee. Maintain level hips and shoulders; keep the abdominals contracted.

Cues: *(right)* To perform a seated overhead press sit on the ball with good alignment, a neutral spine, and abdominals contracted. Press the arms overhead, keeping the scapulae down.

FYI: For an additional challenge, lift one leg.

SUPINE BUTTOCKS SQUEEZE AND SQUAT

Buttocks and hamstrings; quadriceps, buttocks, and hamstrings

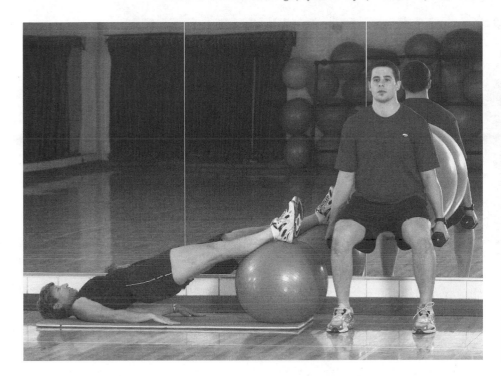 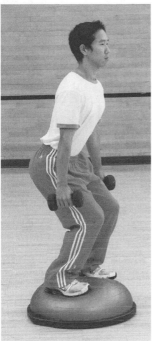

Cues: *(left)* Lying supine with your feet on the ball, contract the buttocks and smoothly press up into a planklike position, abdominals contracted.

Cues: *(middle)* Execute the standing wall squat by standing with the ball against the wall and pressed into the lower back. Place feet far enough away from the wall so that when you squat your knees will form a 90° angle and your shins will be vertical. Your toes, knees, hips, and shoulders should all face the same direction.

FYI: *(right)* A standing squat may also be performed on a BOSU for more difficulty.

SIDE-LYING HIP ABDUCTION

Gluteus medius

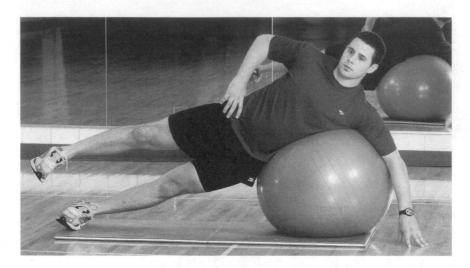

Cues: Lying on one side over the ball, maintain proper alignment with the hips and shoulders stacked and the neck continuing the line of the spine. Perform hip abduction with the top leg.

FYI: You may let the bottom knee rest against the floor or, for greater challenge, keep the knee straight and stack the feet on top of each other.

SIDE-LYING HIP ADDUCTION

Hip adductors, gracilis, and pectineus

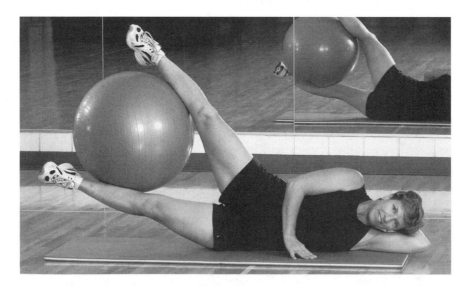

Cues: Lie on your side with the top leg resting on the ball and the ball resting on the bottom leg. The hips are stacked and the spine and neck are in neutral. Moving both legs and the ball upward, adduct the bottom leg.

PRONE PUSH-UP

Pectoralis major, anterior deltoids, and triceps

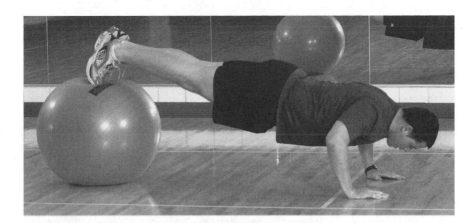

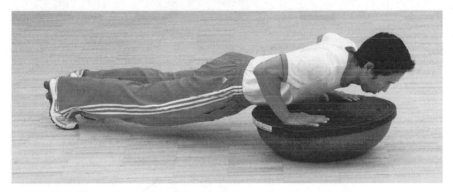

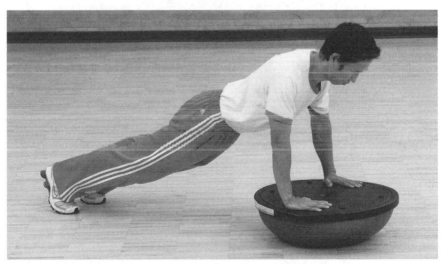

Cues: *(top)* Lie prone on the ball and then walk your hands away from the ball, maintaining a plank position with the abdominals securely contracted and the neck in line with the spine. Begin the push-ups.

FYI: The closer the ball is to your feet, the more difficult the push-ups will be. Try balancing on one leg for a difficult challenge! Push-ups may also be performed with the flat side of the BOSU facing up *(middle and bottom)*.

PRONE REVERSE FLY

Middle trapezius, rhomboids, and posterior deltoids

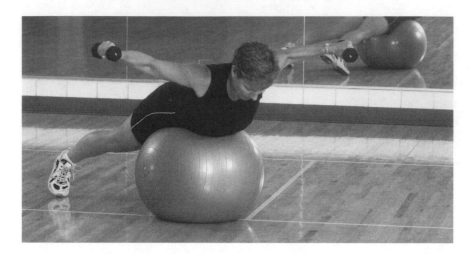

Cues: Lie prone with the ball under the lower ribs and the arms perpendicular to the torso. The elbows are slightly flexed, the wrists are neutral, and the neck is in line with the spine. Horizontally abduct the arms toward the ceiling, retracting the scapulae.

PRONE SHOULDER EXTENSION

Latissimus dorsi and posterior deltoids

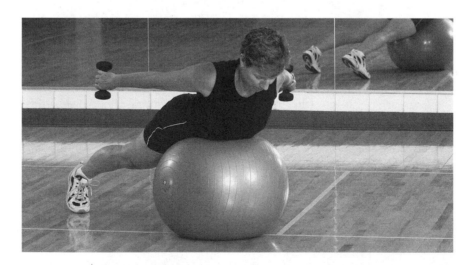

Cues: Lie prone with the ball under the lower ribs and the arms at the sides, elbows straight, wrists neutral, and neck in line with the spine. Lift straight arms up toward the ceiling.

FYI: For additional challenge, lift one leg.

PRONE BACK EXTENSION

Erector spinae

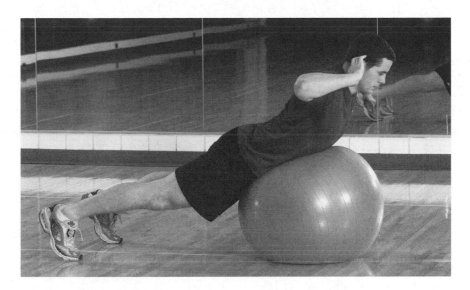

Cues: Lie prone with the hands behind the ears and smoothly extend the spine.

SUPINE ABDOMINAL CRUNCH

Rectus abdominis

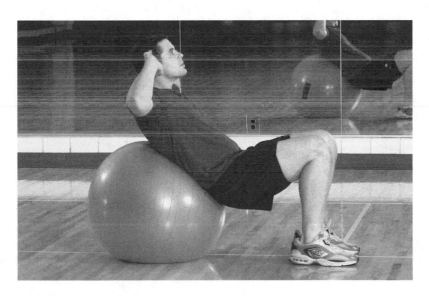

Cues: Lie supine on the ball and perform abdominal curl-ups. Decrease the difficulty by moving into an inclined position or increase the difficulty by moving into a declined position or by lifting one leg.

FYI: Challenge the obliques by performing crunches with rotation.

CUEING METHODS

The type of cueing required for muscle conditioning is different from that required for leading cardio exercise to music. When you are leading step or high-low, for example, good anticipatory cueing is essential so you can let your class know about upcoming moves before they actually happen, helping to ensure that your class moves safely together as a unit. During muscle conditioning, however, anticipatory cues are much less important than alignment, safety, and motivational cues.

Some instructors fall into the monotonous trap of counting every repetition of every strength exercise. There are so many other valuable things to say. We recommend that you save counting for the last set or the last few repetitions. For example, tell your class that they have eight more biceps curls and that you want them to go to the point of fatigue, squeezing their biceps as hard as possible for the last eight repetitions. Then, counting backward from 8, increase the intensity in your voice and add a motivational cue or two to encourage participants to achieve muscle overload by the last repetition. Remember, motivational cues are used liberally by experienced instructors. You can do it!

Additionally, the muscular conditioning segment is an ideal time to face your class, because complex choreography is not an issue. Facing your class is more personal and more direct than facing the mirror and generally provides you with better visibility of your students' alignment. After demonstrating proper form and alignment for the first few repetitions of an exercise, walk around your class to check everyone's form and give personalized modifications when needed. This is an excellent time to address participants by name and give encouragement! The following sections discuss the basic types of cues for muscular conditioning.

Alignment Cues

Here's an example of providing useful alignment cues during the squat: "Be sure your knees are behind your toes and your weight is directed back toward your heels. Point your tailbone toward the back wall. Tighten up those abdominals and lift your chest!" Visual and tactile cues are also very useful for promoting proper alignment. When describing knee alignment in the squat, try visual cueing, as follows: point to your knees and use the wrong, right technique—first demonstrate incorrect knee alignment, drawing an imaginary line from the hyperflexed knee to the floor. Then reposition your knees to demonstrate correct alignment. You can also visually cue by placing your finger over your tailbone to show how it should point toward the back wall. Touch your abdominals to indicate abdominal support. Alignment can be thought of as joint alignment. If you are at a loss as to what to say or show, verbally and/or visually describe the alignment of all the joints. Even in a simple biceps curl, students need to be mindful of their lower-body alignment. How should their knees be positioned? What about their pelvis or their spine, shoulders, neck, and wrists?

Safety Cues

A safety cue educates your participants on how to make the exercise safer and prevent injury. For example, during the squat you could say, "Keeping both hands on the thighs or performing alternating front raises in which you keep one hand on the thigh helps protect your lower back. Maintaining an abdominal contraction while squatting also supports the lower back and guards against injury."

Motivational Cues

Motivational cues can make the difference between a mediocre workout and a great workout. Tell your participants, "Great job!" "I really like how all of you are keeping your knees in good alignment!" "You people are terrific!" "All right!" Many instructors cue on every (or almost every) repetition of a muscle conditioning exercise. Here are additional cues you can use to offer encouragement: "Squeeze!" "Contract!" "Press." "Breathe!" "Oh yeah!" "Release." "Make it look like work!" "Consciously tighten that muscle!" "Go!" "You can do it!"

Educational Cues

The following list includes examples of cueing that we use during strengthening segments to optimize educational opportunities:

- Perform this exercise slowly, smoothly, and with control.
- Breathe in, and as you begin the movement, perform the work, lift the weight, or pull against the resistance—exhale!
- The number of repetitions is not as important as tuning in to the area you are working.
- If you feel any pain, twinges, or joint discomfort, stop!
- Correct form is more important than the number of repetitions or the amount of weight.
- You can do one side until fatigued; then switch to the other side or alternate sides each time.
- If you are new to class, change sides or stop when you get tired, even if the rest of the class keeps going.
- Even though we are doing many repetitions, this type of exercise will not remove fat from this area. To remove fat, you need aerobic exercise. This exercise will help you tone and shape muscles and will allow you to tuck in, pull up, and contour your body.

Looking closer at verbal and physical cues will help you understand that there is more than one way to communicate and direct movement. Verbal cues include cueing movement with appropriate terminology and instruction as previously discussed. For example, when you are teaching a standing outer thigh leg lift to strengthen the gluteus medius, you should do the following:

- Ask participants to contract the stabilizers (abdominals, gluteus maximus).
- Give appropriate alignment cues joint by joint.
- Remind participants that the range of motion of the movement is around 45°, so lift with the side of the heel. If the toe comes up, that's hip flexion, which works the quadriceps and hip flexors.
- Keep the movements slow and controlled and alternate sides to promote better participant comfort and muscle balance.
- Always be encouraging when giving any cue; try to word all corrections in a positive way. Instead of saying, "Don't lock your knees" or "You're locking your knees," say, "Bend your knees slightly, OK?" or "Would you mind softening your knees a bit? That will help reduce both knee stress and back stress and keep you safe."

Physical, hands-on (tactile) cues are another way to give participants feedback on their form. When you give physical cues, walk around the room and observe participants from different angles. Gently placing your hands on a participant's shoulders to remind him to relax his shoulder blades is an example of a physical or tactile cue. Before touching, be sure to ask the participant's permission. Do not touch if the participant seems uncomfortable in any way.

CHAPTER WRAP-UP

Outlined in this chapter are the variables that are common to most muscular conditioning and flexibility segments of group exercise. Knowing muscle anatomy and joint actions, selecting exercises and equipment, and demonstrating and cueing specific exercises and stretches with good alignment are all important when teaching class. The information, skills, and exercises discussed in this chapter are fundamental for a skilled group exercise leader. Muscle conditioning and flexibility are key components of fitness, and we highly recommend that all group instructors become adept at leading these important class segments.

▶ Assignment

Prepare in writing a stretch and strengthening exercise for each major muscle group (calves, shins, abductors, adductors, anterior and medial deltoids, pectorals, hamstrings, lower back, quadriceps, middle trapezius, rhomboids, abdominals, latissimus dorsi, biceps, and triceps). List ROM, joint action, muscles involved (use proper terminology), and at least three cues for each exercise. You may put these on note cards or any format that will help you study for the stretch and strengthening practical exam.

■ Practice Drill

Pick an exercise that is easy to cue (e.g., biceps curl) and see how many alignment, safety, and motivational cues you can come up with. Then practice adding visual cues to your verbal ones.

PART III

Group Exercise Modalities

Step Training

By the end of this chapter, you will

- understand how to warm up for step training;
- be able to teach basic moves and patterns for step;
- be able to build basic combinations and choreography for a step class;
- be able to teach a 2-minute step routine with appropriate content, alignment, technique, cueing, using appropriate music; and
- be able to identify proper alignment, technique, and safety recommendations for step training.

Cardio step classes have been popular since their inception in 1990; approximately 44% of fitness facilities currently offer cardio step programs (IDEA 2007). Step classes promote cardiorespiratory fitness, muscle endurance, coordination, and balance and come with several health benefits (see "Step Training Research Findings" on page 180). Many participants enjoy the rhythmic sound, exact patterning, and high energy of a step class. Expand your options as a group exercise leader by learning how to teach a motivating step class. The main points on the group exercise class evaluation form that relate to step training are listed on page 178.

WARM-UP

Warm-ups for step training should follow the recommendations outlined in chapter 5: They should use a combination of dynamic movements and stretches to prepare the heart, lungs, and major muscles for vigorous activity. However, an optimal step warm-up also incorporates the bench, thus specifically readying the body for the workout to follow. This is achieved by using a floor mix—that is, a mixture of step and low-impact moves. A simple floor mix pattern is shown in table 8.1.

■ Background Check

Before working your way through this chapter, you should do the following:

Read

- chapter 5: Warm-Up,
- the music section in chapter 4, and
- the choreographic technique sections in chapter 4.

Practice

- the music drills in chapter 4 (page 52) and
- the cueing drills in chapter 4 (pages 69-73).

Group Exercise Class Evaluation Form Essentials

Key Points for the Warm-Up Segment

- Includes appropriate amount of dynamic movement
- Provides rehearsal moves
- Stretches major muscle groups in a biomechanically sound manner with appropriate instructions
- Gives clear cues and verbal directions
- Uses an appropriate music tempo (118-128 beats per minute) or motivating music that inspires movement

Key Points for Cardiorespiratory Segment

- Gradually increases intensity
- Uses a variety of muscle groups (especially hamstrings and abductors)
- Minimizes repetitive movements
- Promotes participant interaction and encourages fun
- Demonstrates movement options and gives clear verbal cues
- Gradually decreases impact and intensity during cool-down following the cardiorespiratory session
- Uses music volume and tempo (118-128 beats per minute) appropriate for biomechanical movement

Table 8.1 Floor Mix for a Step Warm-Up

Move	Foot pattern	Number of counts
Grapevine R (on floor)	R, L, R, tap	4
Tap-up, tap-down (on step)	Up, tap, down, tap	4
Grapevine L (on floor)	L, R, L, tap	4
Tap-up, tap-down (on step)	Up, tap, down, tap	4

R = right; L = left.

Dynamic Movement and Rehearsal Moves

A grapevine is performed on the floor, whereas the tap-up, tap-down is a rehearsal move that uses the step. Combining the two specifically and gradually prepares the mind and body for more intense step moves. Because the warm-up is to be performed at a lower intensity than the cardio-conditioning portion of the class, the number of step moves used and the sequencing of the floor mix are important factors. Avoid continuous stepping in the warm-up because it stresses unprepared joints and can increase the heart rate too quickly. Instead, intersperse low-impact moves with step moves.

Stretching

Ideally, some of your warm-up stretches should use the step; common stretches on the bench include those for the hamstring, hip flexor, and calf muscles (see figure 8.1). The ideal time to increase flexibility is during the final cool-

■ Practice Drill

Design and practice a simple 32-count floor mix combination suitable for a step warm-up, using no more than four moves. For example, you might combine one floor move, one step move, one floor move, and one step move.

down portion of the class. Stretching during the warm-up is performed simply to take all the joints and muscles through their full ROM before beginning vigorous exercise. A warm-up stretch is more about extensibility than flexibility and therefore doesn't need to be held as long (8 counts are usually sufficient). Stretch the areas that are commonly tight and are used heavily in a step class: the calf (both gastrocnemius and soleus), shin, hamstring, quadriceps, hip flexor, low-back, and anterior chest muscles.

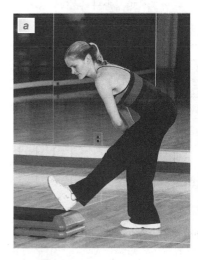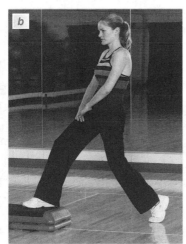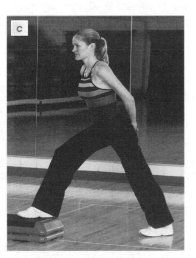

▶ **Figure 8.1** *(a)* Hamstring stretch, *(b)* hip flexor (iliopsoas) stretch, and *(c)* calf (gastrocnemius) stretch.

Step Training Research Findings

Many research studies have shown that step (or bench) training can provide an excellent and predictable cardiorespiratory stimulus that results in important health benefits (Kin Isler et al. 2001; Kraemer et al. 2001). A number of these studies have measured energy expenditure at various step heights and have found that step training meets the ACSM criteria for the achievement of cardiorespiratory fitness (Olson et al. 1991; Stanforth et al. 1991; Woodby-Brown et al. 1993). Research shows that intensity and caloric expenditure increase with step height (Stanforth et al. 1993; Wang et al. 1993; Woodby-Brown et al. 1993). Specific moves and patterns as well as the inclusion of arm movements influence the energy cost (Calarco et al. 1991; Francis et al. 1994; Olson et al. 1991), as does adding propulsion to common step moves (Greenlaw et al. 1995). Some researchers have found that a faster music tempo results in increased energy consumption (Scharff-Olson, Williford, Duey et al. 1997; Stanforth et al. 1991), whereas others have found that holding 2-pound (1 kg) hand weights while stepping does not significantly influence the energy cost (Kravitz et al. 1995; Olson et al. 1991; Workman et al. 1993). Alternating step training with high-low impact (for 45 minutes of cardio) has been shown in one training study to significantly increase high density lipoproteins (HDL) cholesterol (Mosher et al. 2005).

Other studies have measured the impact forces experienced by the feet during step training. Francis and colleagues (1994) found that the feet undergo approximately the same peak vertical forces when stepping on a 10-inch (25 cm) step as when walking at 3 miles per hour (5 kph), which is roughly 1.25 times body weight. However, the lead foot (first foot down off the step) absorbs a greater impact force—1.75 times body weight. This is one reason why it's so important to change the lead foot frequently during step. Other researchers have found that vertical ground reaction forces increase with increasing step height and with the addition of propulsion (Johnson et al. 1993; Moses 1993; Scharff-Olson, Williford, Duey et al. 1997). The forces on the knees during stepping also have been examined (Francis et al. 1994), and researchers have found that greater forces are incurred with an increasing angle of knee flexion. A 24-week study looking at the health benefits of step training found that step training had significant positive effects on bone density in postmenopausal women (Wen et al. 2007), and a study on women aged 50 to 75 years found that balance improved as a result of a step program (Bemben et al. 2006).

One researcher has collected data on step instructors (Kravitz 1994); it was found that instructors have a relatively low percent body fat and favorable upper-body and lower-body strength. Other researchers have examined the effect of step intensity on mood; they found less fatigue and anger in participants who exercised at higher intensities and reduced state anxiety in participants who had just finished step training (Hale and Raglin 2002).

Verbal Cues and Tempo

Cueing during the warm-up is critical. You will be setting the tone for the workout, motivating your class members to get going, and educating them about safety and proper alignment. Your voice should be audible, upbeat, encouraging, and energetic. See chapter 4 for a thorough discussion of the various types of cues. Music tempo in a step warm-up is approximately the same as that in the step cardio segment: 118 to 128 beats per minute.

TECHNIQUE AND SAFETY

Good alignment and technique for step training include maintaining a neutral spine and neck, with the head and eyes up, and keeping the abdominals lifted and contracted. As always, avoid hyperextending, hyperflexing, or twisting the knees (see figure 8.2). Keep all joints facing the same direction and the shoulders down, even, and relaxed. Use a full-body lean when stepping up—visualize one long line from heel to head, and avoid leaning from the hips or waist (see figure 8.3).

◼ Technique and Safety Check

The following are warm-up recommendations for step training:

- Use the step for at least one low- to moderate-intensity floor mix.
- Avoid continuous stepping until the body is thoroughly warm.
- Use the step for some of your short-term static stretches.
- Briefly stretch the areas that are commonly tight or are heavily used in step: the calves, hip flexors, hamstrings, low back, and chest.

You can greatly enhance the safety of your class by not stepping forward off the step; research has shown that stepping forward off the bench rather than stepping backward while facing the bench generates much greater impact forces (Francis et al. 1992). Always step lightly on the platform and avoid pounding the feet. In addition, step to the center of the bench, and make sure the heel doesn't hang off the back; this helps protect the Achilles tendon. When stepping up, extend the knees fully (without hyperextending them). To minimize the risk of patellar tendinitis, always keep the angle of knee

flexion greater than 90°. Stay close enough to the step that you can bring the heels comfortably all the way to the floor when stepping down (landing and rolling through the toe, ball, and heel). Your feet should land approximately one shoe length away from the step. Step down without bouncing. Bouncing when you land on the floor increases the eccentric muscle loading and forceful stretching of the Achilles tendon and may lead to Achilles tendinitis. Encourage your participants to jump up on the step instead! Avoid forcing your heels down to the floor during lunges and repeaters. In this case, use the ball of the foot to make contact with the floor and keep the heel lifted. Forcing the heel down may increase the risk of Achilles tendinitis due to the forceful stretching and eccentric loading of the tendon. When performing pivot turns on the step, unload the lower leg by simultaneously hopping so that the foot is not in contact with the step during the actual turn.

◼ Practice Drill

Design a warm-up segment that incorporates the step to provide short-term stretches for the calf and hip flexor muscles. Precede the calf stretch by limbering the ankle (lifting and lowering the heel) and precede the hip flexor stretch by limbering the pelvis and hip

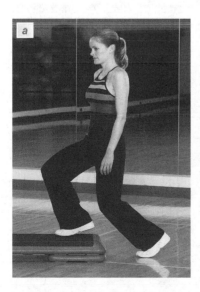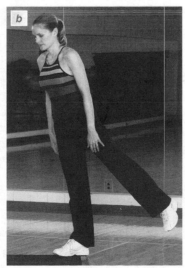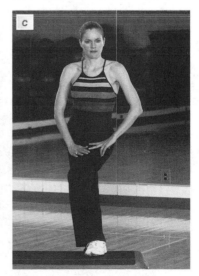

▶ **Figure 8.2** Avoid *(a)* hyperflexion, *(b)* hyperextension, and *(c)* twisting of the knees.

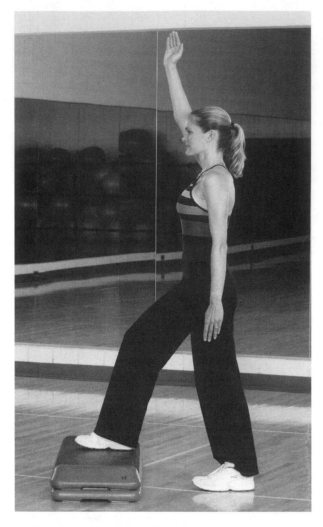

▶ **Figure 8.3** Good alignment on a step.

Help participants choose the proper step height. Step heights greater than 8 inches (20 cm) should be reserved for exercisers with long legs or advanced fitness levels (see table 8.2). It's also a good idea to change the lead leg frequently to minimize repetitive stress to the leg stepping down off the bench. Finally, keep the tempo of your music slow enough that all participants are able to step safely with good technique and alignment. Several organizations recommend step speeds no greater than 128 beats per minute. Music tempo can be a challenging issue in clubs where participants are used to stepping at much faster speeds. However, research clearly shows that effective workouts are possible at speeds less than 128 beats per minute, and these slower speeds have the added benefit of decreased impact forces and enhanced safety for participants. Look where you are stepping by glancing

down occasionally with your eyes while keeping your head up. Avoid high numbers of moves that stress the musculoskeletal system, such as repeaters with more than five repetitions. Limit lunges and other propulsive moves to 1 minute or less, depending on your participants. Avoid using hand weights while stepping; while caloric expenditure increases are minimal, the risk of injury is significantly greater (Olson et al. 1991; Step Reebok 1997; Workman et al. 1993).

 See the DVD for a step warm-up. This warm-up is also outlined in appendix F.

BASIC MOVES

There are six basic locations around the bench from which to perform step moves. The six basic approaches to the step are front, side, end, corner, top, and astride (see figure 8.4).

■ Technique and Safety Check

To keep your classes safe, observe the following recommendations.

Remember to
- maintain a neutral spine and neck, with the head and eyes up;
- keep the abdominals lifted and contracted;
- keep all joints facing the same direction;
- keep the shoulders down, even, and relaxed;
- use a full-body lean when stepping up;
- step to the center of the platform;
- keep the angle of knee flexion greater than 90°;
- help participants choose the proper step height; and
- change the lead leg frequently.

Avoid
- hyperextending, hyperflexing, or twisting the knees;
- stepping forward off the step;
- pounding the feet; and
- using step speeds greater than 128 beats per minute.

Table 8.2 Guidelines for Step Height and Step Speed

Participant level	Step height	Step speed
Novice (new to exercise)	4 in. (10 cm)	118-122 bpm
Beginner (regular exerciser who has never done step)	<6 in. (15 cm)	<124 bpm
Intermediate (regular stepper)	<8 in. (20 cm)	<126 bpm
Advanced (regular, skilled stepper)	<10 in. (25 cm)	<128 bpm

Adapted from the 1997 Revised Guidelines for Step Reebok.

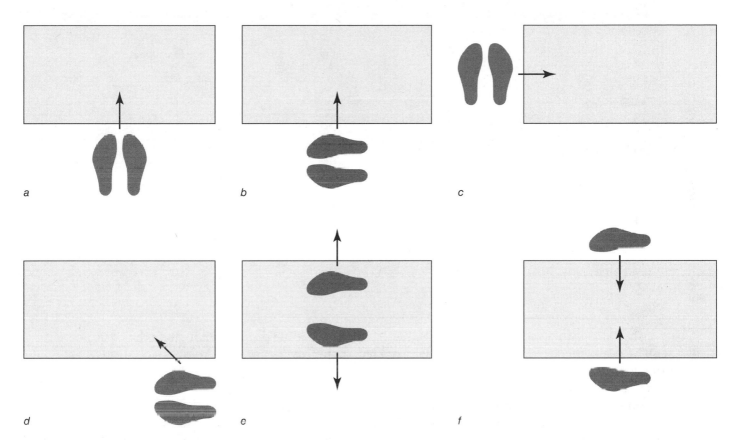

▷ **Figure 8.4** Step locations: *(a)* front, *(b)* side, *(c)* end, *(d)* corner, *(e)* top, and *(f)* astride.

■ Practice Drill

Take a step class and write down the instructor's approaches to the bench. How many of the six approaches were used? Did they flow well? Put together two lower-body moves that share the same approach. Practice alternating these two moves so that you create a simple combination on the step.

Lower-Body Moves

Using a step in group exercise presents many options for basic lower-body movements. The DVD accompanying this text presents the basic lower-body moves in step training; table 8.3 also lists these moves. Those moves near the bottom of the list may be more difficult to teach, may be more complex, or may require different approaches and are better suited for a more experienced instructor. Lower-body moves on the step are all 4-count moves unless otherwise noted.

 See the DVD for basic lower-body step moves.

Table 8.3 Step Moves for Instructors

Move	Typical approaches
Basic step	Front, end, corner
V-step	Front
Tap-up, tap-down	Side, end, corner, front
Lift step (knee lift to the front, side, or back; a kick to the front, side, or back)	Front, side, end, corner, astride, top
Turn step	Side
Over-the-top	Side
Repeater	Front, side, corner, end, astride (8 counts)
Lunge	Top (2 counts), can face front or side
Straddle-down	Top
Straddle-up	Astride
Across-the-top	End
Corner-to-corner	Corner
L-step	Front, end, side
A-step	Corner, side
Charleston	Front, corner, side
Over-the-top pivot	Side

Most of the moves and patterns in table 8.3 can be performed with either a single lead or an alternating lead. A single lead means that the move is executed in such a way that the same foot continues to lead. An example is a V-step with no tap-down: up with the right foot, up with the left, down with the right, down with the left, up again with the right foot, and so on. In a V-step performed with an alternating lead, however, a tap-down is performed on the 4th count, which changes the lead foot: up with the right foot, up with the left, down with the right, down tap left, up with the left foot, up with the right, down with the left, down tap right, and so on.

Additionally, propulsion, or power, can be added to many moves to increase the intensity if desired. Adding propulsion simply means to jump up on the step, which requires significantly more energy (never jump off the step because doing so increases joint stress—see the technique and safety section on page 181). Good moves

for adding propulsion include the basic step, lift step, over-the-top, across-the-top, L-step, tap-up, lunge, and pivot turn.

Upper-Body Moves

As in high-low impact cardio workouts, there are endless variations of upper-body moves in step. Review chapter 4 for a discussion of unilateral and bilateral, complementary and opposition, and low-, mid-, and high-range arm movements. Common arm moves and step patterns include:

- Bilateral biceps curls with the basic step
- Externally and internally rotated shoulders (out, out, in, in) with the V-step
- Overhead press (clap on 4th count) with the turn step
- Bilateral shoulder circumduction with over-the-top
- Chest presses with lunges facing front

■ **Practice Drill**

Practice the short combination you designed in the previous drill (see page 183), this time adding simple upper-body moves.

It's generally easiest for participants if you teach the lower-body movements first. Add the arms only when everyone is comfortable with the lower-body patterns.

BASIC COMBINATIONS AND CHOREOGRAPHY TECHNIQUES

The elements of variation discussed in chapter 4 provide an unlimited number of variations for step moves and patterns. You can vary your moves by changing

- the lever,
- the plane,
- the direction (and, in step, the approach),
- the rhythm,
- the intensity (add propulsion), and
- the style (see pages 57-59 in chapter 4).

For example, let's see how a hamstring curl (knee lift to the back) performed with a front approach to the step can be varied. Begin by performing the hamstring curl and then (1) increase the lever, which results in hip extension; (2) change the plane for a side-out (long lever leg lift to the side); (3) add the element of direction by angling the body diagonally to alternating corners; (4) change the rhythm by performing a hesitation move before each alternating side-out; (5) increase the intensity by adding propulsion (jump up) on each side-out; and (6) play with the style by performing a funky "shimmy" movement with the shoulders on the hesitation and then dorsiflexing the foot and pressing the heels of the hands down on the side-out.

Drilling the elements of variation can result in entirely new moves and even new combinations! It's easiest to transition smoothly when one move begins where the previous move finished (i.e., when the end point and starting point of the two moves connect). Moves that share the same approach usually connect well; for example, both over-the-top and tap-up, tap-down can be performed from the side approach and thus they flow together.

Teaching to Music

It is essential to teach with the music in a step class. Because almost all step moves are 4 or 8 counts, participants will naturally want to initiate moves on the 1st downbeat of 8-, 16-, and 32-count phrases. Find some step music with a strong beat and practice finding the beats until hearing the downbeat and the musical divisions into counts of 4 becomes second nature for you. Teaching on the beat and with the music keeps you and your students from becoming frustrated and discouraged; your patterns will be easier to follow and more enjoyable. Many students, although they may not be able to articulate why, instinctively feel that something is wrong when an instructor is not on the downbeat. Refer to chapter 4 for a thorough discussion of beats, downbeats, measures, and 8-, 16-, and 32-count phrases.

32-Count Blocks

As in high-low impact choreography, step choreography usually consists of blocks of 32-count combinations. These blocks can be repeated

■ **Practice Drill**

Begin performing one basic move and add (or subtract) an element of variation. Perform each move you create at least four times (16 counts) before adding or subtracting another element of variation. Make your transitions smooth and natural by finding moves with connecting end points and starting points (see the section on smooth transitions in chapter 4). Challenge yourself by changing first an element of variation for the upper body, then one for the lower body, and then one for the upper body, building a linear progression.

over and over, expanded or reduced, or linked together to create long, complex combinations. Movements within the blocks can be layered for increasing complexity or changed using the elements of variation (see chapter 4 to learn about the different choreographic techniques). Here's an example of a 32-count block in step training:

1. Facing front, perform three basic steps, leading right (12 counts; to increase complexity, add a different arm movement with each basic step).
2. Perform one half-time squat with the right foot on the bench (face the left side for the squat, then face the front on the return; 4 counts).
3. Repeat to the other side, leading left (for a total of 16 counts).

This first block could be linked to another 32-count block:

1. Facing front, perform two alternating knee lifts (8 counts).
2. Complete one three-knee repeater (8 counts).
3. Perform two alternating knee lifts (8 counts).
4. Complete one three-knee repeater to the other side (8 counts).

You could alternate these two blocks with each other, or you could link them to more blocks to create a longer combination.

 See the DVD for two sample 32-count step practice drills, one easier, one more difficult.

■ Practice Drill

Using a favorite premixed step tape or CD with a strong beat (see chapter 4 for a list of companies that produce step music), put together two 32-count blocks of simple choreography. Be sure to start your routine at the top of the phrase, which is the 1st downbeat of the 32-count phrase.

Repetition Reduction

Repetition reduction is another important technique in skillful step teaching. As discussed in chapter 4, to use repetition reduction you repeat each move several times until participants are comfortable, and then you gradually reduce the number of repetitions. This technique can result in a complex combination that requires everyone to concentrate! Here's a relatively simple example:

1. Start with four alternating V-steps and four alternating knee lifts.
2. Reduce to two alternating V-steps and two alternating knee lifts.
3. Reduce further to one V-step and one knee lift.

Holding Patterns

A holding pattern is simply a move (such as a basic step or an over-the-top) that is repeated over and over for a brief time to allow both the instructor and the participants to collect their thoughts and return to the desired intensity level. Performing a holding pattern provides an ideal time for you to communicate with your students giving alignment, technique, educational, or motivational cues as necessary.

Step Intensity

Compared with traditional cardio floor choreography, step training has workloads that are easier to measure because of the known variable of the step height. As you might suspect, the higher the step, the greater the intensity and the higher the vertical ground reaction forces (Johnson et al. 1993). Students should use a step that provides a sufficient cardiorespiratory challenge but also allows them to move with good form and alignment and minimize the risk of injury. Higher platform heights have been associated with knee discomfort that is attributable to the increased angle of knee flexion (Francis et al. 1994). It is recommended that beginner steppers start with a 4-inch (10 cm) platform and gradually progress to a higher step as they become more conditioned and familiar with proper step biomechanics (Aerobics and Fitness Association of America 2002).

Intensity is also affected by the specific step moves and sequences being used, as well as by increased lever length, elevated arm movements, increased traveling, and a greater number of propulsion moves. Moves that involve more traveling over and around the step or more vertical displacement, such as lunges, have been found to have a greater energy cost than moves that involve less knee flexion and extension, such as basic steps. The energy costs of common step moves are listed in table 8.4.

The music speed can affect the intensity, although most experts do not recommend using a music tempo greater than 128 beats per minute because of the increased risk of injury. At faster tempos, participants have a more difficult time completing their movements with full ROM and may end up compromising their alignment and stepping technique. Compromised technique increases the likelihood of injuries such as Achilles tendinitis (see the section on technique and safety on page 182).

TRAINING SYSTEMS

Step classes can be formatted in several ways, including step supercircuits, step intervals, step alternated with high-low impact intervals, double step (participants use more than one step), and various step fusion options (e.g., step combined with slide or glide, step combined with Pilates, or step combined with stability ball training). Following are descriptions of step circuit and step interval formats.

Step Circuit

In a step circuit or supercircuit class, several minutes of step may be alternated with several minutes of muscular conditioning to create a complete workout (Kraemer et al. 2001). Here's a sample step circuit: warm up for 10 minutes; step for 4 minutes; perform weighted squats, pliés, and lunges on the floor for 4 minutes; step for 4 minutes; perform weighted latissimus dorsi and deltoid exercises for 4 minutes; step for 4 minutes; perform standing chest exercises such as wall push-ups plus upper-back exercises with tubing for 4 minutes; step for 4 minutes; perform biceps and triceps exercises with weights or tubing for 4 minutes; step for 4 minutes; postcardio cool down for 4 minutes; work abdominals and low back on the floor for 5 minutes; and stretch on the floor for 5 minutes. Total circuit time is 60 minutes.

Step Intervals

In this type of class, power intervals are randomly or regularly interspersed throughout the step session. The power interval typically lasts 30 to 60 seconds and consists of a simple move or pattern repeated over and over. Participants are given intensity options that allow them to work at very high levels during the interval if desired. A good example of a power interval is as follows: Facing front, perform two lift steps (knee lift

Table 8.4 Energy Costs of Step Moves

	Basic step	Traveling with alternating lead	Over-the-top	Knee lift	Lunges	Repeaters
$\dot{V}O_2$max (ml · kg^{-1} · min^{-1})	26.2	35.5	26.6	28.7	32.7	32.0
METS	7.5	10.1	7.6	8.2	9.3	9.1
HR	141	167	143	147	162	157
RPE	9.5	12.1	11.0	10.8	11.9	11.9

METS = metabolic equivalents; HR = heart rate; RPE = rating of perceived exertion.

Adapted from Calarco et al. 1991.

with a tap-down) with the right foot leading for 8 counts and follow with four jumping jacks on the floor for 8 counts. Repeat the two lift steps with the left foot leading for 8 counts, and then do four more jumping jacks for 8 counts. Then demonstrate this simple combination with at least three intensity options: (1) without jumping—the jacks become low-impact toe touches to the side, (2) with a jump-up on the step (arms low) during the lift steps and regular jacks on the floor, and (3) with a jump-up on the step (arms high) and fly or cheerleader jacks on the floor with the arms circumducting. Allow your students to select the intensity option that requires more work than during the regular step portion of class but is still appropriate for them.

CHAPTER WRAP-UP

The basic teaching strategies for step include providing a warm-up that incorporates rehearsal moves (generally in the form of a floor mix) and teaching a combination in small parts, usually in 8- or 16-count blocks. Drill these parts, using the principle of repetition, until participants have learned the movements. Teach the lower body first and then add the upper body. Then teach the 32-count block, using repetition reduction until participants have learned the movements. Layer your combination with the elements of variation, changing the lever, plane, direction or approach, rhythm, style, or intensity. Repeat this process with the next 32-count block, and add more blocks onto your first block as desired (A + B + C + D). Use holding patterns between blocks to enhance your communication with your class and to avoid brain strain. Practice these teaching techniques so that you become a creative and effective step instructor.

▶ **Group Exercise Class Evaluation Form Key Points**

■ Gradually increase intensity. After the warm-up, when you are beginning the cardio segment, gradually increase intensity until you reach the peak part of the cardio stimulus. In other words, do not perform plyometric intervals, lunges, and other high-intensity moves near the beginning of the cardio segment.

■ Use a variety of muscle groups and minimize repetitive movements. Avoid performing high numbers of any move in a row, as doing so can lead to overuse injuries and muscle imbalances. Follow four knee lifts on the step with four hip extensions on the step, for example.

■ Demonstrate good form, alignment, and technique on the step. You must be a good role model for your students, because they will unconsciously copy your form and alignment. Stand tall, move with precision, and avoid bouncing down off the step.

■ Use step music appropriately. Use a recommended tempo (118-128 beats per minute) that allows all participants to complete full ROM safely and with control. In addition, keep practicing to get better at moving on the beat, initiating new moves at the beginning of phrases, and using the 32-count phrase.

■ Give clear cues and verbal directions, including anticipatory cues, safety and alignment information, directional cues, and motivational cues. Remember that for big anticipatory cues you usually count backward starting with "4," as in, "4, 3, 2, knee lift." That way, your class members will perform the knee lift together on the downbeat of the next phrase.

■ Promote participant interaction and encourage fun. Have students call out their names, greet their neighbors, and occasionally count down with you. Ask questions such as, "Everybody feeling fine?"

■ Gradually decrease intensity during the postcardio cool-down by avoiding high-intensity moves and eventually moving off the step. A simple example is to march for 4 counts on the step and then march for 4 counts on the floor, repeating several times and finishing with marching only on the floor. Incorporate some static stretches while standing, especially stretches for the calves, hip flexors, hamstrings, and low back.

▶ **Assignment**

Prepare a 2-minute step routine that consists of two 32-count blocks. Teach your routine using the techniques of repetition reduction and changing the lead leg. Prepare an outline of the routine on paper to hand in and one to utilize when you perform this routine in class (this can be on a notecard).

Kickboxing

CHAPTER OBJECTIVES

By the end of this chapter, you will

- understand how to warm up for kickboxing;
- be able to teach basic moves for kickboxing;
- know how to build choreographic patterns and recognize other class formats for leading kickboxing;
- be able to identify proper alignment, technique, and safety concerns for kickboxing; and
- be able to teach a 2-minute kickboxing routine with appropriate content, alignment, technique, and cueing using appropriate music.

Kickboxing has grown in popularity as a group exercise modality through the late 1990s and into the 21st century. The term *kickboxing* can encompass a wide variety of martial arts workouts, including aeroboxing, cardio karate, box step, jump and jab, and Tae Bo. New trends include kickboxing fusion classes and the incorporation of other martial arts disciplines into the fitness setting, including tai chi, Krav Maga, Forza, and capoeira. The goal of most students in a kickboxing class is to promote their health and fitness; most aren't taking the class with the intention of actually fighting. Therefore, the basic moves in a group kickboxing class are slightly modified from classical martial arts styles to enhance safety and reduce the risk of injury. We recommend that you go beyond basic group exercise training and certification and pursue additional training specific to kickboxing if you plan to teach this format. A well-taught kickboxing class can be a great workout and can also be fun and highly stimulating for you and your students (see "Kickboxing Research Findings" on page 191). The main points on the group exercise class evaluation form that relate to kickboxing are listed on this page.

■ Background Check

Before working your way through this chapter, you should do the following:

Read

- chapter 5 on warming up and
- the music section of chapter 4 (pages 50-55).

Practice

- the music drills in chapter 4 (page 52) and
- the cueing drills in chapter 4 (pages 69-73).

Group Exercise Class Evaluation Form Essentials

Key Points for Warm-Up Segment

- Includes appropriate amount of dynamic movement
- Provides rehearsal moves
- Stretches major muscle groups in a biomechanically sound manner with appropriate instructions
- Gives clear cues and verbal directions
- Uses an appropriate music tempo (125-135 beats per minute) or motivating music that inspires movement

Key Points for Cardio Segment

- Gradually increases intensity
- Uses a variety of muscle groups (especially hamstrings and abductors)
- Minimizes repetitive movements
- Promotes participant interaction and encourages fun
- Demonstrates movement options and gives clear verbal cues
- Gradually decreases impact and intensity during cool-down following the cardiorespiratory session
- Uses music volume and tempo (125-135 beats per minute) appropriate for biomechanical movement

Kickboxing Research Findings

A number of studies have examined the effectiveness of kickboxing for cardiorespiratory training (Adams et al. 1997; Albano and Terbizan 2001; Anning et al. 1999; Bellinger et al. 1997; Bissonnette et al. 1994; Franzese et al. 2000; Greene et al. 1999; Kravitz et al. 2000; O'Driscoll et al. 1999; Perez et al. 1999; Scharff-Olson et al. 2000). These studies have found that kickboxing can provide a workout that is sufficient to develop cardiorespiratory fitness. Significant findings from these studies include the following: (1) increasing the music speed from 60 to 120 beats per minute during punching increased the cardiorespiratory response; (2) combining punches with vigorous lower-body moves such as shuffles, jacks, and squats resulted in a better cardiorespiratory stimulus; and (3) there was no significant difference in terms of energy cost between shadowboxing and boxing with a heavy bag. One study found that the average caloric expenditure was 7 calories per minute if the routine was predominantly leg moves combined with upper-body moves; routines using only the upper body are discouraged if the goal is weight management or cardiorespiratory fitness (Ergun et al. 2006). Another study noted that kickboxing elicited a lower $\dot{V}O_2$max than treadmill running elicited at similar heart rates (Wingfield et al. 2006).

Other researchers have examined injuries in kickboxing classes (Buschbacher and Shay 1999; Davis et al. 2002; McKinney-Vialpando 1999). A relatively high rate of injury (29.3% of participants and 31.3% of instructors) was found in the study by Davis and colleagues (2002), which included 572 participants. This study also found that the risk of injury increased dramatically when the frequency of kickboxing was increased: 43% of participants who took four or more classes per week reported injuries versus 25% of participants who took only one or two classes per week. McKinney-Vialpando (1999) found that the faster the music speed, the greater the postexercise pain, and the higher the kicks, the greater the incidence of pain. Axe and crescent kicks were also found to cause pain in 22% of the study participants.

WARM-UP

Kickboxing warm-ups follow the warm-up recommendations outlined in chapter 5 and thus include dynamic movement, rehearsal moves, and appropriate stretching. Alignment cues and a safe music speed are also very important in a kickboxing warm-up.

Dynamic Movement and Rehearsal Moves

The biggest difference between a kickboxing warm-up and other kinds of group exercise warm-ups is the inclusion of dynamic rehearsal moves specific to kickboxing. Remember that a rehearsal move is a low-intensity version of a movement that will be used later in the high-intensity cardiorespiratory portion of class. These moves prepare the body for the kickboxing workout to follow and include punches, jabs, hooks, and kicks, all performed at a slower speed than that used during the actual workout. You should focus on teaching proper form and technique while your class practices these basic movements. When teaching beginners, you may even consider teaching the basic punches and kicks without music to help your students learn proper form and alignment.

Following is a simple warm-up combination that uses rehearsal moves:

1. Using the ready position, punch four times with the right arm—you should be punching once every 4 counts (16 counts).
2. Repeat with the left arm (16 counts).
3. Perform four step touches (16 counts).
4. Do four hamstring curls (16 counts).
5. Repeat.

■ **Practice Drill**

Create your own kickboxing warm-up. Pair a basic upper-body move, such as a punch, jab, hook, or uppercut, with a basic lower-body move, such as a march, step touch, or grapevine.

Stretching Major Muscle Groups

Another important aspect of a kickboxing warm-up is the increased focus on limbering and stretching the muscles that will be heavily used in the routine that follows; these include the calf muscles, hip flexors, inner thigh muscles, hamstrings, low-back muscles, and muscles of the anterior chest and shoulder complex. (For specific stretches, see chapter 7.) It is particularly important to include dynamic movements and full range of motion movements. Stretches held briefly for 3-5 seconds are necessary for these muscles because of the high number of repetitive drills found in a typical fitness-based kickboxing class. As always, the warm-up is an ideal time to stress proper alignment—emphasize alignment in the punches and kicks as well as in the static stretches. Because the incidence of injury in kickboxing classes is relatively high (Davis et al. 2002), a proper warm-up and careful teaching of the basic moves are essential.

Verbal Cues and Tempo

Focus on delivering precise anatomical and educational cues when detailing alignment. Briefly review several joints or areas of the body. For example, when holding a calf stretch you can say, "Hold the head high, with ears away from the shoulders, neck in line with the spine, shoulders down and back, and abdominals in. Your body should form one long line from head to heel; stretch the heel down with the toes facing straight ahead and the hips square." Keep your cues positive, telling your class what to do rather than what not to do. Remember that pointing to or touching parts of your body can be an effective way to cue alignment visually.

A music tempo of 125 to 135 beats per minute is appropriate for most warm-ups. This tempo is fast enough to elevate heart rate, core tem-perature, and breathing rate but not so fast that participants will become winded or will fail to complete the moves.

TECHNIQUE AND SAFETY

Safety is always a primary concern for instructors, especially in kickboxing, where the incidence of injury has been shown to be approximately 30% (Davis et al. 2002). The back, knees, hips, and shoulders have all been reported as injury sites. You should understand the common mechanisms of injury at these sites and take steps to avoid increasing your participants' risk of injury.

In the United States, 80% of people report experiencing low-back pain at some point in their lives (Frymoyer and Cats-Baril 1991). A stable spine during kicks and punches is key to preventing back problems in a kickboxing class. The abdominal and back muscles must be dynamically and statically trained to develop spinal stability, and participants must understand the concept of a neutral spine. Excessive hip flexor involvement from too many kicks can contribute to low-back pain because the iliopsoas muscles attach on the lumbar spine. To prevent this problem, stretch the hip flexors in both the warm-up and the cool-down portions of your class.

You can reduce the incidence of knee pain in kickboxing by teaching good kicking technique. Emphasize performing active retraction, or knee flexion, immediately after the knee extends in a kick. Snapping or ballistically extending the

■ **Technique and Safety Check**

Following are recommendations for the kickboxing warm-up:

- Use at least one combination that incorporates kickboxing rehearsal moves.
- Increase the speed and intensity of the kickboxing moves gradually.
- Thoroughly prepare the hamstrings, calves, hip flexors, inner thighs, low-back, anterior chest, and shoulder muscles with both dynamic movements and light static stretches.

knee with excessive momentum can overstretch the knee ligaments and create knee instability. Torque or sudden twisting moves in which the foot is anchored but the knee turns overstretch the collateral knee ligaments and thus are another mechanism of knee injury. Always keep the toes aligned in the direction of the knees.

Hip pain can result from a lack of muscle balance around the hip joint. Use the hip flexors and extensors as evenly as possible, as well as the hip adductors and abductors and the hip internal and external rotators. Provide plenty of appropriate stretches for these muscles, avoid excessive repetitions of kicks, and always teach a thorough warm-up.

Reduce the incidence of shoulder pain by teaching good punching technique (retracting the arm immediately after each punch) and by training the external rotator cuff and posterior deltoid muscles with specific exercises to counterbalance all the forward motion involved in punching. Shoulder pain is more likely to occur when the shoulder girdle isn't properly stabilized. Instruct participants to punch with the scapulae down, and give isolation exercises for the middle trapezius and rhomboids (scapular retractors) as well as plenty of stretches for the anterior chest muscles. Too many kickboxing classes without proper stretching, muscular conditioning, and body awareness can result in a hunched back and rounded shoulders (excessive kyphosis). With proper instruction, however, you can help your students avoid this type of poor posture and thus avoid injuries.

BASIC MOVES

Although the standard kickboxing moves can be performed in a variety of different martial arts styles (which are listed on page 194), we recommend modifying some of these traditional moves to allow for proper joint alignment and to decrease the risk of injury.

Initial Positioning

All kickboxing moves start from one of two basic positions: the ready position (body faces forward with feet parallel) or the staggered position (body is slightly angled to the side with one foot back).

■ Technique and Safety Check

To keep your kickboxing classes safe, observe the following recommendations.

Remember to

- provide a thorough and appropriate warm-up;
- teach proper execution of punches and kicks;
- ensure that beginners master the basic moves before progressing;
- angle the fist in a three-quarter turn away from full pronation during punching;
- maintain muscle balance;
- maintain proper alignment, especially during kicks;
- cross-train;
- provide plenty of stretches for the hip flexor, hamstring, calf, low-back, upper trapezius, and chest muscles;
- provide strengthening exercises for the middle trapezius, rhomboid, posterior deltoid, abdominal, and low back muscles;
- give equal numbers of punches and kicks on both sides and kick in both front and back; and
- start with only one kickboxing class per week and gradually increase the number, if desired, up to three classes per week.

Avoid

- a snapping motion when kicking and punching,
- advanced and high kicks for all but the most skilled participants, and
- music speeds greater than 138 beats per minute.

In both positions, the elbows are flexed and the fists are close together to protect the face and neck (the forearms should make a V). The core muscles (abdominals and lower back) are engaged at all times, and the shoulder blades are slightly protracted (causing a slight rounding of the upper back and shoulders). The knees are slightly flexed (see figure 9.1).

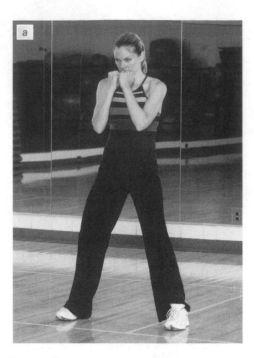 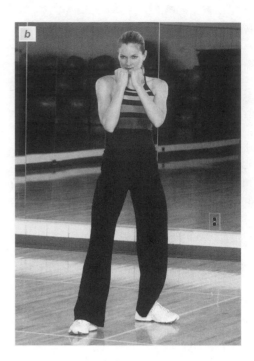

▷ **Figure 9.1** *(a)* Ready position and *(b)* staggered position.

Martial Arts Styles

- American boxing
- Thai kickboxing
- Karate
- Judo
- Taekwondo
- Aikido
- Kung fu
- Jujitsu
- Krav Maga
- Capoeira

Basic Punches

There are four basic punches in kickboxing: the jab, the cross-jab or cross-punch, the hook, and the uppercut. In fitness settings, these punches are performed with a concentric contraction in both directions in order to protect the upper-body joints. In other words, there are two phases to a punch:

1. The punch itself, during which the elbow extends (the triceps contracts) and the fist moves away from the body

2. The retraction phase, during which the elbow flexes (the biceps contracts) and the fist is pulled quickly back into the body

Concentric contraction in both directions prevents the elbow from hyperextending during shadowboxing (punching air) and helps protect the elbow and shoulder joints. Additionally, when punching it is safer to modify the full palm-down, pronated position of a classic punch into a slightly angled three-quarter turn of the wrist, with the thumb slightly higher than the littlest finger (Buschbacher and Shay 1999). You should be especially careful when incorporating equipment such as weighted gloves, focus mitts, or punching bags into your classes. Weighted punches and contact punches greatly increase the risk of muscle strains, ligament sprains, surface abrasions, and jamming and dislocation of the wrist and finger joints. Reserve weighted and contact punching for your advanced classes.

The jab is a straight punch to the front. If you are in the ready position, the torso rotates; if you are in the staggered position, the torso doesn't need to rotate (see figure 9.2).

The cross-jab is typically performed from the staggered position, with the heel of the back foot up so that the whole body can pivot as the punch is thrown. As the spine and hip rotate forward,

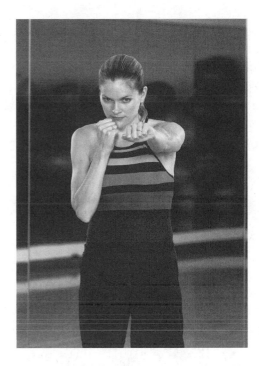

▶ **Figure 9.2** Jab.

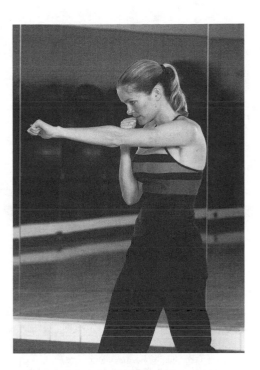

▶ **Figure 9.3** Cross-jab.

the cross-jab crosses the midline of the body and the shoulder follows through (see figure 9.3).

In the hook, the elbow is lifted and the shoulder joint is abducted at approximately 90°. The fist and arm curve around, following a horizontal line in front of the shoulders or face. Keep the fist pronated (palm facing down) or in the recommended midpronated (palm facing the body) position and the elbow flexed. The torso and hip should rotate in the direction of the punch (see figure 9.4).

In the uppercut, the elbow stays flexed but is kept down near the rib cage. The fist is supinated with the palm facing the body. You should allow the shoulder to extend and the arm to move behind the torso (elbow remains flexed) before throwing the actual punch. Tilting the pelvis, lifting the heel, and slightly rotating the torso will increase the power (see figure 9.5).

Basic Kicks

The four kicks used in a typical kickboxing class are the front kick, back kick, side kick, and roundhouse kick. To decrease the risk of injury to the knee joint, you should immediately follow the knee extension phase of your kicks with a quick retraction of the leg. In other words, performing an almost reflexive and conscious knee flexion can

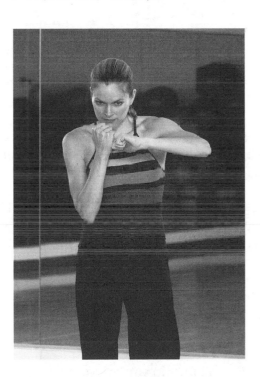

▶ **Figure 9.4** Hook.

help prevent ballistic knee hyperextension when kicking air. To perform proper kicks, your participants must have a strong supporting leg and core (torso) as well as adequate flexibility and balance. Most martial artists take years to perfect their kicking technique, and they begin performing

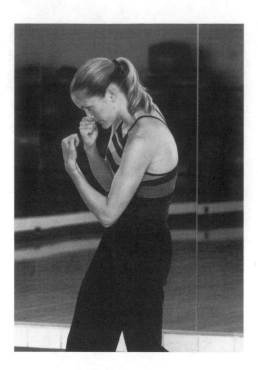

▶ **Figure 9.5** Uppercut.

■ **Practice Drill**

Practice the four basic punches slowly in sequence. Perform one punch every 4 counts: jab right, cross-jab left, hook right, uppercut right. Repeat with jab left, cross-jab right, hook left, and uppercut left. Choose a favorite song that is approximately 130 beats per minute to put on while practicing.

advanced kicks such as the crescent, axe, hitch, and spin hook only after extended study. Discourage beginners and participants who are less fit from attempting repetitive and advanced kicks too soon. Also, reserve head-high kicks for advanced participants, because these kicks require great flexibility, strength, balance, and coordination, and they increase the risk of hamstring pulls and back pain. You will probably need to demonstrate kicks at waist height or lower to reduce the risk of competitive students exceeding their ROM while kicking. It's also a good idea to break down the kick movement for your students. Lead them slowly through the move as follows:

1. Flex the hip.
2. Extend the knee (avoiding hyperextension).
3. Quickly flex the knee.
4. Extend the hip and return the leg to a neutral standing position (see figure 9.6).

In the front kick, the kicking leg moves directly to the front while the body remains squared, with the hips and shoulders facing forward. The kicking hip flexes but the spine remains neutral (no rounding). For advanced participants who have the flexibility and strength to kick head high, a backward lean is permitted; however, participants must maintain neutral spinal alignment throughout the movement. The ankle should be dorsiflexed so that the point of contact for the kick is at the ball of the foot, and the leg should be retracted quickly.

The back kick involves externally rotating the hip of the kicking leg while flexing forward on the standing hip. Again, you should immediately retract the leg after kicking. Maintain a neutral spinal alignment (do not flex the spine) while leaning forward. The point of contact is the heel of the back foot; the ankle should be dorsiflexed (see figure 9.7).

When a participant is performing a side kick, the point of contact is the ball of the foot (again, the ankle is dorsiflexed). Depending on the height of the kick, a side (lateral) lean is acceptable; however, the spine must remain neutral without rounding. The kicking hip internally rotates so that the knee faces forward; the knee extends after the hip is abducted to the desired height (see figure 9.8).

The roundhouse kick involves working from a turned-out (externally rotated) position of both hips. Make certain that your knees and toes are aligned in the same direction so you can avoid unnecessary torque or twisting of the knee and ankle joints. Externally rotate and flex the hip of the kicking leg while performing lateral spinal flexion; imagine you are making contact with the top of the foot (the forefoot) and keep the ankle plantar flexed. Quickly retract the leg to finish the kick (see figure 9.9).

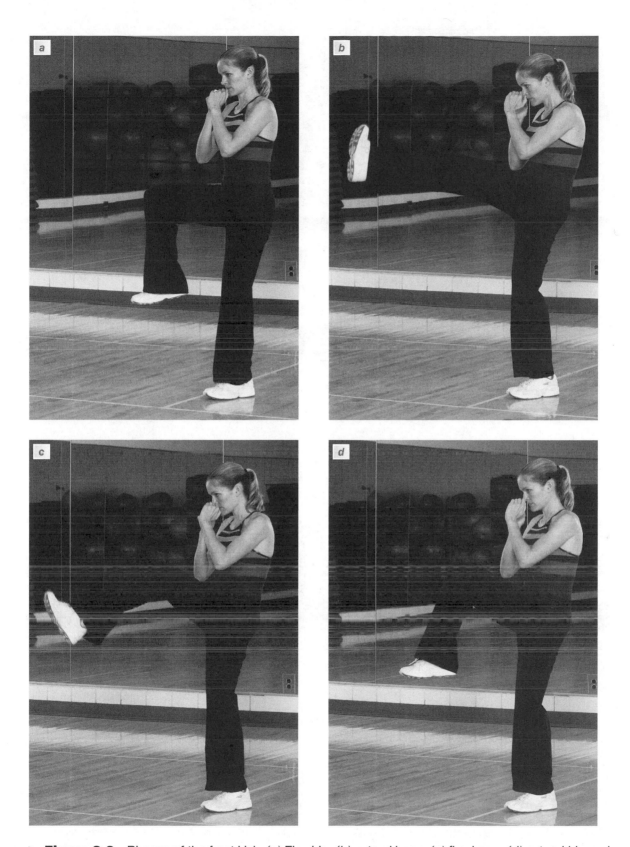

▶ **Figure 9.6** Phases of the front kick: *(a)* Flex hip, *(b)* extend knee, *(c)* flex knee, *(d)* extend hip and return leg to neutral standing position.

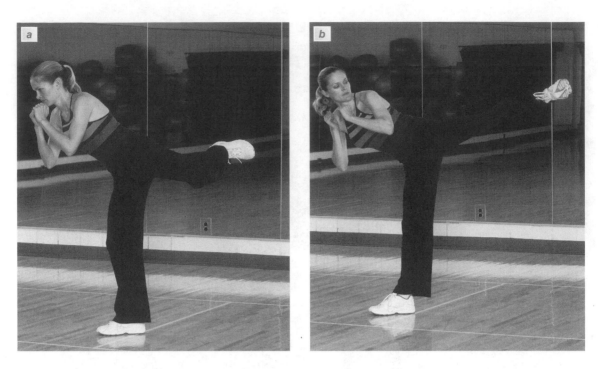

▷ **Figure 9.7** Phases of the back kick: *(a)* standing in hip extension and knee flexion and *(b)* knee extension at waist height.

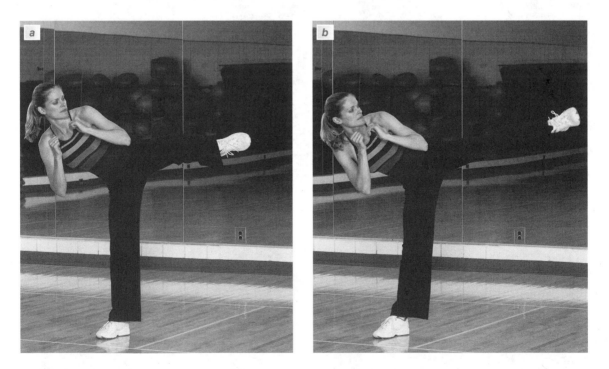

▷ **Figure 9.8** Phases of the side kick: *(a)* standing in hip and knee flexion and *(b)* knee extension at waist height.

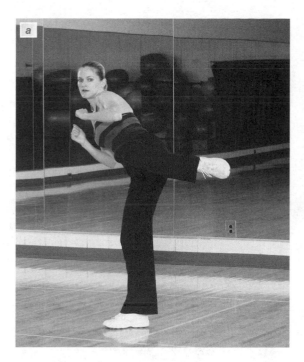 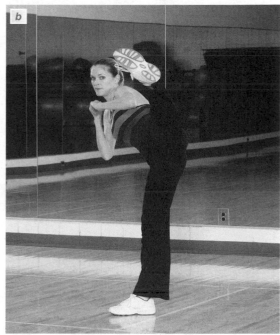

▶ **Figure 9.9** Phases of the roundhouse kick: *(a)* standing hip and knee flexion and *(b)* standing with knee extended.

Other Basic Moves

Other moves common to kickboxing include the boxer's shuffle, jumping rope, the bob and weave, and the lateral slip.

■ The boxer's shuffle is a foot pattern intended to help maintain an increased heart rate and to develop speed and agility; you can use it when developing kickboxing combinations. With your feet hip width apart and parallel, quickly move sideways without crossing the feet.

■ Jumping rope is often used to increase heart rate, power, stamina, and agility. In most kickboxing classes, the jump rope segments are in timed intervals (e.g., 3-5 minutes). During this interval, you can show different moves such as jogging, hopping twice on one foot and then the other, hop kicking with alternating feet, jumping bilaterally, jumping bilaterally while twisting, and jumping jacks, all while jumping over the rope! You can even perform traveling moves such as grapevines and power moves such as jumping high while circling the rope twice around the body (called *salt and pepper*). Participants who haven't yet coordinated the rope movement with

jumping (it takes practice!) can simulate jumping rope by twirling the wrists while holding the arms close to the rib cage. Remind students to land softly and properly, rolling through the toe, ball, and heel and bringing the heels all the way down. Beginners and participants who don't want to perform the high-impact jumping can jog or simply march in place. Jump-rope intervals can be intense, so ease your participants into jumping rope with shorter intervals and be sure to spread the intervals throughout the class.

■ The bob and weave is performed by the upper body and torso while the feet are parallel or staggered; the upper body ducks under an imaginary punch, bobbing from one side to the other.

■ The lateral slip is performed by laterally flexing the spine side to side without bobbing down and up. The feet remain anchored, usually in a parallel position.

 See the DVD for a demonstration of the basic punches, kicks, and movements of kickboxing, include the jab, cross-jab, hook, uppercut, front kick, back kick, side kick, boxer's shuffle, bob and weave, lateral slip, and jump-rope moves.

■ Practice Drill

Choose a favorite song (with a tempo of approximately 130 beats per minute) and practice the four basic kicks on every 4th beat as follows:

- Four right kicks front (16 counts), four left kicks front (16 counts), step touch (16 counts), march (16 counts)

- Four right kicks back (16 counts), four left kicks back (16 counts), step touch (16 counts), march (16 counts)

- Four right kicks side (16 counts), four left kicks side (16 counts), step touch (16 counts), march (16 counts)

- Four right roundhouse kicks (16 counts), four left roundhouse kicks (16 counts), step touch (16 counts), march (16 counts)

BASIC COMBINATIONS AND CHOREOGRAPHY TECHNIQUES

Building combinations in kickboxing is simply a matter of combining the basic moves. Many instructors also enjoy interspersing standard high-low moves such as grapevines, hustles, step touches, hamstring curls, V-steps, and jumping jacks (see chapter 4 for a description of these moves) into the punching and kicking segments. When designing your choreography, use a variety of moves and avoid high numbers of repetitions. Because most kickboxing classes are intended to provide a cardiorespiratory stimulus, you should gradually increase the intensity before you include peak moves and gradually decrease the intensity at the end of class or before participants perform floor work. Peak moves include kicks, jumping jacks, and jump-rope moves. A basic kickboxing combination is shown in table 9.1.

 See the DVD for demonstrations of two kickboxing combinations.

Table 9.1 Sample Kickboxing Combination

Move	Foot pattern	Upper body	Number of counts
Shuffle right	R, L, R, L, R, L, R, pause	Cross jab L on 7	8
Shuffle left	L, R, L, R, L, R, L, pause	Cross jab R on 7	8
Repeat			16
Front kick	R, L kick, L, R, L, R kick, R, L	Ready position	8
Repeat			8
Repeat			8
Repeat			8
Repeat			8
Bob and weave	Staggered position	Ready position	8
Lateral slip	Staggered position	Ready position	8
Repeat bob and weave			8
Repeat lateral slip			8
Jab	Ready position	Jab R, L, R, L (every 4 counts)	16
Hook	Ready position	Hook R, L, R, L (every 4 counts)	16
Repeat entire combination			

R = right; L = left.

■ **Practice Drill**

Using music with a tempo of approximately 125-138 beats per minute, put together your own combination of kickboxing moves. Include punches, kicks, and other basic moves.

OTHER KICKBOXING FORMATS

Some instructors prefer not to teach preplanned choreography on a 32-count block (such as the routine shown in table 9.1). Instead, they may teach a more military or combat style that includes repetitive drills that may or may not use music or follow the musical beat. For example, the class might include 10 minutes of punching (with or without a bag), 3 minutes of jumping rope, 10 minutes of kicking, 3 minutes of jumping rope, 10 minutes of punching, 3 minutes of jumping rope, and 10 minutes of kicking. When using this style, be sure to move in a variety of directions and limit the number of repetitions to avoid overuse injuries.

Other formats include step kickboxing classes (intervals of step alternated with intervals of kick boxing), equipment-based classes (intervals of punching with bags or focus mitts and intervals of kicking shields or bags), and classes with partner drills, circles, and other group formations. Many kickboxing classes move on to push-ups, abdominal work, or other muscular conditioning after the kickboxing portion of class.

CHAPTER WRAP-UP

A kickboxing class can be a fun, energizing, and challenging way to exercise in a group. However, instructors must make safety a priority to ensure an enjoyable experience for all participants. Learn how to throw proper punches and kicks and teach them carefully to your classes, emphasizing correct alignment and technique at all times.

▶ **Group Exercise Class Evaluation Form Key Points**

- Gradually increase intensity. In kickboxing, this means avoiding high-intensity drills, high kicks, and jump rope intervals for the first several minutes of the cardio stimulus. Review the first practice drill in this chapter (see page 190) and see if you can gradually increase the intensity of this combo by increasing the ROM, traveling distance, or impact of the floor pattern.

- Use a variety of muscle groups and minimize repetitive movements. Review your combination from the last practice drill in this chapter (on this page) to be sure you considered muscle balance, variety, and safety.

- Demonstrate good form, alignment, and technique for kickboxing. Keep practicing so that these become second nature to you.

- Use music appropriately. Keep your music speed less than 138 beats per minute for the cardio segment. Music that is too fast makes it difficult for participants to move safely with good alignment. If you choose to teach to the music, move on the downbeat and use 32-count phrases to enhance participant success.

- Give clear cues and verbal directions. Anticipatory cues, discussed in chapter 4, are particularly important when teaching combinations. For example, cue "4, 3, 2, right hook" (the word *hook* is spoken on the last beat).

- Promote participant interaction and encourage fun. Try different room arrangements such as having two groups of participants face each other while practicing punches or having the class stand in one large circle for kicking drills.

- Gradually decrease intensity during the cooldown following the cardio segment; use lower-intensity moves similar to those used in the warm-up. Decrease music speed, ROM, traveling, impact, and overhead arm motions as you return to resting conditions. Walking in place, step touches, and heel digs all can be performed at a low intensity with low arm movements.

▶ **Assignment**

Prepare a 2-minute kickboxing routine that consists of two 32-count blocks. Teach your routine using the technique of repetition reduction and include upper-body and lower-body movements. Make two copies of your routine, one copy to hand in to your instructor and one to use when you perform this routine in class (you can use notecards).

Sports Conditioning and Functional Training

CHAPTER OBJECTIVES

By the end of this chapter, you will

- be able to describe the difference between a functional training class and a sports conditioning class,
- understand safe and effective movements for a sports conditioning or functional training class,
- know what equipment to purchase for a sports conditioning class,
- review current research in sports conditioning and interval training, and
- be able to create a sports conditioning or functional training group exercise class.

Fitness professionals often begin their careers as personal trainers only to find they need some variety in their workday; sports conditioning or functional training classes can provide that variety. Programming schedules often refer to these classes as *boot camp, sports conditioning,* or *cross-conditioning.* They were developed by fitness professionals who sought a less-choreographed approach to the group exercise experience and by personal trainers who figured out that training several clients at one time can be more lucrative and way more fun than one-on-one training. Many instructors take their classes outside or utilize the track in their facility—either way, they move out of the four walls of the traditional group exercise setting. The class format of these classes often appeals to participants who have been involved in a structured sport workout with an athletic team. The setting of these classes often eliminates the need for a microphone and even music. Unlike step and kickboxing, theses classes are not driven by the 32-count phrase. Rather, sports conditioning classes often utilize interval training at a higher

intensity, incorporate movements that are easy to follow and more athletic in nature, and allow participants to work as a team, which creates a sense of group cohesion. If music is played, it is used to motivate and not to set the movement tempo. Fitness facility owners will attest to the value of this type of group exercise as being very important to member retention (Tharrett 2008). This format also appeals to men and thus gets more men into the predominantly female world of group exercise.

SPORTS CONDITIONING VERSUS FUNCTIONAL TRAINING

When people first hear the term *sports conditioning,* they often ask, "What sport are you conditioning for?" It would be nice to include conditioning classes specific to tennis, basketball, golf, and so on in fitness facility programming. Unfortunately, doing so is not practical and would fail to appeal to enough participants

---

Group Exercise Class Evaluation Form Essentials

Key Points for the Warm-Up

- Includes appropriate amount of dynamic movement
- Provides rehearsal moves
- Stretches major muscle groups in a biomechanically sound manner with appropriate instructions
- Gives clear cues and verbal directions
- Uses appropriate music that inspires movement

Key Points for the Cardiorespiratory Segment

- Gradually increases intensity
- Uses a variety of sports conditioning and functional training techniques
- Minimizes prolonged emphasis on any one technique
- Promotes participant interaction and encourages fun
- Demonstrates good form and alignment for all exercises
- Gives clear cues and verbal directions
- Gradually decreases impact and intensity during cool-down following the cardiorespiratory session
- Uses motivating music

to fill such a class. Therefore, the term *sports conditioning,* or *cross-conditioning,* was created to refer to training for sport movements rather than participating in a group exercise format such as water exercise or step (see figure 10.1). Sports conditioning is what most sport-minded participants remember doing to condition for their particular sport or what they remember doing in their physical education classes as they were growing up.

The term *functional training* differs slightly from *sports conditioning* (see figure 10.2). Dr. Astrand coined the term *functional training* in a landmark article titled "Why exercise?" (Astrand 1992). He stated, "If animals are built reasonably, they should build and maintain just enough, but not more structure than they need to meet functional requirements." Dr. Astrand was ahead of his time in predicting that people would soon be focusing more on why they should exercise than on how exercise changes their physique. In a recent article on trends in fitness and wellness, Archer (2007) suggested that people need more of a sense of purpose for why they

◼ Background Check

Before working your way through this chapter, you should do the following:

Read

- the section covering the functional training continuum in chapter 3 to get an idea of exercise modifications for various fitness levels,
- the section on monitoring intensity from chapter 6, and
- the section on the sports conditioning warm-up in chapter 4 as well as watch the demonstration of the sports conditioning warm-up on the DVD.

Practice

- monitoring intensity using RPE,
- movement options that will be utilized in the cardiorespiratory segment, and
- participant interaction as discussed in chapter 6.

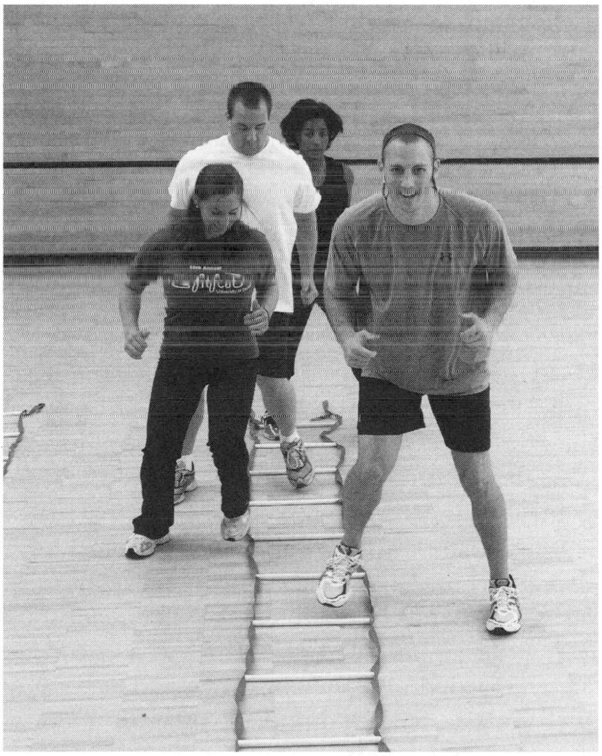

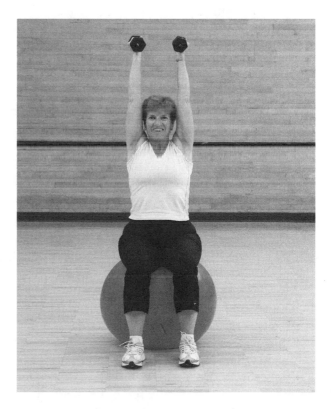

▶ **Figure 10.1** Sports conditioning using ladders to enhance footwork.

▶ **Figure 10.2** A functional training exercise for older adults.

exercise and predicted that soon there will be a blending of fitness and wellness. Rather than exercising for aesthetics and to improve how we look, we will be exercising to improve our lives. In fact, a recent *Newsweek* article (Carmichael 2007) touted that exercise does more than build muscles and prevent heart disease—it also boosts brainpower. This article reviewed several studies showing that people who exercise experience less disease overall and score higher on intellectual tests. John Ratey's (2008) book on Spark reiterates these findings and suggests that if your brain is to function at full capacity your body needs to move. This book and the Newsweek article dispell the myth of the dumb jock and demonstrate the value of exercise not only for physical wellness but also for mental wellness. The term *functional training* is often used to explain this movement from aesthetics to purposeful exercise.

Baby boomers are especially concerned about their functional movement. Life expectancy has reached an all-time high in the United States; however, Americans spend the last 10 to 13 of their years with declining functional ability. They are not able to take care of themselves and thus lose their quality of life in their later years. A study on functional abilities of older adults (DeVreede et al. 2005) showed that training on variable resistance machines that isolate movements does not improve the daily functioning of older adults. In contrast, when older adults performed functional tasks such as sit-to-stand exercises, their quality of daily living did improve. This study suggests that when people exercise they need to consider what exercises they are performing and why they are exercising. As fitness instructors, if our purpose is to enhance our participants' abilities to perform activities of daily living, we may need a whole new functional approach to how we teach exercise.

Muscles know no age so it is important to note that any form of strength training for older adults is effective, especially if they have not been doing any training at all. Therefore, functional training is not the only form of training that makes a difference in the health and wellness of older adults. It is simply the new focus and a new way to think about strength training. Cress and colleagues (1999) found that daily living improved for older adults who strength trained regularly. A meta-analysis on strength training by Rhea and coworkers (2003) supported this conclusion and also found that adding progression to a resistance training program helps to optimize the benefits of strength training. Westcott and Baechle (2007) found that a short circuit routine for older adults makes a difference in their functional lives. Any form of strength training, no matter a person's age, will improve life. It's important to reiterate that muscles know no age. They are just waiting for us to use them so that we can live better—not just longer, but also better. A focus on functional training and progressive weight training brings us to the purpose of why we exercise, which is to improve our quality of life. Thus functional strength training can bring a sense of purpose into our traditional strength-training routines.

Functional training also has roots in the area of sport-specific training. This form of functional training was created by fitness professionals who desired to enhance the performance of athletes. Wolfe (2001) describes functional training as the art of training movements and not muscles. He feels that this paradigm shift is what is needed to make a difference in the performance of athletes as well as the performance of activities of daily living. According to Wolfe, when your exercise programs exclusively use machines or isolated, repetitive movements, you are not training your client's functional needs. You have to incorporate balance and speed and work the body through the various planes of movement (sagittal, frontal, transverse) rather than focus on single-plane movements that strengthen the body in one direction. A practical example of a single-plane movement is performing a seated biceps curl with a dumbbell. This exercise strengthens only the biceps; however, if you lift a box using the strength of your biceps and end up hurting your back, you have failed to train your system to utilize the strength of your biceps. Instead of having functionally strong biceps, you just have strong biceps. Doing a standing biceps curl with resistance bands strengthens the core in addition to the biceps and allows the biceps and core to be overloaded at the same time. This standing curl with resistance bands is more functional than a seated curl using dumbbells.

Santana (2002) has defined functional training by describing the various movement patterns that people use in their daily lives. His theory on functional training states that because in our daily lives we stand and locomote, raise and lower the centers of our bodies, push and pull, and rotate with many movements, our exercise movements ought to mimic these basic daily patterns. This philosophy is in line with the idea that our participants need to take what they ben-efit from our group exercise experience into their lives. If we overload movements and even name movements after functional daily activities, we will help integrate the importance of fitness into our daily lives. Figures 10.3 through 10.6 give several ideas on how to integrate functional activities into a group exercise class.

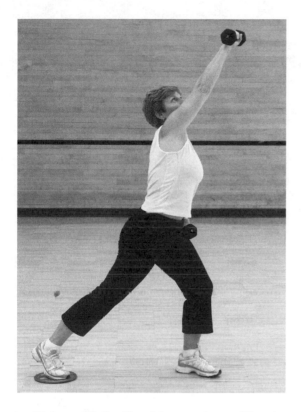

▶ **Figure 10.3** Cue this exercise as "Reach into your cupboards!" rather than "Do an overhead press."

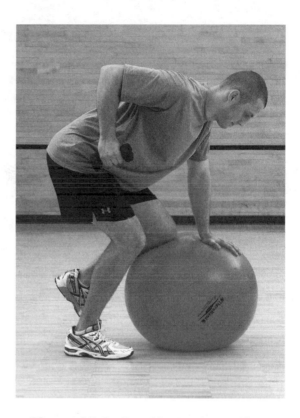

▶ **Figure 10.4** Cue this exercise as "Start the lawn mower!" rather than "Perform a bent-over row."

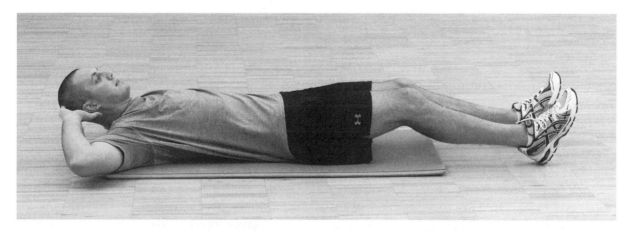

▶ **Figure 10.5** For this exercise, cue your participants, "Keep the legs straight for this abdominal exercise. Because we walk around all day with our legs straight, when we keep our legs straight for this crunch, we are training the abdominals for functional living."

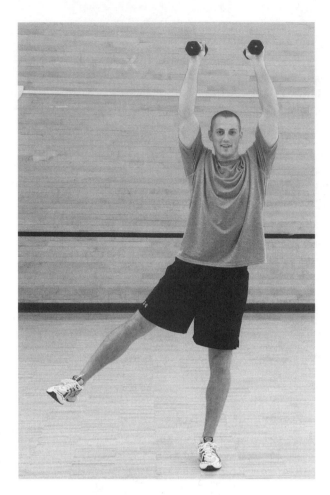

▶ **Figure 10.6** For this exercise, cue your participants, "Alternating hip abduction in a standing position helps you strengthen your gluteal muscles for standing. Because your gluteal muscles keep your hips in line when you walk and run, it's important to strengthen them in an upright standing position."

EQUIPMENT

Choosing how to teach your sports conditioning, boot camp, or functional training class ultimately depends on your personality, your teaching philosophy, and your clients' response to various motivational techniques. Your background as a group exercise leader and perhaps as a personal trainer will also influence how you teach your class (Vogel 2006). It is rare to find any two classes that are formatted the same way. Many sports conditioning classes utilize the equipment available within a group exercise program. For example, McMillan (2005) decided

Sports Conditioning Equipment

Indoors

- Agility ladders
- Steps
- Slideboards
- Cones
- Jump ropes
- Medicine balls
- Dumbbells and weighted bars
- Exercise tubes
- Stability balls or BOSU balance trainers
- Hula hoops

Outdoors

- Running trails or tracks
- Stairs
- Benches
- Hills
- Playground equipment
- Cement walls
- Fitness trail stations
- Logs
- Sand

to turn her step class into a sport step class. She noticed that many participants had drifted away from traditional step classes because such classes contain complex movements that require a lot of skill. To appeal to a different audience, McMillan called her classes *Power Step* and *Sport Step*. She made her movements sport movements by doing things such as adding a reach toward the ceiling to the basic step to mimic rebounding in basketball. She also changed a basic shuffle across the step to a man-to-man defense move. Changing a few simple moves and using creative cues made all the difference in her class. McLain (2005) used a different approach and created an outdoor boot camp class. He held the class in neighborhoods rather than fitness facilities. His goal was to create a club without walls by taking programs out of the facility. This concept is what many health educators are suggesting that fitness professionals undertake. Rather than making participants go to a facility, it is time for professionals to go to the people. There are issues with this concept, such as liability concerns and obtaining appropriate informed consent, but ultimately this program was a success for McLain, and it definitely enhanced the image of the club he represented.

Some programs purchase equipment or provide outdoor facilities to enhance the sports conditioning experience. The equipment you use will depend on what is available to you. Many fitness professionals prefer to use little or no gym equipment, relying on body weight, plyometrics, and props that are available through the facility or outdoors. The highlighted section on page 206 provides equipment ideas for a typical sports conditioning class and many pieces of equipment are shown in figure 10.7.

SAFE AND EFFECTIVE EXERCISE

One of the great advantages of a sports conditioning class is the flexibility it provides you as the instructor. You are free to include whatever sport-specific exercises you like. As you choose your exercises, however, make sure each class includes a warm-up and cool-down and addresses the components of sports conditioning. These include the following:

- Agility (including acceleration, deceleration, and change of direction)
- Balance (including static and dynamic)
- Cardiorespiratory training (including aerobic and anaerobic)
- Neuromuscular training (including coordination and reaction time)
- Core strengthening (including exercises that build strength for the many movements the core participates in each day)
- Muscular strength and endurance (including body weight and external resistance)
- Flexibility (including dynamic flexibility)

As for positioning yourself and your participants, you also have many options. With sports conditioning classes, standing in front of the participants is not the norm. Here are some other positioning ideas:

- Circle: You stand in the middle of a circle that the participants form around you.
- Circle: The participants form a circle and you stand still as they move by you.

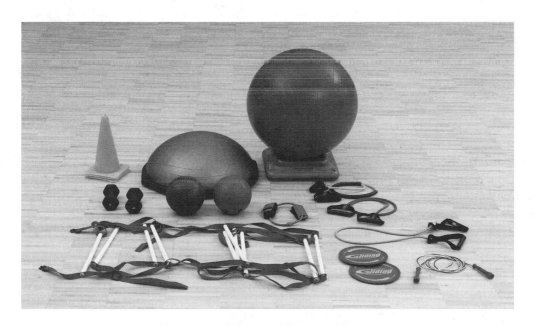

▷ **Figure 10.7** Sports equipment for indoors.

- Groups: The participants form 2 to 3 groups when they perform various drills.
- Open or traditional: The participants spread out across the room or outdoor space but do not form lines.
- Relay: One participant at a time performs the exercise.

 See the DVD to get an idea of what sports conditioning equipment you can utilize in your classes. Notice how the instructor in this demonstration teaches the class differently from the traditional high-low impact, step, or kickboxing classes.

BASIC MOVES

Let's review specific exercise ideas that address the basic components of a sports conditioning class. Note that these exercises also include suggestions for participant positioning.

 See the DVD for demonstration of a sports conditioning warm-up.

Agility

Using an open format or a relay format with participants standing next to each other in one line, have participants run forward 10 feet (3 m), touch a cone, run back, run forward 20 feet (6.1 m), touch a cone, run back, run forward 30 feet (9.1 m), touch a cone, and sprint back. This activity is like the shuttle run many of you experienced in your physical education classes, in which you picked up an eraser rather than touched a cone. If you have 2 to 3 people in the relay line, they will get a rest as other participants run, and so this would be an interval exercise for them. The relay format also can build team camaraderie, as it encourages participants to cheer on their team members as they perform this agility drill. Repeat the drill 3 to 4 times, as team members will improve as they learn the activity.

Balance

Ask your participants to form a circle. Encourage them to jog or walk forward and then ask them to stop and stand on their right leg for 30 seconds when they hear a whistle blow. Have them begin

another movement such as the grapevine and then stand on the left foot for 30 seconds the next time they hear the whistle. Have participants change directions and perform this drill again. Instead of asking participants to balance on one leg, you can have them hold yoga poses such as the tree, warrior, and so on (see figure 10.8). Incorporating balance movements into cardio segments is a good way to interval train by combining components of sports conditioning with the health-related components of fitness.

Cardiorespiratory Training

Our lives are a blend of aerobic and anaerobic movements. We walk from our cars to the front doors of our office building and then take the stairs up to work. Sports are also a blend of the

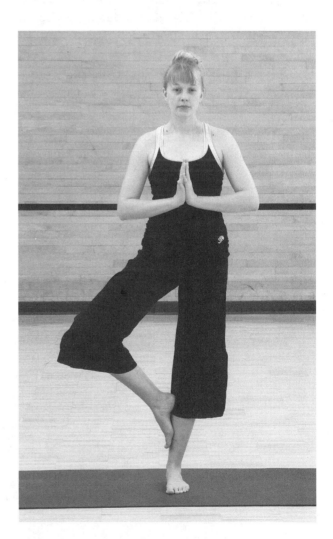

▶ **Figure 10.8** Holding a tree pose (a yoga movement) in a sports conditioning class.

aerobic and anaerobic. We serve a tennis ball, run to get it, and then rest when the point is over. Short bursts of exercise combined with longer aerobic movements make up many sports conditioning drills. Place a bench at the end of your exercise area and have your participants stand at the opposite end. Ask the participants to walk or jog to the bench, walk up 10 flights of stairs (up, up, down, down for 10 counts), and then walk or jog back. You can change this format and have them walk or jog for 10 seconds, 20 seconds, 30 seconds, or 40 seconds; you can also increase or decrease the number of times they step up on the bench. If you are performing this drill outdoors, you can have participants walk or jog on a track and then go up and down a nearby set of stairs. These types of movements fit well in both functional and sports-specific training.

Neuromuscular training

Drills using ladders or jump ropes are a good way to develop coordination and reaction time. Ask participants to line up in groups of three and then walk through a ladder series, alternating right and left legs with one foot in each ladder square. You will need enough ladders to accommodate your groups of three. Place a couple of jump ropes at the end of the ladders and ask participants to jump rope with both feet while they wait their turn to go through the ladder again. You can instruct participants going through the ladders to hop on one leg per square, to hop on both legs per square, or to utilize any other combination of movements. These neuromuscular movements require the mind and body to work together. They are a great way to build both mental and physical outcomes for physical activity training.

Core Strengthening

Building core strength is essential for any group exercise class. The core (i.e., the abdominal, gluteal, and low-back musculature) supports most standing activities, and since humans spend much of their lives standing on two feet, strengthening the core muscles will improve posture and also athletic performance. It is important to strengthen the core while in a standing position for both functional and sports conditioning exercises. Try adding an abdominal and low-back series to a circuit or to the end of the muscular conditioning segment: Perform 1 to 20 curl-ups on the floor with the legs straight (participants who experience low-back pain can bend at the knees to isolate the rectus abdominis). Alternate lifting one leg 6 inches (15 cm) off the ground to increase the workload against the core stabilizers. Perform 10 to 20 oblique curl-ups by lifting the shoulder toward the opposite knee. Finish with plank exercises to work the transversus abdominis (see figure 10.9). Move into a prone position and perform some back extensions to balance out all the spinal flexion used to work the abdominal muscles.

Muscular Strength and Endurance

Chapter 7 reviewed muscular strength and conditioning exercises using body weight or external resistance or both. Many of these exercises

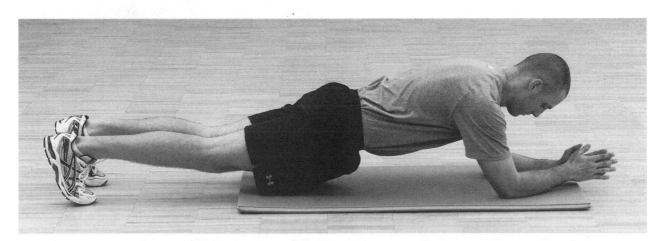

▶ **Figure 10.9** The plank position is a core-strengthening exercise often utilized in sports conditioning classes.

are utilized in sports conditioning or functional training classes. There are a few guidelines you should follow when selecting exercises. To maintain muscle balance, whenever you pick a pushing exercise, you should also select a pulling exercise. For example, if you incorporate an exercise that works the pectorals (pushing muscles), you should also include an exercise that works the rhomboids (pulling muscles). For comfort, work larger muscle groups (such as the quadriceps) before working smaller muscle groups (such as the shins) so that the larger muscle groups can recover while you work on smaller muscle groups. If your focus is on functional training, concentrate on working the muscle groups that do not get used as much throughout the day. For example, when performing daily activities, people often lift items with their biceps. Therefore, your class should focus more on the triceps muscle, which is assisted by gravity all day and rarely gets utilized with daily activity. Try calling a triceps dip off a bench a *get-out-of-your-chair exercise* rather than a *triceps dip* so participants see the connection between their workout and their daily movements (see figure 10.10). Refer to table 3.2 for an overview of functional exercises for health.

Flexibility

Chapter 7 reviews stretching exercises for each muscle group. Many of these stretches are appropriate for sports conditioning or functional training classes (see figure 10.11). Refer to table 3.2 for an overview of the muscles that are recommended for stretching in a functional exercise class. Stretching the muscles that are utilized throughout the day will enhance overall relaxation. Since interval training is often used in a functional training or sports conditioning class, flexibility exercises are often performed in between intervals. For example, after your participants finish a high-intensity walking or jogging interval, lead them in calf stretch against the wall while waiting for the next cardiorespiratory interval to begin. While incorporating stretching throughout the workout is effective, spending the last 5 minutes of class stretching on the ground, where the body is relaxed against gravity, improves flexibility and provides a chance for participants to recover completely from the workout

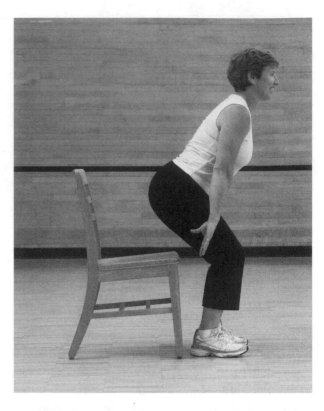

▶ **Figure 10.10** A get-out-of-your-chair exercise for functional training.

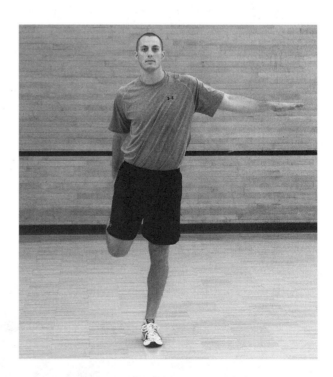

▶ **Figure 10.11** Stretching the quadriceps is a great functional stretch since the quadriceps is a strong muscle used in many daily and sport activities.

▪ Technique and Safety

When teaching any sports conditioning or functional training class, you must make sure that you show exercise modifications for different levels of fitness. You cannot assume that all participants have the same fitness level. Cueing options for movement modifications is the key to leading a successful class. Instructors who demonstrate the intermediate option while suggesting advanced and beginner options will create a sense of comfort that allows all participants to have a good experience. The accompanying DVD dedicates an entire segment to cueing modifications for various participant levels. Notice how the instructor demonstrates the intermediate option in the DVD segment.

before leaving. Remember to hold stretches for 15 to 60 seconds during this segment.

 See the DVD to observe an instructor giving exercise modifications to participants of varying fitness levels.

Let's discuss how you can modify the basic locomotor patterns for various fitness levels. Most of the locomotor patterns we all learned in our physical education classes were high impact and high intensity. These movements are fine when you are young but may become too stressful on the body as we age. Table 10.1 takes these basic locomotor patterns and presents intermediate and low impact and intensity

options for them. Lead the class in the intermediate modifications but demonstrate the other options so participants can choose which level of impact and intensity is right for them.

MUSIC FOR SPORTS CONDITIONING AND FUNCTIONAL TRAINING CLASSES

Step and kickboxing classes require mixed music in which the music tempo is uninterrupted. Music for a sports conditioning or functional training class can be taken right off an iPod, as there is no need to have a consistent music tempo. Music is utilized to enhance the experience of the workout. For example, using the theme song from *Rocky* for cardio intervals can motivate participants to be strong like Sylvester Stallone when he portrayed Rocky. The music on the *Jock Jam* CDs used on ESPN or for introducing sport teams can take participants back to their glory years when they themselves were introduced with their athletic teams. Music helps you as the instructor by providing motivation beyond your encouragement and instruction. Music needs to fit the workout segment in order to help with motivation. For example, a song matched to a muscular conditioning and flexibility segment may be less intense with less bass so that participants are able to hear the specific instructions for the exercises. Some segments, such as a relay race or competition, may be better without music

Table 10.1 Modifications of Basic Locomotor Patterns for Sports Conditioning and Functional Training Classes

High impact and intensity	Moderate impact and intensity	Low impact and intensity
Skipping	Walking with alternating slight hop	Walking using large arm movements
Jumping in place	Tapping side to side with a jump in the middle	Tapping side to side
Running	Walking 10 steps followed by running 10 steps	Walking using large arm movements
Sliding	Sliding without the jumping or carioca	Carioca without jumping
Knee lift with a hop	Knee lift with alternate hopping	Knee lift without hopping
Galloping with both legs hopping	Galloping with only back leg hopping	Galloping with both feet performing a low-impact gallop

so the participants can interact with one another. Matching music to workout segments is a challenge for the instructor. Poll the participants and see what music they like or even ask them to bring in motivating music they would like to hear while exercising. With a sports conditioning or functional training class any music will work, so this class is a good opportunity to get participant input on the music.

Research Findings on Sports Conditioning

- Intermittent bouts of exercise can result in the same energy expenditure as continuous exercise for a cardiorespiratory segment (Darling et al. 2005).

- Golfers improved their swing and their daily living activities after participating in three 90-minute functional training sessions for 8 weeks (Thompson 2007).

- High-risk participants undergoing treatment for heart disease improved their $\dot{V}O_2$max and quality of life by performing high-intensity interval work. (Wisloff et al. 2007).

- Healthy, moderately trained individuals improve fitness and health to a greater degree when participating in interval high-intensity training instead of continuous, moderate-intensity training (Helgerud et al. 2007).

- Circuit weight training that does not include aerobic stations can elicit a cardiorespiratory response that meets the minimal ACSM guidelines for cardiorespiratory fitness (Gotshalk et al. 2004).

CHAPTER WRAP-UP

A sports conditioning or functional training class offers a unique opportunity to improve a participant's enjoyment in a sport or to enhance a participant's

daily living activities. Exercise participants are seeking group exercise that is more purposeful, which is why this format of group exercise is gaining in popularity. Rather than focusing on improving their looks, participants are growing more concerned with how they perform their daily routines as well as how they engage in leisure pursuits. A sports conditioning or functional training class is a very purpose-driven experience that will make a difference in the health and wellness of participants.

▷ Group Exercise Class Evaluation Form Key Points

- Include an appropriate amount of dynamic movement. For the warm-up, use dynamic movements such as walking in a circle.
- Provide rehearsal moves. Introduce rehearsal moves by showing a modification of one of the basic locomotor patterns.
- Stretch the major muscle groups in a biomechanically sound manner with appropriate instructions. Stretch the major muscle groups throughout the workout and especially at the end.
- Give clear cues and verbal directions.
- Use appropriate music that inspires movement.
- Gradually increase intensity during the cardiorespiratory segment.
- Use a variety of sports conditioning and functional training movements.
- Minimize prolonged emphasis on any one locomotor pattern or sports conditioning component.
- Demonstrate good form and alignment for all exercises and participate with clients.
- Promote participant interaction and encourage fun. Use relay race formats and so on to engage your participants in your class.
- Gradually decrease impact and intensity during the cool-down following the cardiorespiratory session.

▷ Assignment

Write a thorough outline for a 10-minute sports conditioning or functional training class that includes a 2-minute warm-up, a 6-minute combination cardio and strength segment, and a 2-minute cool-down that includes stretching. List the specific exercises you will perform and why you selected them, and include the titles of your music pieces. Be prepared to share your workout if you are selected to present it in class.

Stationary Indoor Cycling

CHAPTER OBJECTIVES

By the end of this chapter, you will

- understand proper bike setup, riding alignment, and safety;
- understand how to warm up for stationary indoor cycling;
- be familiar with basic indoor cycling class techniques and music;
- be able to format different indoor cycling classes;
- understand cueing and coaching techniques on and off the bike; and be able to teach a 4-minute indoor cycling segment with appropriate content, technique, cueing, and music.

Stationary indoor cycling (known by such trademarked names as *Spinning, Cycle Reebok,* and *Power Pacing*) is another popular modality for group exercise. Many clubs and facilities designate a room just for indoor cycling, complete with specialized indoor bikes, sound systems, and microphones and even videotapes, disco or strobe lighting, and candles. Unlike more traditional forms of group exercise such as kickboxing or step, indoor cycling classes may be held in darkened rooms without mirrors. The focus is less on how you look or how you compare with others in the room and more on how you experience the workout. As some instructors like to say, "It's about the ride, or journey, itself and not the final result." Because there are no choreographed moves that all participants must do at the same time, it's much easier for indoor cyclists to personalize their workouts. Hence, indoor cycling classes easily accommodate several different fitness levels, with elite cyclists working next to deconditioned novices. Stationary indoor cycling can provide an excellent cardiorespiratory workout, burning 400 to 550 kilocalories per 45-minute ride, not counting the warm-up and cool-down. Many fitness facilities require specific training and certification to teach a cycling class (see the special section on indoor cycling organizations and certifications on page 217). Teaching a stationary indoor cycling class can be fun and exhilarating for both you and your participants! The main points on the group exercise class evaluation form that relate to stationary cycling are listed on this page.

WARM-UP

A stationary indoor cycling warm-up generally follows the warm-up recommendations covered in chapter 5. It consists primarily of dynamic movements, rehearsal moves, and some light preparatory stretching, all taught with skillful cues at the appropriate tempo.

■ Background Check

Before working your way through this chapter, you should

- read chapter 5 on warming up and
- read chapter 6 on cardiorespiratory training.

Group Exercise Class Evaluation Form Essentials

Key Points for the Warm-Up Segment

- Includes appropriate amount of dynamic movement
- Provides rehearsal moves
- Stretches major muscle groups in a biomechanically sound manner with appropriate instructions
- Gives clear cues and verbal directions
- Uses an appropriate music tempo

Key Points for the Cardiorespiratory Training Segment

- Gradually increases intensity
- Uses a variety of cycling techniques
- Minimizes prolonged emphasis on any one technique
- Promotes participant interaction and encourages fun
- Demonstrates good form and alignment for indoor cycling and gives clear verbal cues and directions
- Gradually decreases intensity during cool-down following the cardiorespiratory session
- Uses music volume and tempo appropriate for biomechanical movement

Dynamic Movement and Rehearsal Moves

The focus of a group cycling warm-up is on gradually increasing the intensity to elevate heart rate, ventilation, and oxygen consumption—all preparations for the cardiorespiratory workout to follow. Have participants sit upright on the bike and keep their spine in neutral alignment while cycling to loosen up their legs. Bikes should be adjusted so there is light resistance and just enough tension on the flywheel for participants to stay in control. A typical indoor cycling warm-up lasts approximately 4 to 8 minutes; intensity may be gradually increased toward the end of the warm-up by changing either the resistance or the pedaling speed.

Stretching Major Muscle Groups

We recommend performing some light preparatory stretching and dynamic movements for the upper body while cycling during the warm-up. These moves and stretches should include rolling the shoulders backward, stretching the

Indoor Cycling Organizations and Certifications

Mad Dogg Athletics, Inc.
2111 Narcissus Ct.
Venice, CA 90291
800-847-SPIN
www.spinning.com

Cycle Reebok
800-REEBOK-1
www.reebokuniversity.com

Nautilus, Inc.
16400 SE Nautilus Drive
Vancouver, WA 98683
360-859-2900
www.nautilusinc.com

Keiser
800-888-7009
www.keiser.com

Indoor Cycling Research Findings

Many studies have examined the cardiorespiratory and metabolic responses to group indoor cycling. Virtually all researchers have found that a stationary indoor cycling workout can provide a stimulus sufficient to meet ACSM guidelines for the development and maintenance of aerobic fitness, and most have reported high levels of caloric expenditure, up to 550 kilocalories per 45-minute ride. Several investigators also measured responses to various positions and activities found in a typical cycling class. Standing, climbing, high-resistance settings, and jumping maneuvers elicited the highest heart rate, RPE, oxygen consumption, and caloric expenditure (Chinsky et al. 1998; Flanagan et al. 1998; Francis et al. 1999; Williford et al. 1999). Williford and colleagues (1999) found that speed play and vigorous jumps or lifts may produce transient maximal effects. Several recent studies have examined the effects of cadence on performance at specific workloads. Mora-Rodriguez and Aguado-Jimenez (2004) concluded that a very high pedaling cadence (>120 rpm) reduces performance in well-trained cyclists. In studies of elite cyclists, Foss and Hallen (2004) and Lucia and coworkers (2004) found that when cadence increases along with workload, work efficiency (defined as a low level of oxygen consumption at any given workload) also increases. And in one study (Francis et al. 1999), energy cost was found to be unrelated to cadence; in other words, higher pedaling speeds did not appear to increase caloric expenditure as long as the workload was maintained. John and Schuler (1999) reported that the 6- to 20-point Borg RPE scale may be inaccurate when used by novices during group cycling; thus, these participants may require either heart rate monitors or more detailed instruction regarding the RPE scale. Novice cyclists were also found to have movements and muscle recruitment patterns that were less refined than those of trained cyclists; researchers surmised that the neuromuscular system was not yet sufficiently adapted in new cyclists (Chapman et al. 2004).

pectoralis major (chest), and stretching the upper trapezius (neck) to counteract the rounded, hunched posture so often seen in cycling classes (see figure 11.1). Most instructors reserve lower-body stretching for the end of a cycling class, when everyone is very warm and psychologically ready to relax and hold the static stretches. Stopping the rhythmic rehearsal movements of cycling to perform lower-body static stretches would have the negative effect of decreasing heart rate and oxygen consumption, exactly the opposite of the warm-up purpose. Therefore, we suggest waiting to stretch the lower-body muscles until the end of class.

Verbal Cues and Tempo

The warm-up is an ideal time to teach proper alignment and riding technique as well as review intensity guidelines. Teach your class about neutral spine and scapulae and proper neck, elbow, and wrist alignment. Give pedaling pointers, such as, "visualize your feet spinning in separate perfect circles" or "feel each foot moving

front to back with each revolution" or "create a perfect balance between your right foot and left foot." Additionally, many participants need instruction regarding proper intensity. Now is the time to address heart rate issues, perceived exertion, cadence, and the concept of listening to your body and working at the level that is right for you. Some instructors suggest that participants silently create an intention, or a personal focus, for the workout ahead. Finally, make certain that all participants can hear you; be sure music volume and microphone volume are well balanced.

An appropriate music tempo is one that allows participants to work comfortably at a low to medium intensity during the warm-up. There are no set guidelines for music speed, and participants can pedal either on or off the beat in three ways: (1) One leg completes a downstroke on every other beat (slow), (2) one leg completes a downstroke on each beat (faster), and (3) both legs complete a downstroke on each beat (very fast, or double time). Because of the variability in how music is used, rigid tempo guidelines are

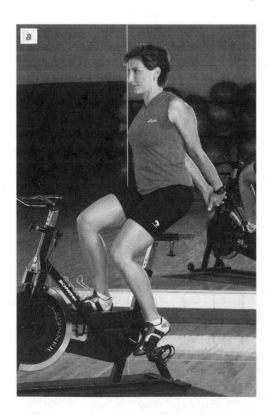
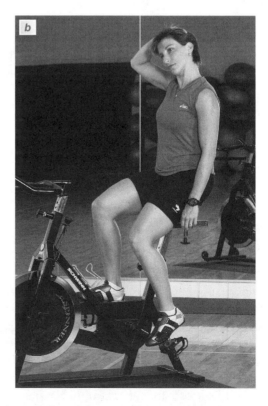

▶ **Figure 11.1** Upper-body stretches for indoor cycling: *(a)* pectoralis major stretch and *(b)* upper trapezius stretch with neck laterally flexed.

somewhat meaningless. Instead, select warm-up music that is motivating, is fun to listen to, and encourages a comfortable pace at a low to moderate intensity.

TECHNIQUE AND SAFETY

Before beginning a cycling class, make certain that each participant is properly aligned and adjusted on the bike. You should be available for at least 15 minutes before class to assist participants with bike setup, to answer any questions, to get to know new participants, and to set up your own equipment (including music and microphones). The three main bike adjustments are the seat height, the fore and aft seat position, and the handlebar height. The correct seat height depends on the cyclist's leg length; the longer the leg, the higher the seat. In general, when the rider is seated on the bike with the balls of the feet on the center of the pedals, there should be a slight bend in the knee of the extended leg when pedaling. Experts suggest this knee flexion should be anywhere from 5° to 30°. If the seat height is too low, inadequate leg extension may cause knee problems, especially in the front of the knee. If the seat is too high, the rider's hips will rock back and forth; in addition, the risk of knee hyperextension is increased, which may cause pain at the back of the knee. Most beginning participants err on the side of setting the seat too low in an effort to minimize saddle soreness. Encourage students to wear padded bike shorts or use gel-padded bike seats, and let them know that saddle soreness usually disappears after the first few sessions. Proper seat height is the key to healthy knees!

For proper fore and aft positioning, adjust the saddle so that the cyclist's front kneecap is aligned directly above the center of the pedal when the pedal is forward and the crank is horizontal (the nine o'clock position). Cycling with the saddle too far forward can cause anterior knee problems. The correct fore and aft position also should allow the arms to comfortably reach the handlebars with the elbows slightly flexed.

Handlebar height is mostly a matter of personal preference. Beginners usually are more comfortable with the handlebars higher and the torso more upright. The upright, neutral spine position is definitely recommended for participants with back or neck problems. The lower the handlebars, the more the cyclist simulates a racing position, which creates favorable aerodynamics when cycling outdoors but is obviously unnecessary when indoors. Teach your participants to ride with a relaxed grip and neutral wrists and to vary their hand positions. Additionally, encourage students to wear stiff-soled shoes that remain rigid over the pedal; students should position their feet so that the balls of the feet, not the arches, contact the pedals. Clipping onto the pedals or securely strapping the shoes into the foot cages can enhance pedaling efficiency. Because most bikes are fixed gear and have pedals that continue to rotate after the feet are taken off them, remind your class members to keep their feet on the pedals until the pedals stop moving or to hold their feet away from the bike if they must detach from the pedals before the pedals come to a complete stop (alternatively, many indoor cycling bikes have an emergency brake that can be pressed to instantly stop the flywheel and pedal rotation).

Always maintain neutral spinal alignment on the bike. The rider is in a neutral spine position (also known as *ideal alignment*) when the four natural curves of the back are in their proper relationship to each other. Maintaining this position is easiest, of course, when the rider is sitting upright with the torso perpendicular to the floor. When the rider is seated and riding with a forward lean, the spine should still be in a neutral position, albeit inclined at a 45° angle, depending on the activity. Avoid tucking

---

■ Technique and Safety Check

Stationary cycling warm-up recommendations are to

- gradually increase intensity,
- include some light preparatory stretching and dynamic movements for the upper body,
- teach proper alignment and cycling technique, and
- give intensity information and guidelines.

■ Technique and Safety Check

To help keep your classes safe, observe the following recommendations.

Remember to

- undertake a thorough, appropriate warm-up;
- maintain a neutral spine whether sitting upright, inclined forward, or standing;
- keep the neck in line with the spine;
- adjust the bike properly;
- keep the wrists in neutral and maintain a relaxed grip;
- wear proper footwear and contact the pedals with the balls of feet; and
- stay hydrated.

Avoid

- tucking the hips under and
- hyperextending the neck.

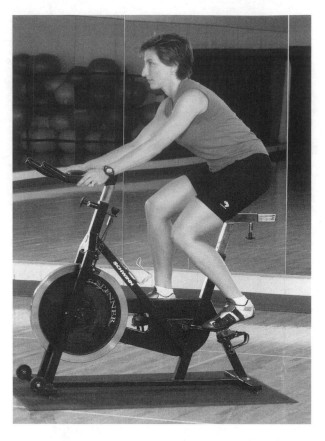

Figure 11.2 Proper seated bike alignment in the inclined position.

the hips under (creating a posterior pelvic tilt), which causes the back to round (or flex) and places much more strain on the structures of the back. The shoulders should be down and slightly retracted; this position is known as *neutral scapular alignment.* Avoid rounding or hunching the shoulders or allowing the shoulders to come up by the ears (see figure 11.2).

 See the DVD for a cycle set-up demonstration.

Remind participants to ride with a full water bottle and a towel. As with any new activity, recommend gradually increasing the frequency of their classes, starting with one or two per week and slowly increasing to three or four classes per week if desired.

BASIC MOVES

The typical indoor cycling class is divided into several segments, or drills, that are usually designed to simulate aspects of an outdoor ride. These segments may be linked to specific songs or cuts of music and are often attached to specific goals for intensity (heart rate or cadence). Segments may include

- seated flats;
- seated climbs (hills);
- standing flat runs or jogs;
- standing climbs (hills);
- seated downhills or flushes;
- rebounds, jumps, or lifts; and
- seated and standing sprints (also known as *spin-outs, fast hammers,* or *power drills*).

Participants are often asked to visualize themselves performing these segments outdoors on various types of terrain. Many instructors create imaginary journeys and scenarios for cyclists to visualize. Images of tropical islands, mountain roads, green forests, sandy beaches, open fields, and grassy meadows can all be conducive to improve the workout and create an enjoyable class experience. Visualization can also be used to improve breathing, alignment, muscle focus, mental awareness, and even self-empowerment! Have participants picture the goal they wish to accomplish and see themselves being successful. This can be a very powerful aspect of a group cycling class.

 See the DVD for instructions on basic cycling moves such as seated flats, seated climbs, and standing climbs.

The seated flat is the most basic cycling technique. Participants can work at a variety of speeds, and the flat road can be used in the warm-up, cardio stimulus, and cool-down phases of class. The seated flat is perfect for cadence drills, alignment and pedaling work, endurance work, and rhythm presses (a pulsating, wavelike movement of the upper body). Recommended cadences for a seated flat ride run the gamut from 80 to 110 revolutions per minute. During the cardio stimulus especially, the seated flat is usually performed in the basic riding position, in which the body is inclined at approximately 45°.

Seated and standing hill climbs are simulated by increasing the resistance on the bike. When performing seated climbs, the rider should shift the hips to the back of the saddle to avoid putting excessive pressure on the knees. When climbing and standing, the rider should move the hands forward on the handlebars and keep the hips in line over the seat (maintaining hip flexion). These segments are usually performed with a slow cadence of 60 to 80 revolutions per minute and can be quite strenuous, with the primary focus on strength. Avoid performing cadences below 60 revolutions per minute with heavy resistance, as this may contribute to back and knee injuries.

In the standing flat run or jog, the focus is on endurance; the resistance is light to medium and the cadence is typically 80 to 95 revolutions per minute. The cyclist's weight is balanced over the lower body while the hands rest lightly on the handlebars. Instructors may require participants to remain vertical or slightly flexed at the hips (keep spine in neutral).

The downhill, or flushing, segment is usually short, lasting 1 to 3 minutes, and is used for recovery after a strenuous uphill climb. The flywheel tension is low, the cyclist is seated, and the breathing rate and heart rate return to more moderate levels.

Rebounds, jumps, or lifts are advanced moves occasionally used to increase intensity. Participants need to be completely familiar with seated and standing positions before attempting jumps. Jumps or lifts are most often taught on the beat at regular intervals: Participants stand up for 8 counts, then sit down for 8 counts. The intervals can be short or long. An entire song or just part of a song may be used for jumping. Keep the lifting and lowering fluid and even, working for smooth knee transitions between sitting and standing. Jumps are usually accomplished without changing the pedal cadence. Be aware that jumping can be hard on the knees. Along with several indoor cycling organizations, we recommend limiting or avoiding jumps in most cycling classes.

 See the DVD for instructions on cadence and resistance, sprints, and rebounds.

Sprints, also known as *spin-outs, fast hammers,* and *power drills,* may be performed while seated or standing. They may be used in intervals or randomly dispersed throughout a segment. During a sprint, the cadence changes to a very fast pace of 100 to 120 revolutions per minute and the resistance is set to light to moderate—just enough to keep the hips from bouncing. Experienced participants may cross their anaerobic threshold and cycle with a near-maximal effort, focusing on speed and power. Be careful when pedaling above 110 revolutions per minute; very little resistance is possible at such high speeds and the flywheel develops such a high momentum that it is basically doing all the work of turning the pedal arms.

■ Practice Drill

Using your favorite music, practice seated flats, seated and standing climbs, standing runs, jumps, and sprints. Work on positioning your body in ideal alignment as you experiment with these positions and riding techniques (see figure 11.3).

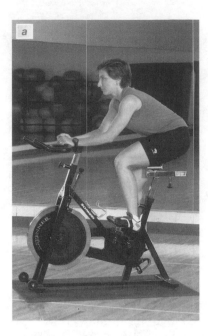
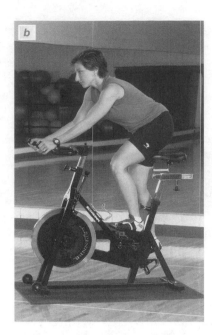
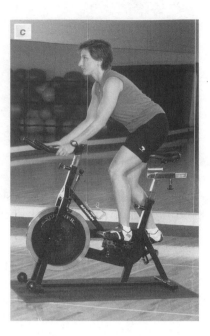

▷ **Figure 11.3** *(a)* Seated climb, *(b)* standing climb, and *(c)* standing run on the bike.

FORMATTING INDOOR CYCLING CLASSES

Formatting a stationary cycling class is simply a matter of combining the basic moves or drills. These combinations become the ride profile, which is the structure, or organization, of the cycling workout. Always prepare your ride profile, with the accompanying music selections, in advance. However, be ready to modify your plan depending on the fitness and skill levels of the individuals in class; the profile is only a guideline and will be subject to change. Each class will be different, and participants will have different needs. If you teach indoor cycling classes regularly, eventually you will accumulate many different class profiles and a large selection of music from which to choose. You can be spontaneous and creative! Always gradually increase the intensity at the beginning of class and gradually decrease the intensity at the end of class. A sample 45-minute profile is shown in table 11.1.

The music you choose for your cycling class is key to making your class a success. Unlike group exercise formats that require music to be metered into even 32-count phrases for choreography purposes, group cycling can be paired with virtually any style of music you choose. Songs may have an even number of beats or not. You can choose from pop, disco, rock and roll, rhythm and blues, jazz, reggae, rap, Latin, country, folk, gospel, classical, new age, world, and movie sound tracks. Find music that makes everyone smile and want to work. It's usually best to include several different kinds of music in your workout so you can fit varying participant preferences and can match the various class segments and moods you'll be creating. Connecting the music with the segments, mood, intensity, and journey can be the most fun yet challenging aspect of teaching an indoor cycling class.

Some instructors prefer to cross-train with their cycling classes. One way to do this is by varying the focus of the classes held throughout the week. For example, the class might focus on strength (hills) on Monday, on endurance on Wednesday, and on speed on Friday. Another approach is to combine indoor cycling with a different exercise modality such as treading, rowing, muscle conditioning, Pilates, or yoga. In this type of fusion format you might lead cycling for 30 minutes followed by yoga for another 30 minutes. The Keiser Power

Table 11.1 Sample Ride Profile

Segment	Body position	Resistance	Cadence (rpm)	Intensity (%HRmax)	Music tempo	Music selection	Duration (min)
1. Warm-up	Seated	Light	80-90	65%	Moderate	New age	5
2. Climb	Standing	Moderate	70	80%	Slow	Rock and roll	4
3. Climb	Standing	Heavy	60	85%	Slow	Rhythm and blues	4
4. Flat road	Seated	Moderate	90	75%	Moderate	Rock and roll	6
5. Flat road	Standing	Moderate	90	75%	Fast	Latin	4
6. Jumps	Seated or standing	Moderate	90	75%	Moderate	Pop	4
7. Climb	Seated	Heavy	60	85%	Slow	Funk	6
8. Downhill	Seated	Light	100	70%	Slow	Classical	2
9. Sprints	Seated or standing	Moderate	110	85%	Moderate	Rock and roll	5
10. Cool-down	Seated	Light	80	60%	Moderate	Pop	3
11. Stretch	Off bike				Slow	New age	>2

Pace cycling program recommends using free weights, rubber tubing, and bands to incorporate muscle-conditioning exercises into the bike workout itself.

INTENSITY

Another important training issue is intensity. One of the benefits of group indoor cycling is that participants work at their own level, and the pressure to conform to the group is much less than it is in a traditional cardio class with mirrors. Even so, you must give your students target heart rate zones, RPE guidelines, and cadence goals and help them learn to assess themselves.

Many indoor cycling instructors strongly recommend the use of a heart rate monitor. Using heart rate monitors has a number of advantages as well as some disadvantages. Heart rate monitors can be very useful if students know their actual training zones, as they might if they have had a graded exercise stress test (see the section on monitoring exercise intensity in chapter 6). The monitors make it easy to keep track of

heart rate at any time during the class and do not require participants to stop moving in order to check their intensity. They can also provide an incentive to work harder when motivation falters. Unfortunately, most exercisers who use heart rate monitors do not know their actual training zones and assume that the standard suggested training zones are accurate, when in fact standard heart rate formulas are suitable for only 75% of the population (McArdle et al. 2006). In the other 25% of the population, the target heart rate zones are either overestimated or underestimated, sometimes significantly. Another limitation of the heart rate method involves the effects of medications (many either decrease or increase the heart rate). No one heart rate formula will fit every participant, so it's wise to use other methods as well. Help your students establish a workout intensity zone—a heart rate training zone, a perceived exertion zone, or both.

During the workout, you can suggest that your students work at a low level (at the low end of their target heart rate zone or at an 8-12 on the 6-20 Borg RPE scale) during the warm-up, cool-down, and downhill segments; a moderate level (at the middle of their zone or 12-14 RPE) during seated flats and standing runs; and a high level (at the top of their zone or 15-18 RPE) during climbs, jumps, and power intervals. Some participants may choose to push past their anaerobic threshold during power surges; this should be reserved for advanced students only.

Remind your students that they can modify their cycling intensity by changing

1. their position (sitting instead of standing),
2. their resistance, or
3. their pedaling cadence.

Cadence is a widely used method for establishing intensity. It is possible to purchase cadence computers that attach to a bike's handlebars to monitor cadence and, usually, heart rate, distance in miles or kilometers, and estimated caloric expenditure. Without such a device, cadence can be counted manually by tapping the thigh on each revolution. A slow cadence is 60 to 80 revolutions per minute (rpm), a moderate tempo is 80 to 100 revolutions per minute, and a fast cadence is 100 or greater revolutions per minute. Being able to suggest cadence goals for each segment enhances your ability to guide and coach participants through a class. Let students know that even though you'll be giving intensity suggestions and goals, they still must exercise at their own pace. In addition to knowing the suggested cadence, many participants appreciate knowing how long each segment will last, so consider making announcements such as, "we'll be working hard on the next hill for 5 minutes," before leading into the more difficult sections.

Include a thorough cool-down at the end of class. Gradually decrease the intensity to little to no resistance while continuing to ride so that your participants' heart rates, breathing rates, oxygen consumption, and caloric expenditure can return toward normal values. We recommend statically stretching all major muscle groups at this time as well. Many instructors prefer to stretch the upper body while slowly cycling on the bike and then dismount to stretch the lower body. In addition to the upper-body stretches, be sure to include stretches for the hamstrings, quadriceps, hip flexors, calves, buttocks, and low back (see figure 11.4).

 See the DVD for a demonstration of a cycling cool-down.

CUEING METHODS

Leadership skills are all-important in an indoor cycling class. In many other group modalities (e.g., step, kickboxing, sports conditioning), instructors must be concerned with getting all participants to move together at the same time. Obviously, this is not necessary for group cycling. Instead, you must focus on motivating, coaxing, encouraging, and setting the mood with your voice and your cues. Use plenty of motivational cues such as, "You can do it!" "Altogether!" "Drive it forward!" Pull your class through difficult segments with positive affirmations such as, "We are strong!" "We are committed!" "You can climb this mountain!"

Helping your students set goals for their workouts is another effective strategy to help them succeed. Ask them during the warm-up to create a focus or an intention for the class. Then remind them of their focus during the challenging segments. For example, you can tell them, "Hang onto that goal!"

Indoor cycling classes are perfect for promoting a sense of teamwork within the class. One popular method for doing so is to divide the class into two or three pods, or small teams, and have the teams take turns sprinting or drafting in a race.

Remember to use visualizations during cycling classes. Many instructors suggest that riders picture themselves following the yellow line straight down the highway while feeling the wind in their faces or smelling the clean ocean air. Some instructors create an entire trip within their class, taking their participants to Hawaii, down the beach, or through rolling hills.

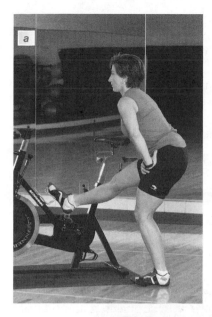
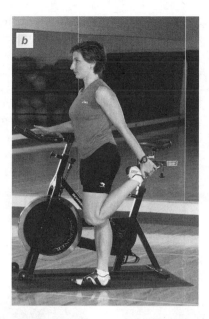
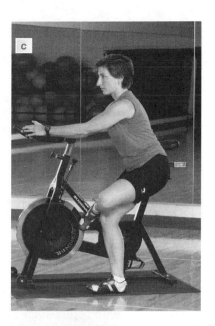

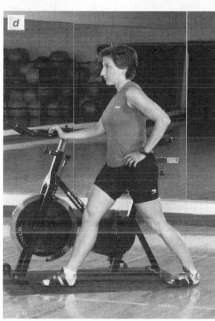
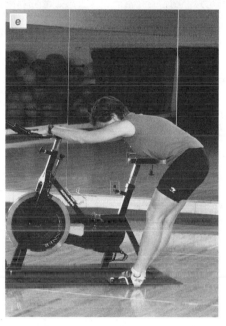

▶ **Figure 11.4** Stretches for *(a)* hamstrings, *(b)* quadriceps, *(c)* buttocks, *(d)* calves, and *(e)* low back.

Take advantage of the opportunity to get off the bike and teach. Walk through your class to check form and alignment and to support and encourage participants when the going gets tough. A simple "Hang in there!" to a fatigued class member can make all the difference.

Participants usually enjoy making noise while riding; you might try getting them to count the number of jumps they're making or try asking them to call out refrains to familiar songs you are playing. Theme classes are a great way to build camaraderie and fun; try picking your music around a special event, theme, or holiday. You can play scary music on Halloween, seasonal music for Christmas, love songs on Valentine's Day, or patriotic music on Memorial Day or the Fourth of July. For times when there aren't any holidays coming up, you can create a Motown music day, disco day, or beach music day. Encourage your students to relax and party!

CHAPTER WRAP-UP

In this chapter we covered indoor cycling, including proper positioning on the bike and cycling safety issues. We also covered warming up, basic moves, programming, intensity recommendations, and cueing for stationary indoor cycling classes. Mastering this information is fun and rewarding and can expand your teaching horizons!

▶ Group Exercise Class Evaluation Form Key Points

- Gradually increase intensity. In a cycling class, you should do this during the warm-up.
- Use a variety of cycling techniques, such as seated flats, standing runs, and seated and standing climbs.
- Minimize prolonged emphasis on any one technique (for example, avoid spending excessive time on hill climbs).
- Promote participant interaction and encourage fun.

- Demonstrate good form and alignment for indoor cycling. Be sure to help set up your participants properly on their bikes.
- Give clear cues and verbal directions, including intensity instructions, affirmations, visualizations, goal setting, and team building.
- Help students to monitor their intensity during the cardio segment, either with heart rate checks or perceived exertion checks.
- Gradually decrease intensity during the postcardio cool-down and include some static stretches at the end of class.
- Use music appropriately.

▶ Assignment

List 15 motivational cues and affirmations appropriate for coaching a cycling class. Prepare a 45-minute indoor cycling profile with music suggestions similar to those in table 11.1. Include music authors in the music selection section.

Water Exercise

CHAPTER OBJECTIVES

By the end of this chapter, you will

- know the benefits of water exercise,
- understand the properties of water and Newton's laws of motion,
- be able to give exercise examples using specificity of water training principles,
- understand appropriate use of equipment specific to water exercise, and
- be able to modify the group exercise class evaluation form for water exercise.

As we strive to make the exercise experience more purposeful and fun for our participants, we need to consider water exercise. Water exercise is growing in popularity in the United States as the population ages and participants seek nonintimidating and nonimpact exercise. Vogel (2006) believes that despite the emerging popularity of water exercise, many fitness consumers still view it as a specialized or overly gentle activity. As these consumers become aware of the many facets of water exercise, however, they will be more likely to view it as an effective way to enhance health and wellness.

Currently pools are viewed as a place for getting a cardiorespiratory workout by swimming. Unfortunately, pools are expensive to maintain when used only for lap swimming. In a water exercise class, more than 25 participants can work out in the pool and enjoy the benefits of the water's resistance. Water exercise can be the most effective form of group personal training if the right equipment is available. We need to think of our pools as giant resistance machines. In fact, research tells us that pools can be great for muscular strength and conditioning. Tsourlou and colleagues (2006) studied the training effects of a 24-week aquatics class on muscular strength in healthy elderly women and found that the water provided an alternative to traditional resistance training as well as enhanced the social environment for this population. Both pools and strength and conditioning areas can provide overload to train the muscles. In the strength and conditioning area, variable resistance machines overload the muscles by using weights that are designed to move against gravity. In the pool, the viscosity and other properties of water overload the muscles. Thus water exercise can improve muscular strength and endurance just as weight training does (see "Water Exercise Research Findings" on page 230).

Group water exercise classes often see many newcomers seeking instruction for water exercise. Many participants who try water exercise for the first time find that the pool environment allows them to set their own pace and intensity and to rest when necessary. On the other hand, people who need a more intense workout find that the resistance that water provides acts in all directions (and not just in the direction of gravity), no matter what the movement. In some ways, water exercise is safer than land-based activity—falls don't carry the same threat of injury, and joints receive less stress from impact.

Group Exercise Class Evaluation Form Essentials

Key Points for the Warm-Up Segment

- Includes appropriate amount of dynamic movement
- Provides rehearsal moves
- Stretches major muscle groups in a biomechanically sound manner with appropriate instructions
- Gives clear cues and verbal directions
- Uses music that fits the movement

Key Points for the Cardiorespiratory Segment

- Gradually increases intensity
- Uses a variety of water exercise techniques
- Minimizes prolonged emphasis on any one technique
- Promotes participant interaction and encourages fun
- Demonstrates good form and alignment and gives clear verbal cues
- Gradually decreases intensity during cool-down following the cardiorespiratory session
- Uses music appropriately

Furthermore, water cools participants as they work out, so sweating is not a problem (Sanders et al. 1997).

Water is particularly kind to people who are overweight and also to women (Brown et al. 1997), who are genetically programmed to carry more "stored energy" and thus more body fat. When overweight participants enter a traditional group exercise class, they are often intimidated by the mirrors and the fact that people can see them. In a water exercise class, the body is covered up by water and extra body fat actually makes the person more buoyant. Nagle and coworkers (2007) found that aquatic exercise in combination with walking can serve as an alternative to walking exercise alone for overweight women who are losing weight, and so aquatic exercise can improve functional health status. The current obesity pandemic in the United States will continually increase the popularity of water exercise in this country.

As the focus of exercisers shifts from aesthetic fitness to functional fitness, use of the water for exercise will increase because it is one of the best environments to accomplish functional and specific resistance training (Bravo et al. 1997; Simmons and Hansen 1996; Suomi and Koceja 2000). Sport scientists know that to improve sport performance, muscles must be trained with movements that are as similar as possible to the desired movements or skills required in a specific sport. A movement performed in a sport can be replicated in water for added resistance. Water exercise is also a wonderful medium

■ Background Check

Before working your way through this chapter, you should do the following:

Read

- chapter 3 on the core concepts in class design and
- chapter 7 on muscular conditioning.

Practice

- monitoring intensity using RPE (see chapter 6),
- and showing various movement options for different intensity levels, and
- participant interaction as discussed in chapter 6.

Designing a Water Workout

According to Weltman (1995), $\dot{V}O_2$max is not the best predictor of endurance performance on both land and water. He believes that the blood lactate response to submaximal exercise is a better indicator of endurance. Studies (Brown et al. 1997; DeMaere and Ruby 1997) on water exercise have verified that blood lactate responses to an exercise in the water are greater than responses to the same exercise performed on land. The resistance of the water creates an anaerobic response to exercise that is similar to what happens physiologically during resistance training on land. A large increase in blood lactate levels, especially in deconditioned participants, can be uncomfortable and lead to exercise adherence problems. Thus, because of the resistance properties of water, interval training has been recommended for water exercise, especially for beginners. A person does not go into a weight room and continuously lift weights. Rests are incorporated between muscle groups or sets to allow the blood lactate to be recycled within the body. Resistance exercises are usually performed in sets. The first set marks the move and increases ROM. The second set then provides maximum muscular overload. Frangolias and colleagues (2000) determined that when participants train in water, eventually they adapt to the environment and stop showing increases in blood lactate levels. In other words, once participants gain the strength to overcome the resistance of the water, they won't see the big increases in blood lactate levels that they first saw when they began exercising in water. Progressive overload is important to the success of a water exercise class because it provides a way for participants to keep improving (see properties of water section on progressive resistance, page 231).

Water Exercise Research Findings

■ When the chest cavity is immersed in water, heart rate decreases, and so it is not appropriate to utilize land-based target heart rates when monitoring exercise intensity (Craig and Dvorak 1968; D'Acquisto et al. 2001; Svedenhag and Seger 1992).

■ Training from water exercise can carry over to improve function and health on land (Bushman et al. 1997; Davidson and McNaughton 2000; DeMaere and Ruby 1997; Eyestone et al. 1993; Frangolias et al. 2000; Gehring et al. 1997; Takeshima et al. 2002; Tsourlou et al. 2006).

■ When running in deep water, women experience less physiologic stress than men experience (Brown et al. 1997).

■ Aquatic exercise can serve as an alternative to walking exercise alone for overweight women who are losing weight (Nagel et al. 2007).

■ Running in deep water is an adequate method of cardiorespiratory training whether it is being used for an injured runner or as a different form of training (Loupias and Golding 2004).

■ Pool exercises targeting activities of daily living can improve performance of these activities on land (Sanders et al. 1997; Templeton et al. 1996; Jentoft et al. 2001).

■ Interval training in the water is recommended for beginners to reduce local muscular fatigue, increase duration, and make the workout more enjoyable (Frangolias et al. 1996; Michaud et al. 1995; Quinn et al. 1994; Wilbur et al. 1995).

■ Water exercise has a greater anaerobic demand (in untrained water exercise participants) and therefore provides muscular strength and endurance training throughout the entire session (Brown et al. 1997; Evans and Cureton 1998; Frangolias and Rhodes 1995; Michaud et al. 1995; Wilbur et al. 1996).

■ Reducing the speed of movements performed in water is essential. Movements in water should be approximately one-half to one-third slower than movements on land (39% slower) for equivalent energy expenditure (Frangolias and Rhodes 1995). Allow students to adjust their speed based on their RPE (Gehring et al. 1997; Hoeger et al. 1995).

■ Once participants are trained, they can be challenged with increasing resistance just as is done in strength and conditioning programs. Equipment overload (usually provided by surface area) and speed adjustments need to be applied progressively (Mayo 2000).

for injury rehabilitation and provides a way to gradually progress to functioning on land (Sanders & Lawson 2006). From a health perspective, skills that enhance proper posture are critical to daily functioning. Many movements performed on land do not functionally train the muscles for improved posture. For example, performing supine curl-ups on land does not really prepare the abdominals to be strong in a functional, upright position—rather, these curl-ups strengthen the abdominals in a forward, flexed position. In the pool, simply walking through the natural resistance provided by water works the abdominals in the upright position and thus strengthens the abdominals specifically to

improve daily functioning (Kennedy and Sanders 1995). Performing basic locomotor patterns (i.e., walking and running) using the water's resistance enhances functionality as the body stabilizes itself against resistance, plus there is little load on the body's lower-extremity joints. Thus, water exercise provides specific resistance in an upright, functional position while at the same time unloading the musculoskeletal system (Norton et al. 1997). Finally, many land-based activities such as tai chi and Pilates can provide solace and relaxation by moving into the water (Archer 2005). Overall, water exercise is slowly moving from its traditional clients (older adults and younger adults with injuries) to newer markets that include athletes, younger adults, and mind–body enthusiasts (Vogel 2006). The main points on the group exercise class evaluation form for water exercise are listed on page 228.

PROPERTIES OF WATER

Let's examine the properties of water that make water exercise different from land exercise. Then we can move on to studying Newton's laws of motion as they apply to water. Knowing the principles that govern movement in water is important to maximizing the success of your water exercise classes.

Viscosity, or the friction between molecules, causes resistance to motion. Water is more viscous than air, just as molasses is more viscous than water (Aquatic Exercise Association 1995). Because water is more viscous than air, it provides greater resistance to motion than air provides. When you walk forward in the water, the viscosity (cohesion and adhesion of the water molecules) creates a block of water you must move with you. This block of water, often called a *drag force,* adds overload that increases energy expenditure.

Buoyancy is a force experienced in water that is analogous to experiencing the force of gravity on land. Buoyancy pushes the body upward and has the opposite effect of gravity. An object's buoyancy depends on its density relative to its size; the relative density of an object determines whether it will sink or float (Bates and Hanson 1996). Thus body composition, because it affects body density, affects a participant's buoyancy. Participants with greater amounts of body fat (or stored energy) have greater buoyancy. On the other hand, participants with less body fat have a greater relative density and thus are less buoyant. Leaner participants may need the assistance of buoyant devices when exercising in deep water. For example, a very lean athlete running in deep water requires a different flotation device from the one used by a female with average body fat. Buoyancy will also affect ROM when exercising in water. In an exercise such as standing hip abduction (figure 12.1), buoyancy will push the leg toward the top of the water. If the leg goes beyond the 45° ROM of the hip abductors, the quadriceps and not the

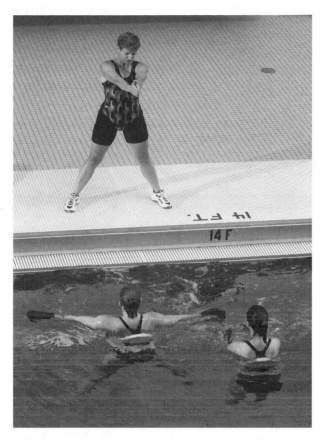

Figure 12.1 When leading participants in hip abduction, cue them to keep their ROM to 45° so they do not allow buoyancy to cause hip flexion at 90°.

hip abductors will act as the primary mover of the exercise. Thus you must keep ROM in mind when cueing your participants. In this case, you must remind your participants to keep the hip abduction movement to 45°.

Progressive resistance is created by varying speed, surface area, travel, and work against buoyancy to gradually increase muscular overload to achieve training effects. Being able to vary the plane of motion during a resistance exercise, which is difficult to do in a traditional group exercise class, is one of the most important benefits of water exercise. For example, if a participant horizontally adducts the pectoral muscles by performing a basic dumbbell fly while standing on land, gravity forces the deltoid muscles to be the prime mover (since the deltoids must work to keep the dumbbells lifted in the air). For this movement to be effective for the pectoral muscles, the participant must lie in the supine position to perform a dumbbell fly.

When the participant performs a dumbbell fly while standing in water, however, the pectorals are the prime mover because the deltoids are assisted by buoyancy. Because in water gravity does not affect the direction of resistance, you can vary movements and planes and also work in an upright functional position. In other words, water exercise allows you more options for upright overload.

A water exercise progression for the pectoral muscles is illustrated in figure 12.3. Always warm up before beginning any exercise progression series. To warm up the pectoral muscles, stand in place and horizontally adduct the shoulder joints in a relaxed fashion, using functional ROM. Then increase the speed or force of the movement, which will push the body backward. Next increase the surface area of the movement by putting on webbed gloves. Increase the speed again. Next begin to jog forward so that you are traveling against the current while performing horizontal adduction of the shoulder joint. Increase the speed of travel. Finally, suspend the body by lifting the feet off the bottom of the pool so that you must drag the surface area of the body through the water. Be sure to contract the trunk stabilizers to add more drag with the body and to stabilize against the effects of buoyancy. This resistance progression can be applied to exercises for all muscle groups.

A general understanding of Newton's laws of motion is essential for providing safe and effective water exercise instruction. Let's take a moment to review these laws while applying them to water exercise.

Creating Progressive Resistance in the Water

- Increase speed or force.
- Increase surface area.
- Increase speed even more.
- Travel against the current.
- Increase speed of travel.
- Add trunk stabilizers (suspend the move).

Inertia is described by Newton's first law of motion. Inertia is the tendency of a body to remain in a state of rest or of uniform motion until acted on by a force that changes that state. When the human body moves through water, it creates inertia currents. The movement of the water currents influences the effectiveness of an exercise. For example, running in circles in water reduces the work of moving, whereas turning around and running against the inertia currents just created increases the work. If a person stands in place in the water, there is little inertia to work against. Therefore, standing in place is less work than moving. Short travel moves such as running 10 feet (3 m) and turning around and running back for 10 feet (3 m) use the inertia currents to create overload. Have beginners do most of their exercises in place to gain balance and skill without having to deal with inertia currents. Once they progress, you can introduce movement through the water.

Acceleration is mentioned in Newton's second law of motion, which states that force equals mass times acceleration. Thus, this law tells us that speed (acceleration) can be used to create resistance overload. For example, if you want to increase intensity while walking in water, you can walk faster without changing your ROM. You will be moving the same amount of water, but it will be harder to move because you are moving faster. When you add acceleration to your moves, you gain power, because power is defined as resistance times speed. Be careful not to compromise ROM when you introduce acceleration; shortening the ROM makes the muscle movement more isometric and results in greater pain due to lack of blood flow. Using full ROM is the optimal way to train muscles.

Action and reaction are tied together in Newton's third law of motion, which states that for every action there is an equal and opposite reaction. For example, when we reach out in front with extended arms and push the water behind us, our body moves forward. The action is the arm movement and the reaction is the body movement. Use this concept to analyze what you want and what you can get out of a movement. For example, when you adduct the shoulder (a latissimus dorsi movement) in deep water, the concept of action and reaction means that your body will pull up slightly. You can use this reaction to overload the shoulder muscles instead of allowing the body to come up. By holding the body steady, you will be resisting the action and reaction law and therefore performing more work. You can do the same in shallow water by bending your knees to bring your arms beneath the water. Determine the reaction direction of the action and then work against it for overload or with it for recovery.

WARM-UP

Warming up for a water exercise class is slightly different than warming up for a land class. In water, dynamic ROM exercises replace static stretching movements. For example, in a land class, the hamstrings are warmed up and then stretched statically. In a water class, hip flexion and extension exercises both warm up and stretch the quadriceps and hamstrings because there is not any eccentric muscle contraction due to the lack of gravity. If participants are in cool water that is below 86 degrees Fahrenheit (30 degrees C), a vigorous warm-up may be appropriate to promote thermoregulation of the body. If the pool temperature is 86 degrees Fahrenheit (30 degrees C) or above, which is considered thermoneutral, it is not necessary to

move vigorously to keep the body warm. Full-ROM exercises are appropriate and encouraged in a water exercise warm-up.

Land and Water Differences

One of the reasons why exercising in water is comfortable and relatively pain free is because movement in water requires very little eccentric muscle contraction (you can, however, add equipment that requires eccentric muscle contraction). Eccentric muscle contractions are often associated with delayed onset muscle soreness (Byrnes 1985). Coupling the fact that movement in water involves predominantly concentric muscle contractions with the fact that activity in water is nonimpact in nature makes the pool a very comfortable workout environment. To become an effective instructor in water exercise, you need to understand these and other physiological implications of movement in water. Table 12.1 shows the differences between muscle contraction on land and muscle contraction in water for standing shoulder abduction and adduction.

Table 12.1 Standing Shoulder Abduction and Adduction on Land Versus in Water

Environment	Equipment	Joint action	Anterior or middle deltoid contraction	Latissimus dorsi contraction
Land	None	Shoulder abduction	Concentric	None
Land	None	Shoulder adduction	Eccentric	None
Water	None or surface area device	Shoulder abduction	Concentric	None
Water	None or surface area device	Shoulder adduction	None	Concentric
Water[a]	Buoyant device	Shoulder abduction	None	Eccentric
Water[a]	Buoyant device	Shoulder adduction	None	Concentric

Participant should stand upright, with hands at sides and feet shoulder-width apart.

[a]Slow speed to resist buoyancy.

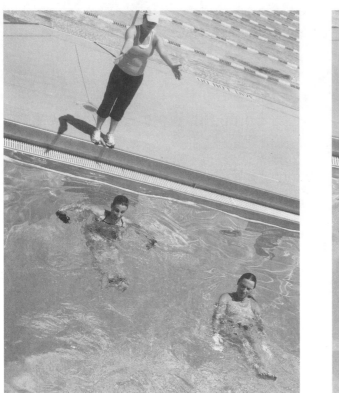
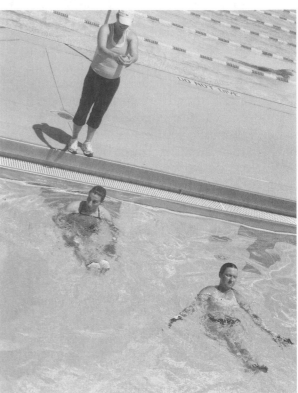

▶ **Figure 12.2** Horizontal shoulder abduction with participants using surface area devices (gloves) to increase the muscular overload.

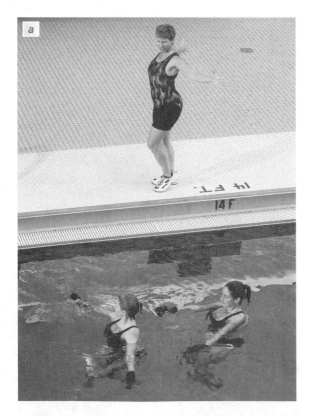
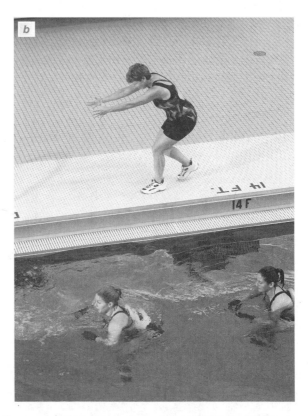

▶ **Figure 12.3** Pectoral progression: *(a)* assisting the breaststroke and *(b)* resisting the breaststroke.

Dynamic Movement and Rehearsal Moves

Following are samples of dynamic rehearsal moves that target specific muscle groups. Have participants perform each of these movements through their full ROM. Keep increases in tempo to a minimum.

Figure 12.3 shows a pectoral progression using a breaststroke. At first, the participant marks the move performing horizontal shoulder adduction in place, next the participant moves backward to assist the move (12.3a). Then, to overload the movement, the participant jogs forward to create resistance against the breaststroke (12.3b).

Figures 12.4 through 12.8 show total-body movements that can be used to thermoregulate the body by increasing core temperature through energy expenditure. In these movements, participants can travel against and then with the inertia currents.

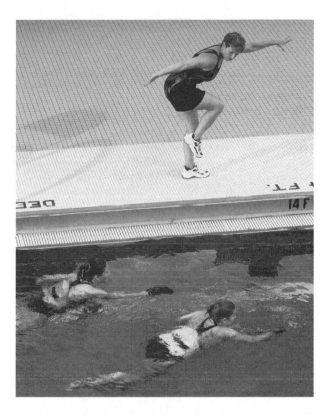

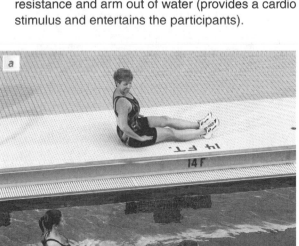

▶ **Figure 12.4** Parade wave with external resistance and arm out of water (provides a cardio stimulus and entertains the participants).

▶ **Figure 12.6** Rock climber in which resistance is created by pushing the hands down in the water (works the gluteal and triceps muscles).

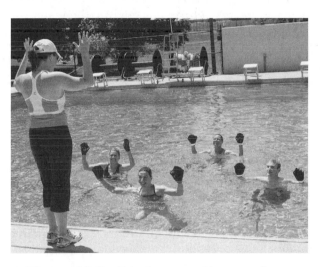

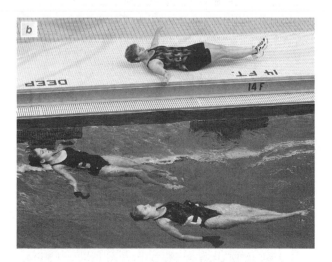

▶ **Figure 12.5** Seated flutter kick with (a) backward movement and (b) change in surface area (works the quadriceps and abdominal stabilizers).

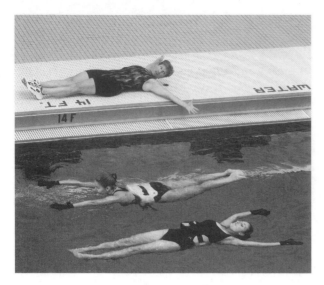

▶ **Figure 12.7** Lie supine, tuck the knees, and stretch out in a prone superman position (works the abdominal muscles).

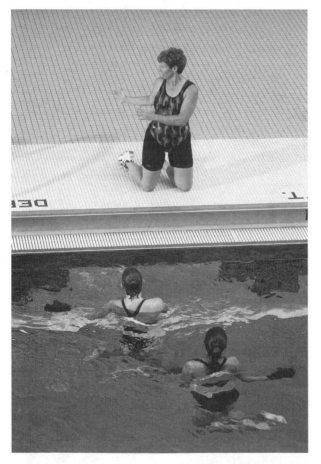

▶ **Figure 12.8** Washing machine in deep water. Use buoyant devices in shallow water (works the obliques and rotator cuff muscles).

Stretching Major Muscle Groups

Taking the muscles through their full ROM replaces static stretching in water exercise. The muscles do not have to work against gravity, and so when a muscle contracts, the opposing muscle is automatically stretched. Therefore, you do not need a stretching segment when teaching a water exercise class.

Visual Cues and Tempo

Teaching from the deck is very important in water exercise, because visual cues are as important as verbal cues. We recommend that you demonstrate all moves and allow participants to learn all moves before they get into the water. In terms of music, water exercise is a lot like indoor cycling: Use the music to set the mood and not necessarily the tempo. If you move on the beat all the time, you will not progress participants properly. Use the tempo of the music as a gauge. For example, start with the beat and then ask participants to work faster than the beat for 15 seconds.

TECHNIQUE AND SAFETY

Before teaching a water exercise class, make sure a lifeguard is present so you can focus on

---

■ Technique and Safety Check

Following are recommendations for your water exercise warm-up:

- Make sure to use appropriate speed when demonstrating movements on the deck.
- Emphasize full ROM with each movement.
- Keep participants moving and check for water temperature comfort.
- Point out individual muscle groups to the participants and use total-body movements to keep the body warm.
- Demonstrate how to use music tempo as a gauge by moving on the beat, moving faster than the beat, and moving slower than the beat.

your instruction. You cannot be responsible for both safety and instruction. However, do discuss safety issues, especially for participants who are not comfortable in the water. Believe it or not, many people cannot swim. If you are teaching in deep water, make sure the participants have their flotation devices adjusted properly. Review how each piece of equipment should be worn before starting the class. For example, there are different levels of buoyancy belts for deep water exercise. A participant who is lean needs a belt that provides more buoyancy, whereas a participant with more body fat needs less buoyancy. In fact, some participants who have a lot of stored energy (body fat) may not even need a buoyancy belt. Once the class has started, take a moment to remind participants of safety skills, especially when working in deep water. While exercising, some participants may fall forward and not be able to get their face out of the water. Others may fall backward and not be able to get their legs down. Teach recovery skills for these situations, and throughout the workout remind participants to engage their abdominal muscles to stay upright. Inform the lifeguard of any participants who are not comfortable in the water so that the lifeguard can watch them closely. Finally, if you are working in a pool that has a drop-off into deep water, be sure the lane lines separate the shallow and deep areas.

Technique and Safety Check

To help keep your water exercise classes safe, observe the following recommendations.

Remember to

- encourage full-ROM movements before speeding up,
- use different movement planes,
- encourage participants to maintain a neutral spine and neck and keep the head and eyes up,
- encourage participants to keep abdominal muscles lifted and contracted,
- strive to work all major muscle groups and identify them to participants to increase body awareness,
- make sure a lifeguard is on duty and water safety practices are introduced,
- demonstrate movements visually on deck so participants understand what to do, and
- encourage individuality and proper progression throughout the workout by allowing participants to work at their own levels.

Avoid

- following the tempo of the music for the entire class,
- speeding up your deck demonstrations to land speed, and
- getting in the water with participants before performing visual deck demonstrations.

BASIC MOVES

Understanding the basic water exercise movements will help you create your water exercise routine. There are three different water depths to teach in:

1. Deep water, in which you use a flotation device
2. Transitional water, in which your feet are on the pool floor but your lungs are submerged
3. Shallow water, in which the water depth is below the xiphoid process

When teaching in the shallow depth, there are three different ways to use the water:

1. Rebound a move and jump, which creates more impact and more intensity.
2. Stay neutral with the shoulders at the water surface and use the resistance of the water with less impact.
3. Suspend the move, which is more difficult but has the least impact.

Understanding the basic moves by muscle group will get you started on water movement combinations. The basic total-body movements are illustrated in figures 12.9 through 12.12. These movements use large muscle groups to increase energy expenditure and are also very functional. For example, the mall walk is a basic walking movement named after a popular leisure activity—shopping! Another total-body move, the cross-country skier, mimics the motion of cross-country skiing. Any time a functional movement can be brought into a water activity, participants will benefit and find that the same movement is easier to perform on land.

Basic Moves for Total-Body Conditioning

Figures 12.9 through 12.12 illustrate total-body conditioning movements that involve both the upper and lower body. These movements fit well into the muscular strengthening and cardio segments of a water workout. Use acceleration, inertia currents, and progressive resistance to challenge participants.

Basic Moves for Lower-Body Conditioning

Figures 12.13 through 12.19 demonstrate exercises that work the lower-body muscle groups—the quadriceps and hamstrings. They are isolation movements but remain a part of the cardio segment because the body must be supported while performing these isolation movements.

Basic Moves for Upper-Body Conditioning

Figure 12.20 illustrates a reverse breaststroke that works the rhomboid muscle group. At first the body is moved forward to assist the movement (figure 12.20a), and then a flutter kick with the legs is added to resist the movement (figure 12.20b). Participants should move their arms in different planes while working the pectorals or rhomboids, because multiplanar resistance is one of the advantages of water exercise. In the water, the body can move against resistance in

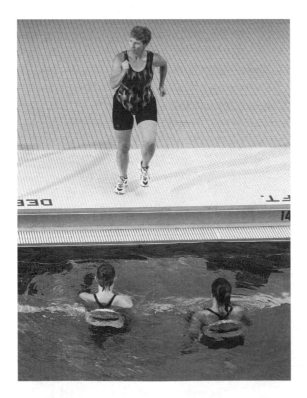

▶ **Figure 12.9** General jogging and walking (works the quadriceps, hip flexors, and hamstrings).

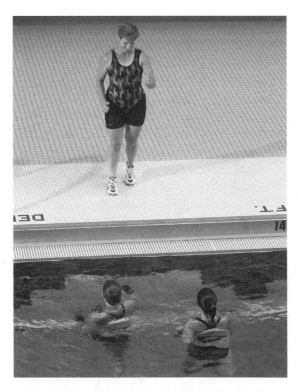

▶ **Figure 12.10** Mall walk (increases the lever length and strengthens the hip flexors).

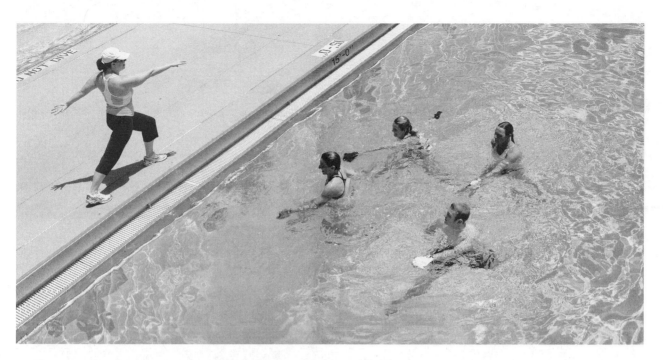

▷ **Figure 12.11** Cross-country skier (works the hip flexors, gluteal muscles, hamstrings, deltoids, and latissimi dorsi).

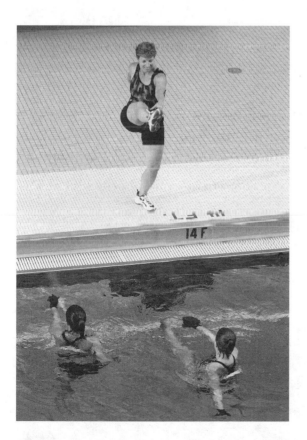

▷ **Figure 12.12** Straight-leg raise with opposite hand and foot (works the hip flexors, latissimi dorsi, and posterior deltoids).

more natural patterns, and the direction of resistance is less important than it is in land-based exercises.

Figures 12.21 and 12.22, along with figures 12.7 and 12.8 from earlier in the chapter, show different warm-up movements that can also be used as total body movements during the strength and conditioning portion of class. Figure 12.21 shows a jumping jack that uses the hip abductors, pectorals, and latissimi dorsi. Figures 12.22, 12.7, and 12.8 emphasize movements that are great for warming up the core and stabilizer muscles of the upper body. Figure 12.22 shows a move that works the abdominal muscles isometrically while the deltoids propel the body into motion. Figure 12.7 shows a movement that works the abdominal and low-back muscles through their full ROM. Finally, figure 12.8 shows how to isolate the oblique muscles in rotation. All of these exercises are excellent dynamic warm up and rehearsal moves for a water exercise class. See appendix G for a sample water exercise routine.

 See the DVD for a general overview of basic movements in water exercise.

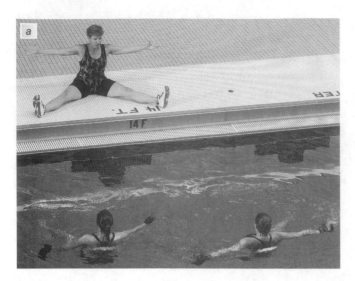
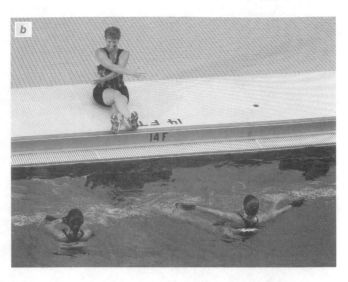

▶ **Figure 12.13** *(a)* Seated V-position with arms and legs in deep water and *(b)* a jumping jack in shallow water (work the pectorals, rhomboids, hip abductors, and adductors).

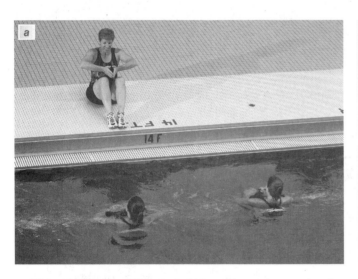
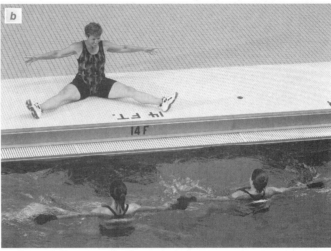

▶ **Figure 12.14** The seated V-position using pectorals and hip adductors creates *(a)* backward motion in deep water and *(b)* suspension in shallow water.

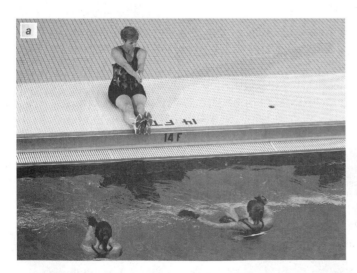
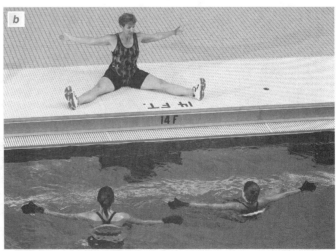

▶ **Figure 12.15** *(a)* The seated V-position using rhomboids and hip abductors creates motion in deep water and suspension in shallow water. *(b)* While sitting, retract the shoulder blades with a long-lever arm and abduct the legs. You will travel forward (works the rhomboids and hip abductors).

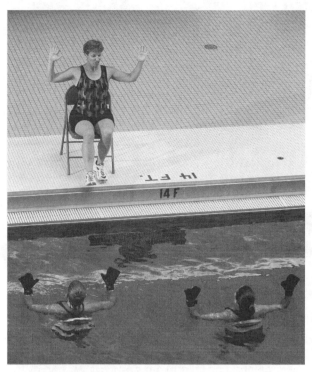

▶ **Figure 12.16** The sit kick—perform knee flexion and extension in deep water and stand on one leg in shallow water (works the quadriceps and hamstrings).

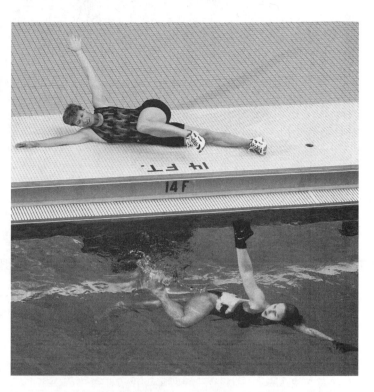

▶ **Figure 12.17** Bicycling in a circle—in deep water, keep the arms out to the side, and in shallow water, use a floatation device under the arms (works the hamstrings, gluteal muscles, quadriceps, and deltoids).

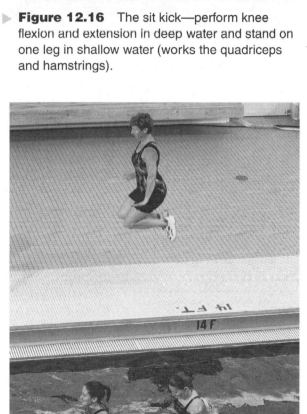

▶ **Figure 12.18** Frustrated dolphin—perform upright double-leg curls in deep water or jog backward in shallow water (works the hamstrings).

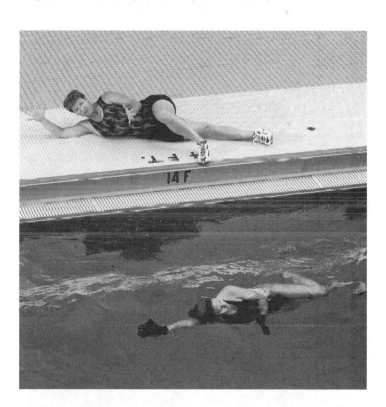

▶ **Figure 12.19** Bicycling in a circle—add overload by opening the hands while circling (works the quadriceps and hamstrings).

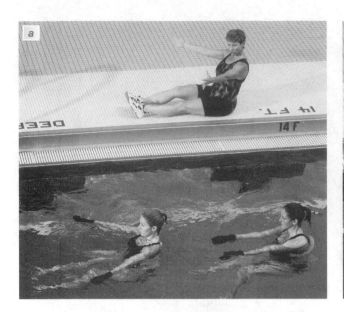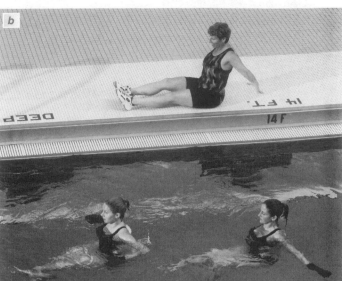

▶ **Figure 12.20** Reverse breaststroke that is *(a)* assisted by pulling the arms down and back and *(b)* resisted by kicking the legs in front (works the rhomboids and trapezius).

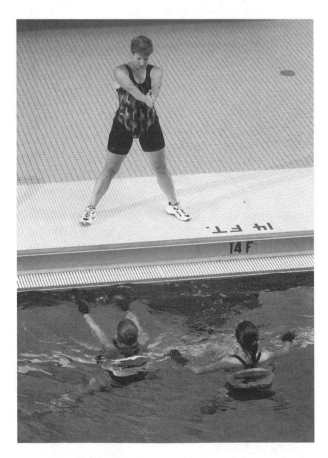

▶ **Figure 12.21** Jumping jack with the legs moving in different planes (works the hip abductors and adductors, pectorals, and latissimus dorsi).

TRAINING SYSTEMS

Because participants who are new to water exercise experience an increase in lactate that is greater than what is experienced when moving on land, we can modify the workout plan to couple interval exercise with continuous movement (Eyestone et al, 1993). Interval training in the water helps participants adapt to the increased blood lactate levels and makes the activity more enjoyable. The premise of interval training is that an individual can produce a greater amount of work if high-intensity bouts are separated by times of rest (Kravitz 1994). Many people find the resistance of the water too challenging for continuous work and so may get more out of their water exercise class through interval training. Following are terms you should know in order to understand interval training:

- **work interval**—The time of the high-intensity work effort.
- **recovery interval**—The time between work intervals. The recovery interval may consist of light activity (sculling only) or moderate activity (easy jogging).
- **work–recovery ratio**—The time ratio of the work and recovery intervals. A work–recovery ratio of 1:3 means that the

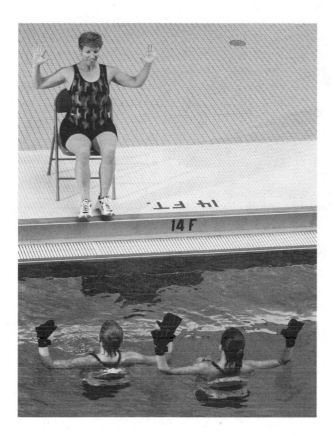

▷ **Figure 12.22** The professional sitter or "mall walk" (works the abdominal stabilizers, deltoids, and hip flexors).

Benefits of Interval Training

- Increased enjoyment due to added variety
- Potential for greater total work in a shorter amount of time
- Improved anaerobic and aerobic power and capacity
- Potential for fewer injuries and less participant burnout
- Increased adherence to exercise

Do not perform interval training during the entire time of your group exercise class. Rather, insert smaller segments of interval training when you can. A sample series of interval training in the water is outlined in table 12.2.

EQUIPMENT

Once participants have been involved in a water exercise class for 6 to 8 weeks, they will adapt to the resistance of the water, and eventually they will need to use equipment to overload the muscles. There are several types of overload devices available. In this section, we discuss surface area devices and buoyancy devices. Using buoyancy devices over long durations and for full-body support (without a belt) can be detrimental to the shoulders when working in deep water because buoyancy assists the deltoids and thus pulls the shoulder joint into a horizontal position. These devices are best used in shallow water, where they are less burdensome to the shoulder joint. Figure 12.23 shows examples of buoyancy devices. Surface area devices are

recovery interval is three times as long as the work interval. An example of a 1:3 ratio is jogging 1 minute and recovering 3 minutes.

- **cycle (repetition)**—A cycle is a work interval combined with a recovery interval. Since a recovery interval follows a work interval, some resources report the number of work intervals as repetitions.

- **set**—The number of cycles performed for an exercise. A series of four work–recovery cycles makes one set of four cycles.

Table 12.2 Interval Training Series for Water Exercise

3 min	3 cycles	40 s recovery and 20 s work
3 min	3 cycles	30 s recovery and 30 s work
3 min	3 cycles	20 s recovery and 40 s work

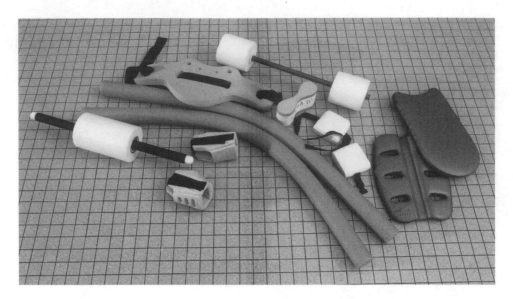

▶ **Figure 12.23** Buoyancy devices.

good in both deep and shallow water. They predominantly elicit concentric muscle contractions of the agonist and antagonist muscle groups. They also overload the movements, as they require a greater amount of water to be moved. Figure 12.24 shows examples of surface area devices.

Encourage slow speeds when working with buoyancy equipment; moving too quickly will cause the equipment to bounce right out of the water, just as a dumbbell on land falls to the ground if it is lowered too rapidly. Buoyancy devices allow eccentric muscle contractions to occur in the water. Stabilizing the core is crucial because the core serves as the base for

many exercises. Water equipment companies are beginning to develop surface area and buoyancy devices that can be individualized to the person, just as a 5-, 10-, or 15-pound (2.3, 4.5, and 6.8 kg) handheld weight can be used to individualize resistance in a land class. Check out the resource list on this page for water fitness products.

CHAPTER WRAP-UP

As exercise instructors, we need to broaden our concept of resistance training and use as many different modes as we can, especially as our participant population grows older and seeks more choices for nonimpact exercise. Water exercise is an effective form of group exercise that minimizes impact. The perception that water exercise is for older adults or people with musculoskeletal injuries has been challenged. Many forms of land-based exercise, including Pilates and tai chi, are finding success in the water. The water provides a sense of peace and relaxation that cannot be replicated on land. Plus, it brings back fond memories of leisure time spent by the pool or on the beach. Connecting leisure and exercise helps enhance long-term adherence to exercise, as it creates a sense of purpose. Use the principles of Newton's laws of motion and the multiplanar movements made possible by the resistance of water to make your class a success. Add fun and enthusiasm and you'll find that your participants repeatedly come back for more.

Water Exercise Resource List

www.sprintaquatics.com

www.aquajogger.com

www.waterfit.com

www.aquatherapeutics.com

www.fernoperformancepools.com

www.aeawave.com

www.waterart.org

www.poolates.com

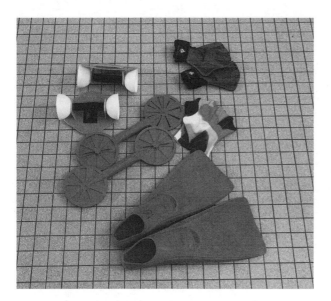

▶ **Figure 12.24** Surface area devices.

▶ **Group Exercise Class Evaluation Form Key Points**

- Include an appropriate amount of dynamic movement. Use total-body movements to get the body warmed up.

- Provide rehearsal moves. Perform 5 to 6 repetitions of moves that work the major muscle groups you will focus on during the workout, and work through the full ROM.

- Stretch the major muscle groups in a biomechanically sound manner with appropriate instructions. In water exercise, there is no static stretching in the warm-up because participants

get too cold. Dynamic, full-ROM movements provide for muscle lengthening and can replace static stretching because of the loss of gravity in water. Some static stretching can be performed at the end of the workout in shallow water or in deep water with a ledge but is not required.

- Give clear cues and verbal directions. Use at least one posture cue when introducing a new movement. Because water speed needs to be one-half to one-third of land speed, slow down all demonstrations of movements on the deck so that they match their speed in the water.

- Use a variety of water exercise techniques. Use the properties of water and Newton's laws to evaluate the effectiveness of movements.

- Gradually decrease the intensity during the cool-down following the cardiorespiratory session. Once you have relaxed and stretched, spend a few minutes in total-body movements to rewarm the body before getting out of the pool—if you are in cool water. If the water is warm, concentrate on relaxation and visualization.

- Use music appropriately. Use motivating music that fits the segment and mood. Following the beat the entire time does not allow for individualization of exercises.

▶ **Assignment**

Attend a group water exercise class. Identify two properties of water and two of Newton's laws of motion you see at work in the class. Write down 10 motivational cues you observe being used in the class. Type a one-page (double-spaced) paper on your observations.

Yoga

CHAPTER OBJECTIVES

By the end of this chapter, you will

- be able to describe the basic philosophy of yoga;
- understand how to begin a yoga class;
- be able to teach basic yoga postures and make proper alignment, technique, and safety suggestions; and
- be able to design a short yoga routine for beginners.

The 5,000-year-old discipline of yoga continues to grow in popularity in most health and fitness settings. The 2007 IDEA Health and Fitness Association Programs and Equipment Survey found that 56% of program directors offer yoga classes in their facility, and together with Pilates classes, yoga classes average 13 sessions per week (Schroeder and Friesen 2007). Learning to teach yoga can be rewarding, can increase your income and career opportunities, and can contribute to your personal growth.

Since yoga is a unique and comprehensive philosophy, encompassing a system of physical movements that differs from systems used in traditional physical fitness, we recommend that you become trained and certified specifically to teach yoga before you begin to lead yoga classes. This chapter is intended to provide an introduction to the basic philosophy, types, and styles of yoga, as well as present a basic yoga routine, complete with postures, alignment information, and breath work. Again, since yoga provides such an ancient, yet deep and profound approach to living and being, we strongly recommend extensive additional training. For information on yoga training and certification, see the list of yoga web sites on page 250.

Group Exercise Class Evaluation Form Essentials

Key Points for the Warm-Up Segment

- Includes appropriate amount of dynamic movement
- Gives clear cues and verbal directions
- Uses an appropriate music selection

■ Background Check

Before working your way through this chapter, you should do the following:

Read

- chapter 7 on muscular conditioning and flexibility training.

PHILOSOPHY OF YOGA

Yoga is not just a system of exercise or stretching, as is sometimes thought in the West. Rather, it is a complete system for living. Yoga can be an ideal way to improve quality of life, as it enhances both physical and psychological well-being. The word *yoga* means to unite, or to yoke together, the mind, body, and spirit; ancient Indian sages (India is the land of yoga's origin) believed that to be whole and fully alive, a person must develop the most vital body, mind, and spirit possible. The practice of yoga encompasses a physical discipline (known as *hatha yoga*) as well as breath work, meditation, positive thinking, healthy diet, and service to others. Ultimately, yoga is intended to be a foundation for self-realization. Yoga is sometimes called the *discipline of conscious living*, as it aims to teach its practitioners that every moment is an opportunity to be deeply present, real, kind, and true. Practicing yoga on a regular basis can help you experience a deep inner stillness and to know joy, bliss, and the truth of who you are. This is why in the Kripalu yoga tradition, yoga is called *the practice of being present* (Faulds 2006).

Five principles govern the practice of yoga:

1. Proper relaxation, which releases muscle tension, conserves energy, and helps release worries and fears.
2. Proper exercise, including the use of yoga postures (known as *asanas*), which systematically aligns and balances all parts of the body to promote strength and flexibility of the muscles and to improve the health of the internal organs.
3. Proper breathing (known as *Pranayama*), which increases the intake of oxygen, recharges the body, and improves mental and emotional well-being. Breath work is said to be the link between mind and body.
4. Proper diet, which in yoga is based on natural whole foods and is well-balanced and nutritious. According to yogic wisdom, a proper diet keeps the body light and supple and the mind calm, increasing resistance to disease.

5. Positive thinking and meditation, which are essential in removing negative thoughts, quieting the mind, and promoting inner stillness.

Aside from the more familiar physical practice of yoga (known as *hatha yoga*), other branches of yoga exist and include the following:

- Raja (royal) yoga. Practitioners on this path focus on self-restraint, moral discipline, concentration, and meditation.
- Karma yoga. A person practicing karma yoga seeks self-transcendence and spiritual freedom by serving others.
- Jnana yoga. Jnana yoga encompasses the

Hatha Yoga Classes

Healing and Restorative

- Excellent for special needs (colds, headaches, indigestion)
- Passive, soothing, nurturing approach
- Utilizes many resting postures
- Often incorporates props
- Involves practice of self-care
- Creates sensitivity to body's needs and inner wisdom
- Appropriate for all fitness levels

Gentle

- More pose (asana) driven than restorative yoga
- Involves relatively easy, basic postures
- Focuses more on flexibility than on muscular strength or endurance
- Provides many opportunities for rest in between poses

Moderate

- Combines basic and moderate poses
- May be organized into a flow routine
- May require significant muscle strength and endurance as well as balance and flexibility
- More driven by form and alignment
- Provides less opportunity for resting between poses

Power

- Organizes poses into a more specific pattern, or flow
- Movement is mostly continuous, with some holding of more difficult postures
- Requires muscular strength, endurance, flexibility, and balance
- Provides very little rest until the final relaxation

Ashtanga

- Very vigorous and athletic
- Transition between postures involves some jumping
- Uses many difficult, strenuous, and advanced poses
- Organizes poses into specific patterns, or forms
- Provides no rest until the final relaxation

Yoga Web Sites

www.yogaresearchsociety.com

www.iayt.org

www.yrec.org

www.iynaus.org

www.kripalu.org

www.yogajournal.com

www.yogateachersassoc.org

www.sivananda.org

www.anusara.com

www.ashtanga.net

www.yogafit.com

www.yogaalliance.com

www.yogilates.com

practice of discernment and wisdom and is said to be the path of the sage.

- Tantra yoga. Practitioners seek self-transcendence through tantra yoga, which is a more ceremonial form of yoga practice.
- Bhakti yoga. Bhakti yoga is said to be the path of love or of having an open heart.

In the West, hatha yoga is by far the most familiar form of yoga. The types of hatha yoga classes that are commonly available in fitness and health clubs are listed and described on page 249. This list of hatha yoga classes is organized on a continuum from the easiest to the most difficult class to perform physically.

Additionally, various styles, also known as *schools* or *traditions*, of yoga have evolved, often around the teachings of a particular guru, or teacher. Popular styles in the West include Iyengar, Bikram, viniyoga, Jivamukti, Kripalu, Sivananda, and Anusara.

A very popular trend in the United States is the yoga fusion class. The most common fusion styles are fitness and yoga (check out www.yogafit.com) and Pilates and yoga (check out www.yogilates.com). Other creative instructors have combined yoga with Spinning, t'ai chi, and step. One of the main benefits of a fusion class is that it introduces yoga to participants who otherwise might not try yoga; on the other hand, yoga purists may be put off by such a class.

BREATH WORK IN YOGA

Many yoga experts believe that breath work is the single most important component of a yoga practice. It is thought that the breath carries *prana* (the Sanskrit word for *life force*), and so the term *Pranayama,* loosely translated as *breath work,* may also be thought of as "life force (life energy) work." Not only does our physical life depend on our breath, but breath is also associated with our emotions and our mind. The breath speeds up when you are excited or nervous and grows shallow when you are experiencing stress. On the other hand, relaxation and peace can be created through deep, slow, relaxed breathing. Ancient yogis realized that by controlling the breath they could affect their minds, emotions, and bodies, and thus breath work remains a crucial component of yoga today.

Most yoga classes begin with some focused breathwork, or Pranayama, and students are reminded to deepen the breath throughout class. Most yoga flows, or routines, are designed to flow with the natural rhythm of the breath, with each move consciously occurring on either an inhale or an exhale so that breath and movement become one. Staying mindful of the breath is a powerful way to stay focused on the present moment; if the mind projects into the future or rehashes experiences from the past, students can be instructed to gently bring it back to the present by concentrating on the sensations and sounds of their own breathing.

The basic abdominal, or diaphragmatic, breath is the foundation of all yogic breathing. Everyone breathes abdominally during deep, restful sleep, but many people forget how to breathe abdominally during waking hours; instead they habitually perform shallow chest breathing. One of the best things you can do when teaching a yoga class (indeed, when teaching any class) is to help your students relearn to breathe diaphragmatically. During the inhale, the diaphragm drops down to allow the lungs to inflate; this causes a displacement of the internal organs, which relax outward.

Thus, the abdomen moves *out* on the inhale. During the exhale, the diaphragm pulls upward, forcing air out of the lungs, and the internal organs move back toward the spine. Thus the abdomen moves *in* on the exhale (see figure 13.1).

Another type of breath in yoga is the Ujjayi breath, known variously as the *ocean-sounding breath* or the *victory breath*. While this breath is very similar to the abdominal breath described above, both the inhale and the exhale are accompanied by an audible sound even though the lips are closed. The sound made on the exhale is very much like a soft, breathy, prolonged sigh; the same breathy sound is also produced while inhaling. The overall effect is somewhat like the sound of ocean waves going in and rushing out. Once this breath is mastered, most people find it very relaxing, deeply soothing, and peaceful.

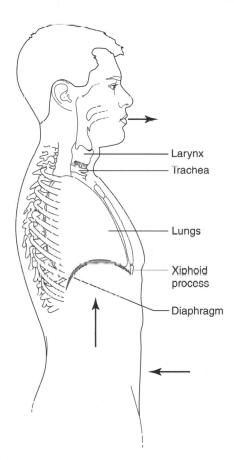

▶ **Figure 13.1** Basic abdominal breathing. The diaphragm relaxes downward and the abdomen relaxes out during inhalation, and the diaphragm pulls upward and the abdomen pulls in during exhalation.

Larynx
Trachea

Lungs

Xiphoid process

Diaphragm

■ Practice Drill

Sit comfortably on the floor or in a chair; make sure your spine is straight. Place one hand on your chest and the other hand on your abdomen. Breathe normally in and out through your nose (keep your mouth closed) and notice which hand moves the most. Gradually deepen each inhale, allowing the hand on your abdomen to have the most movement, while exaggerating and lengthening each exhale.

A primary purpose of this breath is to help focus the mind; it is hard for your mind to race all over the place if you are concentrating on making the Ujjayi sound.

Integral to yoga is the concept of connecting the breath to various movements. Certain moves are always performed on an inhale, while others are done on an exhale. For example, exhaling while forward bending or flexing the spine feels natural since the abdomen pulls in during the exhale, facilitating spinal and trunk flexion. Likewise, spinal extension and backward bending work best while inhaling (see figure 13.2).

WARM-UP

The warm-up in yoga varies depending on the type of class being offered. Almost all yoga classes begin with breathing, Pranayama, centering, or meditation. In an Ashtanga, or a power-oriented yoga class, the initial breathing and centering is traditionally followed by a series of dynamic moves known as the *Sun Salutation*. This Sun Salutation may be repeated numerous times and serves to increase core temperature. In a restorative or gentle yoga class, the warm-up often starts with Pranayama or meditation and then continues with gentle limbering movements such as seated sun breaths, seated side bends, and cat tilts and dog tilts on hands and knees. Many yoga instructors blend techniques from the two types of classes, so that the general warm-up flow may be as follows: breathing, Pranayama, meditation, sun breaths, cat tilts and dog tilts, other limbering moves on hands and knees, downward dog and/or standing forward bend, and then Sun Salutations.

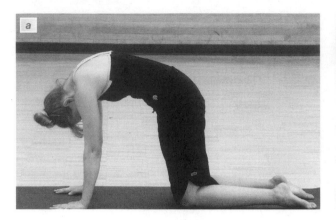
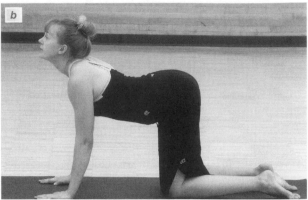

▶ **Figure 13.2** Breathing with movement in the all-fours position: *(a)* spinal flexion on the exhale and *(b)* spinal extension on the inhale.

■ Practice Drill

On your hands and knees, gently and slowly move back and forth through spinal flexion and extension, synchronizing your breath with your movement. Exhale when your head and tailbone are down (spinal flexion) and inhale when your head and tailbone are up (spinal extension). Adjust the speed of your movements to your breathing rate.

The Sun Salutation (known as *Surya Namaskar* in Sanskrit) is a graceful flow of 12 postures. It is intended to be performed without stopping, and the student should alternate inhaling and exhaling on each posture. There are two main ways to perform the basic Sun Salutation (see table 13.1).

 See the DVD for a sample yoga warm-up.

Yoga Research Findings

The benefits of yoga have long been promoted in ancient texts and today are touted by current authors and yoga instructors. These benefits include enhanced physical and physiological fitness, improvements in psychological parameters such as decreased stress and depression, and increased spiritual well-being (this may include increased feelings of peacefulness, compassion, and a sense of oneness with all beings).

Let's examine the scientific evidence on the benefits of yoga. Yoga's influence on physical and physiological fitness has been studied relatively thoroughly, especially in India. A number of very large literature reviews are available, most notably the 2004 literature review conducted by the International Association of Yoga Therapists, which listed hundreds of studies (Lamb 2004). Here are some selected findings reported in these reviews:

■ In a study commissioned by ACE, researchers Porcari and Boehde (2005) found that 50 minutes of power yoga burned approximately 237 calories and elevated participants' heart rates to 62% of HRmax. Posttest measures showed that study participants increased flexibility, balance, and muscular strength and endurance (abdominal and chest).

- A study at Adelphi University found that the metabolic demand (energy cost) of Ashtanga yoga was similar to that of moderate-intensity aerobic dance or walking (Carroll et al. 2003).
- A study by Tran and colleagues (2001) measured improvements in muscle strength, endurance, flexibility, cardiorespiratory fitness, body composition, and lung function after an 8-week training study in which subjects participated in yoga classes two times per week.
- Kristal and coworkers (2005) found that practicing yoga on a regular basis helped study participants maintain or lose weight throughout the midlife years. Since yoga does not burn a high number of calories per session, researchers surmised that the benefit resulted from the increased mindfulness and body awareness of the participants, which led them to make better choices in food quality and quantity.

Yoga has been studied extensively as a therapeutic intervention for a variety of diseases and disorders. Numerous studies have examined yoga's effect on cardiovascular disease (including hypertension and regression of atherosclerosis), respiratory disorders (especially asthma), metabolic disorders (e.g., diabetes), and neurological, musculoskeletal, and psychological problems. Selected findings from a large literature review conducted by Khalsa (2004) include the following:

- Yoga has been found to be an effective modality for relieving low-back pain. For example, a 12-week therapeutically oriented viniyoga program was found to be more effective than conventional group exercise or a self-help program for improving back function and reducing chronic low-back pain (Sherman 2005).

Many other studies have also shown improvements in low-back pain with yoga (Galantino et al. 2004; Jacobs et al. 2004; Williams et al. 2003; Williams et al. 2005).

- Yogic breathing exercises improved asthma symptoms in study subjects (Cooper et al. 2003).
- An 8-day yoga program lowered low-density lipoprotein (LDL) cholesterol and reduced risk factors for coronary heart disease and diabetes (Bijlani 2005). A landmark study in 1990 showed that a program that included yoga and other lifestyle changes could reverse coronary heart disease (Ornish et al. 1990).

One of the hallmarks of yoga is its ability to induce the relaxation response. This relaxed mental state is helpful in therapeutic settings; in fact, yoga therapists specialize in helping patients recover from trauma, depression, anxiety, and other types of psychological stress. Many studies have examined yoga's beneficial effects on psychological health (Arpita 1990; Lamb 2004; Khalsa 2004).

Some researchers have even attempted to identify yoga's influence on spiritual health. Spiritual wellness has been described as "a high level of faith, hope, and commitment in relation to a well-defined world view or belief system that provides a sense of meaning and purpose to existence in general and that offers an ethical path to personal connectedness with self, others, and a higher power or larger reality" (Hawks et al. 1995). One study found that spirituality increased in cardiac patients who attended a yoga and meditation retreat (Kennedy et al. 2002). Questionnaires given before and after the retreat demonstrated that after the retreat participants experienced an increased sense of connection with others, an increased awareness of an inner source of strength and guidance, an increased desire to achieve higher consciousness, and an increased confidence in their ability to handle problems.

In short, yoga has been repeatedly shown to improve not only important fitness parameters but also overall health and well-being.

Table 13.1 Sun Salutation Variations

Step	Sun salutation #1	Sun salutation #2
1	Mountain pose, prayer position (exhale)	Mountain pose, arms overhead (inhale)
2	Mountain pose, arms overhead (inhale)	Forward bend (exhale)
3	Forward bend (exhale)	Monkey pose, head up (inhale)
4	Lunge, right foot back, head up (inhale)	Forward bend (exhale)
5	Plank position (retain the breath)	Plank (inhale)
6	Chaturanga dandasana (exhale)	Chaturanga dandasana (exhale)
7	Upward-facing dog (inhale)	Upward-facing dog (inhale)
8	Downward-facing dog (exhale)	Downward-facing dog (exhale)
9	Lunge, left foot back (inhale)	Monkey pose (inhale)
10	Forward bend (exhale)	Forward bend (exhale)
11	Mountain pose, arms overhead (inhale)	Mountain pose, arms overhead (inhale)
12	Mountain pose, arms at sides (exhale)	Mountain pose, prayer position (exhale)

Both Sun Salutation variations involve a number of harder stretches (e.g., the standing forward bend, downward-facing dog, and upward-facing dog) as well as the plank and chaturanga dandasana, which are strength moves. The fact that more difficult stretches and strength moves are part of the traditional Sun Salutation means that this flow may be problematic for beginners and for participants with special conditions such as low-back pain. When leading such participants, instructors should provide plenty of modifications for the poses of the Sun Salutation or substitute a gentler warm-up.

The following is a simple warm-up flow that does not incorporate the Sun Salutation:

1. Sit in cross-legged easy pose for deep breathing, Pranayama, and/or meditation.

2. Perform three sun breaths (inhale, arms up; exhale, arms down) in this position.

3. Continue with three side stretches. Lift the right arm up on the inhale and lower it on the exhale. Repeat the three stretches with the left arm.

4. Gently twist to the right on an exhale, keeping the spine straight. Inhale and return to center. Twist to the left, exhaling.

5. Remain sitting and stretch the legs straight out in front. Circle the ankles three times in one direction followed by three times in the other. Dorsiflex the ankles, pressing heels away; then press the balls of the feet away. Finish by pointing the toes (plantar flexion). Repeat.

6. Move to hands and knees. Exhaling, flex the spine into the cat stretch, head and tailbone down. Gently and mindfully inhale and extend the spine into the dog tilt, head and tailbone up. Repeat 3 to 5 times, noticing all sensations.

7. Remain on hands and knees and place the spine in neutral, abdominal muscles lifted. Curve the spine to the right (lateral flexion), exhaling. Inhale and return to center. Exhale and curve the spine to the left. Repeat.

8. If comfortable, gently circle the pelvis, allowing the spine to move in all directions; allow the head to move freely.

9. Return to neutral spine and extend the right leg behind, toes curled under on the floor. Gently press the heel backward, feeling a comfortable stretch in the calf muscles. Breathe. Repeat with the left leg.

In this type of warm-up, a primary purpose is to connect mind, body, and spirit, or breath. Participants are encouraged to move in ways that feel best to their bodies in the moment; maintaining an ideal alignment is not the goal here. If students find a particular move uncomfortable, you should prompt them to avoid or modify that move. The goal is to find positions and movements that feel especially good and that help to relieve tension and stress.

VERBAL CUES AND MUSIC

There are several types of cues that may be used when teaching yoga. Generally, yoga instructors try to speak in a soft, calm tone and utilize what may be called "suggestions" instead of direct commands. For example, instead of saying, "Stand tall, shoulders down, chest up, abdominals in, knees soft," a yoga teacher might say, "Lifting the crown of your head up, allow your shoulders to feel heavy. Expand and open your heart while scooping the abdominals in and softening your knees." Imagery cues help participants connect with their bodies, their environment, and their spiritual nature. For example, an instructor may guide participants through the Mountain Pose (Tadasana) by saying, "Feel the soles of your feet pressing down into the earth, and lengthen the crown of your head up to the heavens. Allow your body to be the connection between heaven and earth." Cues that create imagery and cues that help participants develop an inward meditative focus are hallmarks of the yogic style of teaching. Alignment cues are also used liberally, particularly with postures that require ideal alignment to help prevent injury. In the seated forward bend (Paschimottanasana), for instance, an instructor might pause to teach participants about hinging at the hips versus bending at the waist and to explain that hinging from the hip when bending forward helps keep the spine in neutral and reduces the strain on the low back. Many other alignment cues could be given for the head, neck, shoulders, knees, and feet.

Music varies in a yoga class, depending on the style or particular class segment. During the rigorous, repetitive sequences of a power-type class, world ethnic music (often with drums) is frequently used as background, although there is no movement on the beat. During the more introspective opening and ending segments of class, music is soft, soothing, and meditative. Alternatively, some yoga instructors teach part

Common Types of Yoga Cues

Alignment Cues

Example (for the standing position): "Press your shoulders down, away from your ears."

Breathing Cues

Example (for the prone position): "Feel your back rising and falling and your ribs expanding with each breath."

Educational/Informational Cues

Example (for the modified cobra pose): "This is a great posture for helping to counter the force of gravity, which tends to pull us forward, creating rounded shoulders and a hunched back."

Safety Cues

Example (for Utkatasana or chair pose): "Avoid dropping your hips below your knees, as this increases the pressure on your kneecaps and can lead to knee injuries."

Visualization/Image Cues

Example (for a standing or sitting position): "Feel a spiral of energy moving up the spine."

Affirmational Cues

Example (for a seated forward bend): "I am releasing all tension; I am letting go."

Inward Focus and Spiritual Transformation Cues

Example (for the resting or corpse pose): "Resting in the vastness of Being, I surrender to my Higher Self."

Visual Cues

Example: Instructor places a hand over the crown of the head and lifts it up, indicating that participants should lengthen the spine, stand tall, and elevate the crown of the head.

Music Reference List

www.gaiam.com

www.powermusic.com

www.shantiommusic.com

www.spiritvoyage.com

www.yoga.com

---

or all of the class without music. The music reference list on this page lists good Web sites for finding yoga music.

TECHNIQUE AND SAFETY

Because yoga postures, or asanas, range from the very safe and gentle all the way to the extremely difficult and controversial, instructors need to have a thorough understanding of common mechanisms of injury to the major joints so they can make educated choices about what to include in their class. Furthermore, a specific posture may have many modifications, ranging from very easy to very hard, from which instructors must choose when designing their class. We have developed a good model for the concept of progression: the progressive functional training continuum. This model is detailed in our book *Functional Exercise Progressions* (Yoke and Kennedy 2004) and shown on page 40 in chapter 3.

For an example of the functional exercise progression continuum at work, let's examine the cobra pose, or Bhujangasana. You can see in figure 13.3 that as the variations of this pose progress across the continuum from easiest to hardest, spinal ROM increases dramatically and greater and greater amounts of strength are required of the spinal extensors and triceps. The more extreme versions of the cobra pose increase the risk of injury for all but the most advanced, flexible, strong, and adept practitioners of yoga. Therefore, you should not lead the majority of your students through the hardest versions of the cobra; instead, you should be familiar with the easier and safer modifications.

The language, or vocabulary, of yoga includes many difficult postures and positions. In fact, the pretzel-type positions are probably what most people picture in their minds when they think of yoga. However, these more difficult postures are intended to be the result of years of diligent practice; they are at the end of the progression, not the beginning. Difficult postures are for long-term yoga practitioners who have high levels of muscle strength, endurance, flexibility, and balance. Table 13.2 lists some of the more problematic yoga postures and their potential mechanisms of injury.

All the postures listed in table 13.2 can be modified to minimize their injury potential. Before leading participants through these types of postures, the class instructor should provide safety information and cues for modification. For example, when teaching the standing forward bend (Uttanasana), you could suggest that participants start with a yoga block, which shortens the distance between the hands and the floor. By using a yoga block, participants who are too inflexible to place their hands on the floor are still supported (with hands on the block), and their back is therefore protected. A yoga block can be placed vertically, on its side, or flat to match the participant's flexibility. You can suggest that participants keep the block nearby so

---

■ Technique and Safety Check

To help keep your yoga classes safe, observe the following recommendations:

- Provide an appropriate warm-up.
- Encourage participants to listen to their bodies and only do postures in ways that feel appropriate.
- Provide plenty of modifications and show ways to make a pose easier.
- Avoid high-risk, advanced, or controversial postures.
- Give plenty of alignment cues in traditional postures and in classes that are alignment driven.
- Help participants integrate mind, body, and spirit by giving frequent reminders about breathing.

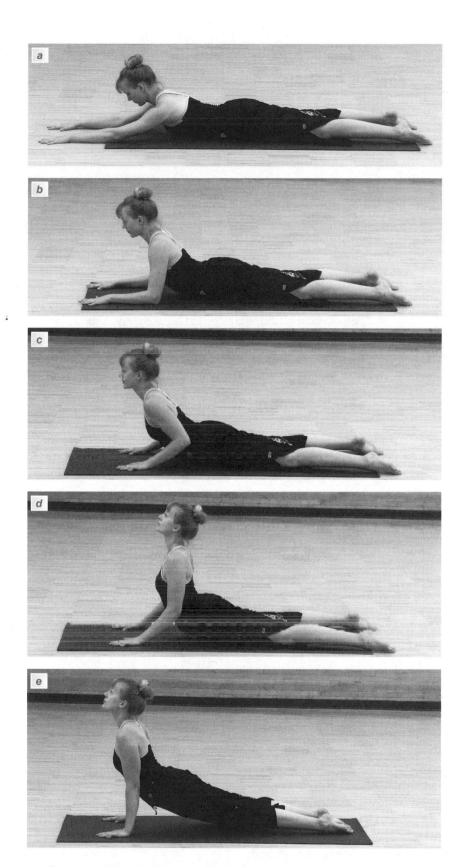

▶ **Figure 13.3** The functional exercise progression continuum for the cobra pose: *(a)* baby cobra, *(b)* sphinx, *(c)* partial cobra, *(d)* full cobra, *(e)* upward-facing dog, and cobra with feet on head.

Table 13.2 Problematic Yoga Postures and Their Potential Mechanisms of Injury

Joint	Posture (asana)	Mechanism of injury
Shoulder	Chaturanga dandasana	Hyperextension of shoulder in a weight-bearing position results in a dislocation force.
	Prayer position, hands behind back	Extreme shoulder internal rotation and overstretch of external rotator cuff muscles.
Cervical spine	Plow pose and shoulder stand	Weight bearing on hyperflexed cervical spine may cause vertebral fracture, nerve impingement, and occlusion of blood vessels; position increases cranial blood pressure and pressure in the eyes.
Lumbar spine	Standing forward bend (if participant is too inflexible to place hands on floor)	Unsupported spinal flexion overstretches the long ligaments of the spine, leading to spinal instability.
	Seated forward bend with hands in air (especially if participant is unable to hinge at the hips)	Unsupported spinal flexion overstretches the long ligaments of the spine, leading to spinal instability.
	Standing forward bend with twist (if participant is too inflexible to place hands on floor)	Unsupported spinal flexion with rotation may cause tearing in the annulus fibrosis of the disks, leading to disk herniation.
	Crescent moon pose	Unsupported lateral spinal flexion overstretches the long ligaments of the spine, leading to spinal instability.
	Upward-facing dog and full cobra pose	Extreme lumbar hyperextension overstretches the long ligaments of the spine, leading to spinal instability.
	Boat pose (V-sit)	Long-lever traction creates a shearing force on the vertebrae of the lumbar spine.
Knee	Deep squats (e.g., malasana)	Hyperflexion in a weight-bearing position places large shearing forces on the knee joint, leading to knee instability and excess compression of the knee cartilage.
	Hero pose, lotus pose, pigeon pose	Knee torque overstretches the ligaments of the knee, leading to knee instability.

they can use it whenever they are performing a standing forward bend. If several inflexible participants are in your class, it is helpful if you also use a yoga block in your demonstration of standing forward bends.

Note that during the Sun Salutation, the spine is at increased risk whenever the practitioner moves back and forth between the standing Mountain Pose (Tadasana) and the standing forward bend (Uttanasana). A teacher concerned about safety might instruct participants to keep their hands at their sides (as opposed to overhead) while moving between the two postures

or to place their hands on their thighs for support while lowering into or lifting out of the forward bend. We strongly recommend that you get competent instruction in yoga safety before becoming a yoga teacher.

BASIC MOVES

Yoga postures, or asanas, can be divided into the following categories: standing postures, backward-bending postures, forward-bending postures, twisting postures, and inverted postures. Also, a relaxation pose is always provided at the end of class. In the following sections, we will discuss a few of these postures; for more instruction, please attend a yoga teacher training course.

 See the DVD for a brief demonstration of common standing and back-bending yoga postures.

Standing Postures

Standing postures are ideal for teaching proper alignment. They also help develop balance and lower-body strength.

Mountain Pose

The mountain pose has several arm variations, including arms at the sides with fingertips actively pointing down, arms reaching straight overhead with fingertips pointing up and shoulder blades down, and hands pressed together in front of the heart in the prayer (Namaste)

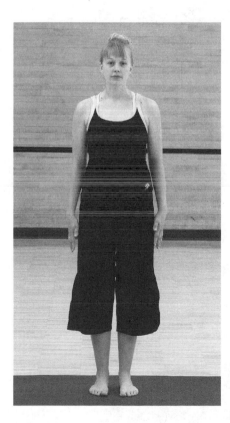

▶ **Figure 13.4** The Mountain Pose (Tadasana) is the classic standing posture from which all other standing postures are derived.

position. In all cases, cue participants to feel the oppositional energy of the pose: Parts of the body are pressing down, while parts of the body are pressing up. The mountain pose is an active, energetic posture; it is much more than mere standing in place.

Stand with feet pressed firmly into the ground, weight evenly distributed. Feet may be hip-width apart for increased stability or may be placed together, big toes touching, for an increased balance challenge. Lift the kneecaps and the thigh muscles; feel the pubic bone lifting upward while the tailbone presses downward. Lift the abdominal muscles and the rib cage. Simultaneously, feel the shoulder blades pressing down. Lengthen the neck and lift the crown of the head. Breathe deeply and fully (see figure 13.4).

Crescent Moon Pose

When teaching beginners or students with back pain, you should start with the modified version of the crescent moon pose. In the modified version, one hand remains down, pressed into the side of the body for support. Performing lateral spinal flexion in this way is safer for the lower back.

Stand in mountain pose and stretch both arms overhead. Press the palms together or interlace the fingers with the index fingers pointing up (so that hands are in steeple or temple position). Inhale and lengthen the spine, the crown of the head, and the fingers upward. Exhale and arc to one side. Imagine your body is between two panes of glass and is unable to lean forward or backward—only to the side. Inhale and lengthen to straighten up; exhale and repeat to the other side (see figure 13.5).

Warrior II Pose

This beautiful pose requires lower-body strength and endurance, particularly if it is held for any length of time. Because of its requirements, the Warrior II pose can heat and energize the body; even so, the upper body should feel calm, balanced, and at peace. This dynamic of work (lower body) and peace (upper body) helps practitioners learn to stay calm and relaxed under pressure.

Proper alignment of the front knee is critical in the Warrior II pose; remind students not to torque, or rotate, the knee. The knee should flex no more than 90°. Participants who wish

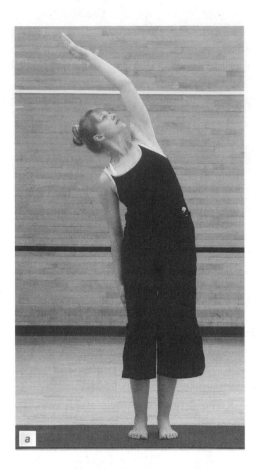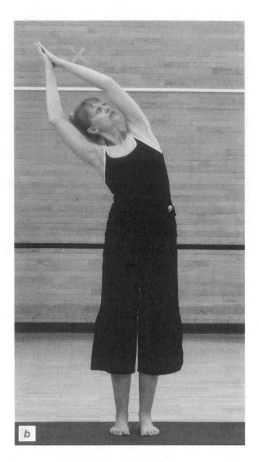

▶ **Figure 13.5** The Crescent Moon Pose (Ardha Chandrasana) *(a)* modified and *(b)* traditional versions.

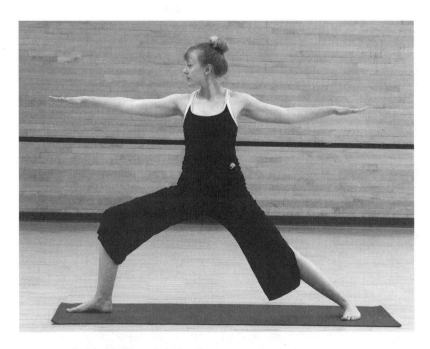

▶ **Figure 13.6** The Warrior II Pose (also known as *Peaceful Warrior* or *Virabhadrasana II*).

to progress the Warrior II pose should step the feet farther apart and bend the front knee to the full 90°. Novice practitioners may keep the feet closer together and bend the front knee less.

Step your feet wide apart and turn the left foot 90° toward the side of the room. Angle your back (right) foot slightly inward, keeping the entire foot on the floor. Bend your left knee in the direction of your second toe, and check to see that it stays straight ahead, twisting neither to the right or the left. Square your hips and torso toward the front of the room, keeping your torso perfectly upright. Straighten your arms out to the sides at shoulder height (parallel to the earth) and reach your fingertips to the sides of the room. Turn your head to the left and gaze out over your left fingers. Feel your abdominal muscles lift and contract, and lift the muscles between the legs. Feel the lines of energy radiating out from the center of the body. Hold the posture and continue to breathe comfortably (see figure 13.6).

Tree Pose

Many variations exist for the Tree Pose; they can be arranged from easiest to hardest along the progressive functional training continuum. A low to intermediate version is shown in figure 13.7. To make the tree pose easier, simply keep the toes of the nonsupport leg on or very near the ground and stand near a wall or barre for support. To make the posture more difficult, place the foot of the nonsupport leg high up on the inner thigh of the support leg, or place the nonsupport leg in a half-lotus position. Arm variations for the tree pose include holding the hands in prayer (Namaste) position in front of the heart, holding the hands in prayer position overhead, and stretching the arms up and opened out overhead.

Stand on one foot with the sole of the foot firmly rooted into the earth. Feel the line of energy from the earth lifting up and through the support leg. Bend the knee of the nonsupport leg and place the foot against your calf, turning out the knee. Engage the abdominal muscles and breathe comfortably, placing the hands in prayer (Namaste) position in front of the heart. Lift the crown of the head and feel energy spiral upward through the spine. To maintain your balance, focus your gaze on a spot directly in front of you or on the floor about 8 feet (2.4 m) in front of the body (see figure 13.7).

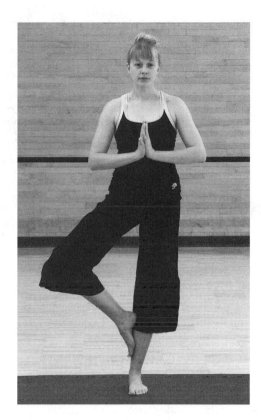

▶ **Figure 13.7** The Tree Pose (Vriksasana) is one of the many balance postures found in yoga. It not only promotes physical balance but it is said to help create a deep sense of peace and inner balance.

Backward-Bending Postures

Postures involving spinal extension and hip extension fall under the category of backward-bending postures. Back bending is very helpful in counteracting the forward pull of gravity experienced in daily living. When done regularly, backward-bending poses improve posture and help maintain a supple, youthful spine. Encourage your students to listen carefully to their bodies when performing these postures; spinal extension, particularly through a large ROM, may not be appropriate for everyone.

Cobra Pose

Perhaps the most famous of the backward-bending postures, the cobra pose is considered controversial for the general population due to its overstretching of the anterior longitudinal ligament of the spine and its potential for excessive vertebral and disk compression. As we

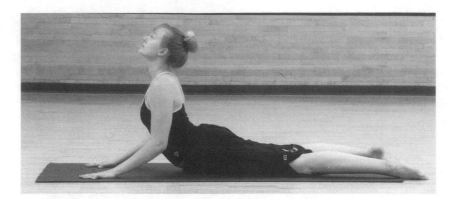

▶ **Figure 13.8** The Cobra Pose (Bhujangasana).

discussed earlier, several variations of the cobra pose exist, including safer and easier modifications (see figure 13.3).

Even though we give cues for the traditional cobra pose in the following paragraph, you should know the basic modifications, including the modified cobra or Sphinx Pose and the baby cobra. In the Sphinx Pose, the forearms are placed on the floor so that the torso is propped up on the elbows; the fingertips are spread wide. In the baby cobra, the spine is only slightly extended, with the arms either straight out in front or splayed wide with the elbows bent. Instructors should make certain to teach and demonstrate these easier modifications if novices or participants with back pain are present in the class.

Lie facedown on your mat, with your hands under your shoulders and your elbows bent. Before lifting up into the cobra pose, energize your body, feeling a line of energy running from your toes, up through your legs, up your spine and all the way to the top of your head. Lengthen and engage the leg muscles and point the toes. Press your sacrum down and slide your shoulder blades down away from your ears. Using your back muscles, raise your torso to a comfortable height, lifting and pressing the chest and heart forward. Allow your head and neck to continue the line of the spine (no cranking, or hyperextending the cervical spine). Spread the fingers wide, slightly bend the elbows, and move the shoulders away from the ears (see figure 13.8).

Prone Boat Pose

We provide cues for an easy version of the prone boat pose in the following paragraph. For an even easier version, lift only one leg and the opposite arm. To progress the pose, simply extend both arms overhead and lift both arms and legs.

Lie facedown on your mat with your arms at your sides and your palms facing down. Lengthen your entire body from head to toes, energizing your muscles. Keeping your head and neck in line with your spine, inhale and lift your upper body and legs off the floor to a comfortable height. Hold for three or more breaths, feeling the body rise and fall with each inhalation and exhalation (see figure 13.9).

Forward-Bending Postures

Commonplace in yoga, forward-bending postures can feel incredibly wonderful to advanced yoga practitioners, who find that hinging at the hips is easy due to flexible hamstring muscles. For participants with less flexibility, however, forward bending can be extremely uncomfortable and potentially injurious to the spine. For this reason, yoga instructors must provide plenty of modifications to make forward bending safer and more enjoyable for all.

 See the DVD for a brief demonstration of common forward-bending, twisting, and relaxation yoga postures.

Head-to-Knee Pose

Props can be very helpful in forward bending; you can suggest to your students that they use a strap or belt around the outstretched foot and/or a blanket or rolled towel under the edge of the buttocks. Both of these devices facilitate flexing at the hips, an important aspect of proper

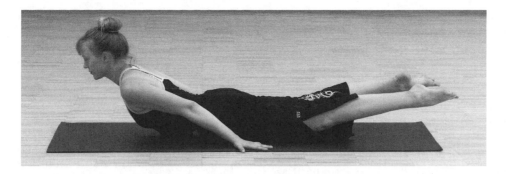

▷ **Figure 13.9** The Prone Boat Pose (Navasana), like many other prone postures, is said to help tone the internal organs as well as strengthen the spinal and hip extensors.

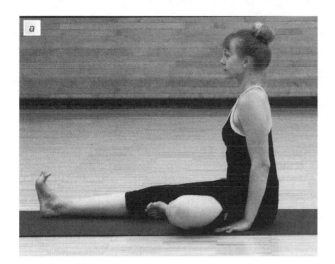

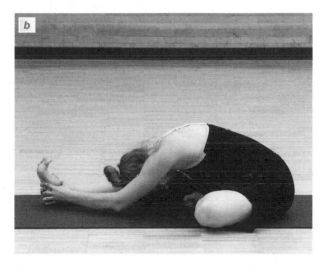

▷ **Figure 13.10** The Head-to-Knee Pose (also known as *Janusirshasana* or the seated unilateral forward bend) is generally easier than bilateral (both legs) forward bending. It provides a very deep stretch for the hamstrings as well as for the gluteus maximus, erector spinae, and calves.

alignment in forward bending. When the hips are able to flex to 90° or more, it is much more likely that the spine will remain in neutral as the practitioner fully enters the head-to-knee pose. A spine kept in or near neutral is in a safer position than one that is fully flexed (especially unsupported) due to overstretching of the posterior longitudinal ligament. When props are unavailable, participants who are unable to flex the hips at 90° and thus exhibit a hunched, flexed spine should be instructed to place their hands behind the hips to help prop the spine into a more upright and neutral position.

Sit on your mat with your right leg extended out in front and your left knee bent with the sole of the left foot pressed against the right inner thigh.

Lengthen through your right leg, feeling the line of energy pressing out through the heel (the foot is dorsiflexed). Start by sitting tall with your spine lengthened in neutral and your hips squared. Feel your weight directly above the sitting bones; your tailbone should be off the floor. Hinging from the hips, keep the waist long and lower your torso over the thigh. Place the hands wherever it feels comfortable: Place them under the calf or ankle, grasp the toes, or (if flexible enough) clasp the hands around the bottom of the foot. Alternatively, you may hold a strap placed around the bottom of the foot. Hold this pose for several breaths, inhaling and exhaling deeply. When exhaling, feel your abdominal muscles lift up against the spine; imagine letting go with each exhale (see figure 13.10).

Child's Pose

While most practitioners find the child's pose very comfortable, those with knee problems may not be able to relax fully due to the deep hyperflexion at the knee joint. Fortunately, there are modifications and props that can make the pose enjoyable for almost everyone. Allow your participants to choose whether they prefer to have the knees closer together or farther apart, depending on comfort. Placing a blanket or doubled-up mat under the knees can keep them from grinding into the floor. If deep knee hyperflexion is a problem, place a blanket or rolled-up towel behind the knee joints to decrease the knee flexion. If knee pain still persists, try placing a yoga block under the sitting bones to minimize weight bearing on the knees. Ankle pain can be eased with a rolled-up towel under the ankle joints. Several upper-body variations exist, including arms extended overhead on the floor (a great latissimus dorsi stretch), arms resting alongside the body with palms up (let the shoulder blades protract and relax), arms folded across the lower back, and hands cupping the sides of the face.

Sit back in a kneeling position with your hips resting toward your heels. Your knees can be closer together or farther apart; see what your body prefers in this moment. Allow your arms to rest alongside your body with your hands near your feet, palms up. Let your forehead rest on the mat and close your eyes. Allow your shoulder blades to feel heavy; feel them separating and relaxing toward the floor on each side. Breathe deeply and feel your back rising and falling and your ribs expanding and releasing. Let your whole body sink toward the earth. Rest in the pose for 5 to 10 breaths (see figure 13.11).

Twisting Postures

Twisting poses are asymmetrical; a spinal twist pulls one side of the body in the opposite direction from the other side of the body. To keep the spine safe, you must lengthen it before twisting. Twisting while the spine is in flexion or extension increases the risk of disk injury. On the other hand, twisting is a natural motion of the spine; moving the spine through a rotational ROM on a regular basis promotes lifelong suppleness and flexibility of the spine.

Seated Spinal Twist

The seated spinal twist can be modified by placing a blanket or rolled-up towel under the edge of the buttocks; it can be progressed by bending the extended knee around and under the body. An advanced progression involves wrapping the top arm around and through the top knee and binding the hands together behind the back.

Sit upright on your sitting bones with your right leg extended out in front, foot flexed. Cross your left leg over the right; bend your left knee and place the left foot on the floor next to your right thigh. Press your left leg in toward your torso; sit tall with your pelvis grounded and your shoulder blades pressed down. Rotate your spine to the left, crossing your right arm over

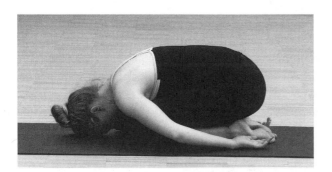

▶ **Figure 13.11** The Child's Pose (Garbasana or Balasana) is a healing posture often regarded as a blissful resting pose; it also provides a relaxing stretch for the erector spinae and gluteus maximus muscles.

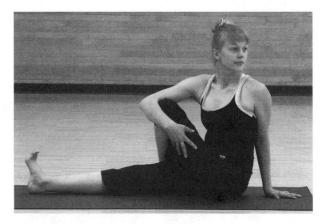

▶ **Figure 13.12** The Seated Spinal Twist (Ardha Matsyendrasana) is a multimuscle stretch. It is said to provide a gentle massage and stimulation to the digestive system.

the left knee (alternatively, you can hug the left knee with your right arm). Allow your left arm to travel behind the body; press your left palm down into the mat. Smoothly turn your head to the left and gaze over your left shoulder at the horizon, chin level. On each inhale, lift your spine higher; on each exhale, gently rotate a bit farther (see figure 13.12).

Supine Spinal Twist

The supine spinal twist is easier than the seated spinal twist. When leading this pose, let your students decide which variation they should use for the most healing effect. Variations include bending both knees to one side (knees can be up close to the armpits or far away, depending on individual comfort), crossing the top knee over the bottom knee and rolling to one side, bending the top knee to the side and keeping the bottom leg straight in line with the body, abducting the arms perpendicular to the body, placing the arms overhead, and placing one hand on the top knee.

Lie on your back and bring both knees to your chest. Gently roll both knees to the left and onto the mat. Allow your arms to open out into a T, perpendicular to your body; your palms should face up. If you like, hold your top knee with your left hand. If comfortable, turn your head to the

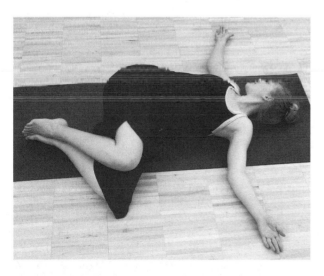

▶ **Figure 13.13** The Supine Spinal Twist (Suptaikapadaparivrttasana) is a multimuscle stretch. It is helpful for sciatic pain, as it opens up the space between the vertebrae where the sciatic nerve passes through, helping to minimize nerve impingement.

right, feeling a stretch in your hips, waist, back, and chest. Relax, breathe deeply, and allow your body to sink into the earth (see figure 13.13).

Inverted Postures

Many inverted postures exist in yoga. In fact, some experts consider a standing forward bend or a downward dog to be a mild inversion. Others consider the legs-up-the-wall pose to be a gentle modification of the shoulder stand and therefore a mild inversion. However, an inverted posture more commonly refers to poses such as the headstand, shoulder stand, plow, or handstand. Most of these postures are advanced and are beyond the scope of this text. If you wish to learn more about these postures and about yoga, please seek a qualified yoga teacher training program.

Relaxation Pose and Ending the Class

A yoga class always ends with a few moments of deep relaxation. This is the time to completely let go of all muscular tension and all cares and concerns. Yogic texts tell us that when we lie in total relaxation the benefits of the yoga class are fully integrated into the body. The traditional relaxation pose is called Savasana.

Encourage participants to get as comfortable as possible. Since they'll be lying in relaxation pose for 5 minutes or more, they may want to put socks and sweaters back on or cover themselves with a blanket. Some facilities provide eye pillows, which are small, sand-filled, scented, silk pillows especially designed to rest over closed eyes and enhance relaxation. If extra blankets are available, you may suggest that participants with back issues place a rolled-up blanket under their knees for additional comfort.

After covering yourself for warmth, lie on your back with your legs slightly apart and rolled out. Allow your arms to lie a slight distance away from your body; let your palms face up. Gently press your shoulders back and down, feeling the earth below. Let your neck lengthen and continue the line of your spine. Slightly tuck your chin. Breathing deeply and slowly, sense your muscles letting go and falling toward the earth. Let your joints relax and open and feel your breath expanding into each cell of your

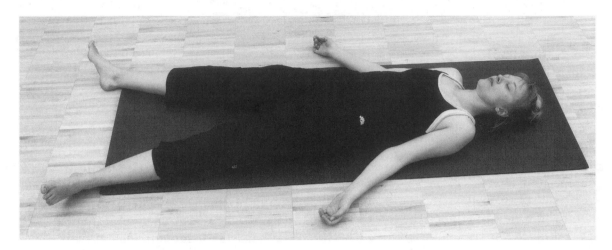

▶ **Figure 13.14** Savasana is the traditional relaxation pose.

■ Practice Drill

Using yoga music that is soft, amorphous, and relaxing or that has a gentle world beat, put together your own short combination of yoga moves, starting with an appropriate warm-up and concluding with the relaxation pose. Practice cueing the basic moves and postures in a way suitable for yoga.

body. With each exhale, let go a little more, feeling a profound peace come over your body (see figure 13.14).

After several moments, have participants roll to one side and rest for a few more breaths, and then gradually return to easy cross-legged sitting pose. It is traditional to finish a yoga class with sitting in meditation, although in many classes the instructor may read an inspirational poem or saying. Finally, the instructor may finish with "Namaste," hands pressed together in prayer position over the heart. *Namaste* is a Sanskrit word meaning, "The light within me honors the light within you." Alternatively, yoga classes may end with chanting *Om,* the sound of the universe, one, or peace.

EQUIPMENT AND CLASS SETTING

A yoga class can be taught with a minimum of equipment. All that is needed is a yoga mat (most yoga mats are relatively thin, allowing a sense of contact with the floor or earth below). However, there are many props that can enhance the yoga experience or help students attain proper alignment. These include straps, belts, ties, yoga blocks, towels, eye pillows, sandbags, and blankets.

Creating the proper environment is crucial for the practice of yoga. The yoga room needs to be quiet, private, and somewhat warm so that it facilitates stretching and relaxation. Many instructors like to set the mood for peace and introspection by burning candles or incense.

CHAPTER WRAP-UP

Yoga has been called a discipline for living. It is a holistic practice that unites body, mind, and spirit. In this chapter we covered some basic yoga philosophy, styles and types of yoga, fundamentals of breath work, yoga research findings, verbal cues, music, props, appropriate environment, technique and safety, warm-up, basic yoga postures, and final relaxation. We hope this chapter will inspire you to explore yoga more fully and to take a yoga teacher training course. You will find many personal benefits from the practice of yoga as well as increase your ability to help others.

▶ Group Exercise Class Evaluation Form Key Points

Yoga does not have a significant cardiorespiratory component. The evaluation form guidelines that apply to yoga come from the warm-up, muscular conditioning and flexibility training, and cool-down sections of the form.

- Connect the breath to the mind and body by performing breathing exercises.
- Give verbal cues on posture and alignment. Every movement in yoga requires correct posture and alignment, and so such cues are critical to leading participants in yoga.
- Encourage and demonstrate good body mechanics. Yoga movements require a visual demonstration by the instructor. Make sure all your demonstrations are appropriate and emphasize proper progressions.

- Observe participants' form and suggest modifications for participants with injuries or special needs as well as progressions for advanced participants. Walk around the room after giving a visual demonstration of the movement so you can observe participants and make sure they are performing the postures correctly.
- Use appropriate music. Usually light background instrumental music is the most appropriate for yoga classes. Keep the volume low so you can also keep your voice low, calm, and soothing.
- Emphasize relaxation. The last 5 to 8 minutes of a yoga class often include a relaxation and visualization segment. This segment is essential to allow participants to relax fully and integrate the yoga postures.

▶ Assignment

Write a 100-word paragraph describing the elements of yogic philosophy. Research one of the styles of yoga and write a 250-word summary of your findings. Be prepared to teach and cue a short warm-up, a standing posture, a backward-bending posture, a forward-bending posture, a twisting posture, and a relaxation pose to a small group.

Pilates

CHAPTER OBJECTIVES

By the end of this chapter, you will

- be able to describe the basic principles of Pilates;
- understand how to begin a Pilates class;
- be able to teach basic Pilates mat exercises and make proper alignment, technique, and safety recommendations; and
- be able to design a short Pilates mat routine appropriate for beginners.

The Pilates system was developed by Joseph H. Pilates (1880-1967) in the first half of the 20th century. At first known to only a small group of dancers and elite athletes in New York City, the Pilates method gradually spread, and since 1990 it has become widely popularized in many cities around the world. According to the 2007 IDEA Health and Fitness Association Programs and Equipment Survey, 68% of program directors at fitness facilities offer Pilates mat classes on their group exercise class schedules (Schroeder and Friesen 2007). Learning to teach Pilates will grow your career opportunities!

THE PILATES METHOD

The Pilates method of body conditioning is comprehensive, encompassing more than 2,000 exercises. This chapter introduces the major concepts underlying the Pilates method, describes the most familiar mat exercises, and discusses basic alignment, technique, and safety concerns. We strongly recommend that you seek additional training and certification in Pilates before teaching a mat class or working with Pilates equipment. For help with training and certification, see the list of Pilates resources on this page.

In his 1945 book, *Pilates' Return to Life Through Contrology,* Joseph Pilates outlined the guiding principles of the Pilates method and detailed 34 mat exercises. We will discuss several of these mat exercises in this chapter. However, many more Pilates exercises can be done on special Pilates equipment. Standard equipment includes the Pilates reformer, cadillac, barrel, and chair as well as small pieces such as the Pilates circle, arc trainer, half barrel, and spine

---

■ Background Check

Before working your way through this chapter, you should do the following:

Read

- chapter 7 on muscular conditioning and flexibility training

---

Pilates Resources

Books

Clark, M., and C. Romani-Ruby. 2001. *The Pilates reformer: A manual for instructors.* Tarentum, PA: Word Association.

Gallagher, S., and R. Kryzanowska. 2000. *The Joseph H. Pilates archive collection: Photographs, writings and designs.* Philadelphia: Bainbridge Books.

Isacowitz, R. 2006. *Pilates.* Champaign, IL: Human Kinetics.

Lessen, D. 2005. *The PMA Pilates certification exam study guide.* Miami, FL: Pilates Method Alliance.

Siler, B. 2000. *The Pilates body.* New York: Broadway Books.

Web Sites

Balanced Body, www.pilates.com

Bodies in Balance, www.bibpilates.net

Peak Pilates, www.peakpilates.com

PHI Pilates, www.phipilates.com

Physicalmind Institute, www.themethod-pilates.com

Pilates Method Alliance (PMA), www.pilatesmethodalliance.org

Polestar Pilates, www.polestarpilates.com

PHI Pilates, www.phpilates.com

Stott Pilates, www.stottpilates.com

Group Exercise Class Evaluation Form Essentials

Key Points for the Warm-Up Segment

- Includes appropriate amount of dynamic movement
- Gives clear cues and verbal directions
- Uses an appropriate music selection

Table 14.1 Core Muscles and Joint Actions

Joint	Muscle	Joint action
Pelvis	Iliopsoas	Hip flexion, anterior pelvic tilt
	Gluteus maximus	Hip extension, posterior pelvic tilt
	Rectus abdominis	Posterior pelvic tilt
	Quadratus lumborum	Lateral pelvic tilt
Spine	Rectus abdominis	Spinal flexion
	Obliques	Spinal flexion with rotation
	Transversus abdominis	Abdominal compression
	Erector spinae	Spinal extension, spinal rotation
	Multifidi	Spinal extension, spinal rotation
	Quadratus lumborum	Spinal lateral flexion
Shoulder girdle	Trapezius	Scapular retraction, depression, upward rotation, elevation
	Levator scapulae	Scapular elevation
	Rhomboids	Scapular retraction, downward rotation
	Pectoralis minor	Scapular depression, protraction
	Serratus anterior	Scapular protraction, upward rotation
Neck	Trapezius	Cervical spinal lateral flexion, extension
	Erector spinae	Cervical spinal extension
	Sternocleidomastoid	Cervical spinal rotation, flexion

supporter. Currently you can find the larger pieces of equipment in Pilates studios, although more and more fitness facilities are investing in specially equipped Pilates rooms that are staffed with teachers specifically trained and certified in Pilates. Generally, training on the Pilates apparatus is done one on one with a Pilates trainer, although some studios offer small group training if enough equipment is available. For example, if a studio has four reformers, a group of four clients may practice Pilates together while led by a qualified Pilates instructor.

The Pilates system of exercise improves muscle strength, endurance, flexibility, balance, and coordination. It is often listed as a mind–body discipline and an ideal way to promote core stability. According to the 2006 position statement of the Pilates Method Alliance, "Pilates exercise focuses on postural symmetry, breath control, abdominal strength, spine, pelvis, and shoulder stabilization, muscular flexibility, joint mobility and strengthening through the complete range of motion of all joints. Instead of isolating muscle groups, the whole body is trained, integrating the upper and lower extremities with the trunk" (Pilates Method Alliance 2006, 2).

The Powerhouse

Joseph Pilates' idea was that the body's core is the powerhouse of strength from which all movements emanate. Most Pilates experts agree that core stability is the ability to keep the pelvis, spine, neck, and shoulder girdle stable while performing various activities. See table 14.1 for a list of key core muscles and their actions.

Many, if not most, of the exercises in the Pilates repertoire challenge the core muscles to contract isometrically against resistance and to stabilize the core joints while the extremities move. Such exercises include the hundred, the leg circle, the single straight-leg stretch, swimming, the seated spinal twist, the side kick, and the leg pull-up.

Mobility Versus Stability

Joseph Pilates believed that a fit body is both strong and flexible and that a healthy spine is both stable and mobile. Accordingly, many Pilates exercises promote spinal suppleness (along with fluidity of motion). Practitioners are taught to articulate the vertebrae of the spine, which means to move one vertebra at a time. Exercises that articulate the spine include the roll-up and roll-down, rollover, and spine stretch. If the spine is supple, it is able to flex fully; this is important for optimal performance of exercises such as rolling like a ball.

Abdominal Hollowing

Abdominal hollowing (also known as *scooping* or the *drawing-in maneuver*) is a hallmark of Pilates exercise. The muscle responsible for abdominal hollowing is the transversus abdominis, which performs abdominal compression. You can use many images to help participants perform abdominal hollowing; you might cue participants to pull the navel to the spine or to pretend they're zipping up a pair of jeans that are a size too small. The ability to draw in the abdominal muscles may help prevent low-back pain, since conscious abdominal contraction can support the spine anteriorly during tasks that involve bending over and lifting heavy objects. Abdominal hollowing has also been advocated as a means to stabilize the spine (Hodges et al. 1996) and to

increase the action of the pelvic floor muscles. Abdominal hollowing may be performed in all positions, including standing, sitting, side-lying, all-fours, supine imprinted, and supine neutral positions (see figure 14.1).

Imprinting

An imprinted spine is one that is consciously pressed into the mat when a person is lying in the supine position. An imprinted spine is no longer in neutral, as the lumbar curve is flattened against the floor and the pelvis is tilted posteriorly. The imprinted position may be optimal for beginners or participants with low-back pain because it provides more spinal stability than a neutral position provides; in addition, the position enables more tactile reinforcement since the participant can feel the spine contacting the mat. Ideally, the imprint and posterior pelvic tilt should be performed by contracting the rectus abdominis and not by tensing the gluteals (see figure 14.2). The imprinted position, while safe and effective for most people, is not comfortable for everyone. Participants who find the imprinted spine uncomfortable should be encouraged to work in a neutral spinal position.

Neutral Spine

While Joseph Pilates did not discuss the concept of a neutral spine, believing instead that the back should be kept flat (forming a plumb line), most contemporary Pilates practitioners have updated Pilates' original ideas to match what we now know about the body, including the benefits of

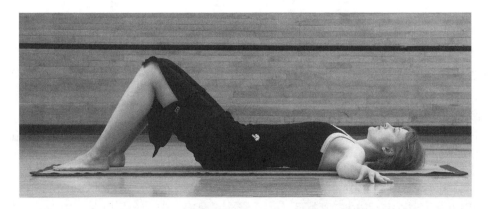

▶ **Figure 14.1** Abdominal hollowing in the supine neutral position.

the neutral spine. A neutral spine is one that is in ideal alignment, with its four natural curves assuming their ideal relationship to each other. The spine is not meant to be flat like a wall. Rather, it is designed to have an inward curve at the cervical spine, an outward curve at the thoracic spine, another inward curve at the lumbar spine, and another outward curve at the sacrum (see figure 14.3). When the spine is in neutral, the neck and the pelvis are also in neutral. Most experts maintain that a neutral spine distributes stress, shock, and impact forces in the safest way possible (Norris 2000; Cholewicki et al. 1997; McGill 2002). A Pilates class is an ideal medium for teaching students about neutral alignment, as the purpose of many exercises is to keep the spine in neutral against a resistance or against the movement of the extremities. Such exercises include the leg circle, corkscrew, spine twist, side kick, leg pull-down, leg pull-up, kneeling side kick, and push-up.

Breathing

Joseph Pilates was emphatic that full inhalations and exhalations are essential to oxygenate the body; each breath cleanses and replenishes the body. He recommended inhaling and exhaling on specific parts of each exercise, as you will see later in this chapter. In general, a full exhale is recommended during spinal flexion movements, as this is more anatomically correct, while an inhalation is often more natural when extending the spine or opening the body. Many experts recommend maintaining abdominal hollowing for the duration of any exercise in which the

---

> ■ **Practice Drill**
>
> Inhale and exhale using the abdominal breath described in chapter 13. On the exhale, when your abdomen naturally pulls in, consciously draw it in, attempting to press your navel even further toward the spine. Feel your abdomen hollow, or scoop inward. See if you can do this move when standing, sitting, lying supine, and lying prone.

spine is stabilized (hollowing helps maintain stability); therefore lateral rib cage expansion is encouraged during breathing. This is in contrast to moving the abdomen out and in, as is done in relaxed abdominal breathing (discussed on page 250 in chapter 13). Allowing the abdomen to relax out and in may have the undesirable result of destabilizing the spine when a person is holding certain positions such as the plank position or is carrying heavy objects.

Setup and Maintenance of Proper Alignment

Many Pilates instructors begin each exercise with a setup. This is simply a teaching technique in which participants are asked to place their bodies in the ideal alignment, or setup, for the upcoming exercise. For example, when teaching side kicks, the instructor may take a moment to fully detail and place students in the optimal starting position, describing the alignment of each major joint, the neutral position of the spine,

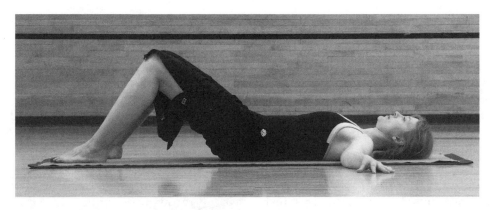

▶ **Figure 14.2** The imprinted spine.

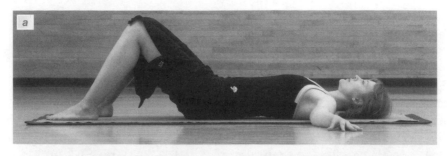

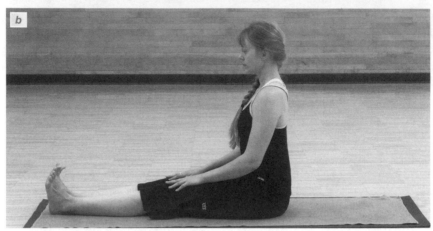

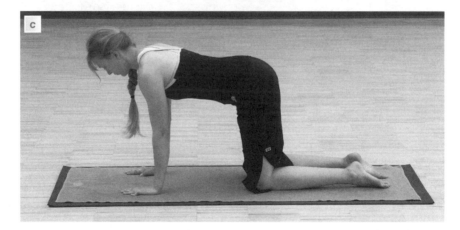

▷ **Figure 14.3** The neutral spine in the *(a)* supine, *(b)* seated, and *(c)* all fours positions.

and the hollowing of the abdominal muscles. Only after being satisfied that all students are in the proper starting position does the instructor actually cue the exercise. Executing all moves with proper alignment is a central concept in Pilates. Moving with concentration, control, and precision at all times is critical. Pilates himself wrote that performing one precise and perfect movement is better than completing many half-hearted ones.

Lengthening

Most Pilates exercises are designed to promote a lengthening sensation throughout the body. In other words, one part of the body energetically reaches in one direction, while another part of the body reaches in the opposite direction. Elongation is felt through the joints and the muscles. Toes, fingertips, and the crown of the head are often cued to reach as far away from center as possible.

■ Practice Drill

Sit in a comfortable position, either in a chair or on the floor. Your spine should be long and in neutral. Take a full diaphragmatic inhale, allowing your abdomen to expand slightly. Exhale, consciously pulling your abdomen in, imagining that your navel is touching your spine. Then, keeping your abdomen hollowed and as far in as possible, continue to breathe for several breaths. Do not allow your abdomen to move with your breathing; maintain abdominal hollowing. Feel as if your rib cage were expanding laterally with each breath and allow your upper back to move with each inhale and exhale. Feel your abdominal wall remaining firm and inwardly contracted during the entire practice.

In many exercises, there is a sensation of stretch even though the working muscles are contracting concentrically. Such exercises include leg circles, rollover, single straight-leg stretch, corkscrew, double-leg kick, spine twist, and teaser.

WARM-UP

In Joseph Pilates' original method for mat exercise, there is no warm-up, at least not according to the standard definition given in chapter 5. The very first exercise in his authentic series is the hundred, which he intended to serve as a warm-up exercise. While the hundred does involve vigorous pumping of the arms (100 times) and is intended to be performed with strong rhythmic inhalations and exhalations, the rest of the body remains stable, lying supine on the floor in sustained spinal and hip flexion. We believe (along with a number of Pilates experts) that more dynamic movement is needed before beginning the hundred in order to safely prepare the body for the Pilates mat exercises that follow.

Since the majority of a Pilates mat class is on the floor, warm-ups, when provided, are also generally on the floor or mat. The warm-up is an ideal time to introduce key concepts such as proper breathing, neutral spine, spinal mobility, abdominal hollowing, imprinting, lengthening, control, precision, and mindfulness. The following is a sample warm-up appropriate for a Pilates class:

1. Seated breathing practice. Sit on your mat with your knees bent, legs together, and feet flat on the floor. Wrap your arms and hands around your legs and let your spine round. Rest your torso on your thighs and relax your head and neck. Breathe deeply and feel your back and posterior and lateral rib cage expand and release with each inhale and exhale. Take 3 to 5 deep breaths.

2. Round and release. Sit on your mat with your legs crossed, spine straight, and hands on knees or shins. Exhale, rounding and flexing your spine, allowing your pelvis to posteriorly tilt, and coordinate the exhale with abdominal hollowing (pull your navel toward your spine). Inhale and lift and lengthen your spine back up to neutral; return your pelvis to neutral as well, sitting well up onto your sitting bones. Repeat this limbering move 3 to 5 times, connecting your breath to the movement and emphasizing abdominal hollowing with each exhale.

3. Side bend and twist. Remaining in the cross-legged position, place your left hand on the floor and reach your right hand up to the ceiling, inhaling. Exhale as you return the right hand to the floor. Repeat three times to the right before repeating the entire move on the left side. Then, sitting quite tall, rotate your spine to the right on an exhale. Inhale as you return to center; exhale as you twist to the left. Repeat three times.

4. Supine imprint and release. Lie on your back with your knees bent, feet flat on the floor, and arms at your sides. Place the pelvis, spine, shoulder blades, and neck in neutral. Exhale and gently press your lower back into the mat, pulling the abdominal muscles into your spine (drawing in/hollowing maneuver). Remember to use the abdominal and not the gluteal muscles for hollowing. Inhale and allow your pelvis and spine to return to neutral (do not overextend your spine past neutral). Repeat 3 to 5 times.

5. Supine articulated bridge. Lie on your back with your knees bent, your feet flat on the floor, your arms at your sides, and your pelvis, spine, shoulder blades, and neck in neutral. Exhale and posteriorly tilt your pelvis, tipping your tailbone upward. Still exhaling, peel your spine off the floor, tailbone first, keeping your head and shoulders down. Inhale at the top of the motion. Exhale and one by one, articulate the spine, lowering the vertebrae back down onto the mat. Inhale to rest. Repeat 3 to 5 times.

6. Supine rib cage placement. Lie on your back with your knees bent, your feet flat on the floor, your arms at your sides, and your pelvis, spine, shoulder blades, and neck in neutral. Inhale and slide your shoulder blades up toward your ears; exhale and press them away from your ears, keeping your scapulae on the mat at all times. Repeat 3 to 5 times. Then inhale and protract your shoulder blades up and away from the mat; exhale and press them firmly down into the mat, retracting them toward each other if possible. Your chest will lift and a space may form under the thoracic spine when the shoulder blades are fully retracted. Repeat 3 to 5 times. Finally, allow your shoulder blades to rest on the mat in neutral (neither protracted nor retracted).

7. All-fours cat tilt and dog tilt. On your hands and knees, exhale and flex your spine up into the angry cat stretch, head and tailbone down, abdominal muscles drawn up and in. Inhale and gently extend your spine, head and hips up. Move back and forth through these two positions 3 to 5 times, allowing your spine to become more supple and limber.

VERBAL CUES AND MUSIC

Cueing in Pilates is perhaps more alignment driven than it is in other forms of group exercise. Remember that two of the underlying principles of Pilates are control and precision. Ideally, each and every exercise is executed with concentration and flawless alignment, every time. Skilled Pilates instructors have a well-developed eye for subtle alignment issues in their students. Knowing the common alignment and technique errors in the standard Pilates repertoire and in their students, competent instructors are ready with effective cues, hopefully preventing the errors before they occur. To that end, it is common to detail, that is, to give many specific alignment cues for each major joint during an exercise, as well as to remind students about breathing, abdominal hollowing, and lengthening. Additionally, instructors need to be able to say the same cue in multiple ways, as each student will respond differently to a cue. For example, if the exercise requires a flexed spine, some participants will flex it immediately upon hearing, "Round your back," whereas others will not respond at all. To reach these students, the instructor might try other cues such as, "Curve your spine," "Make your spine into a C curve," "Pull your ribs and hips toward each other," "Curl your spine into a half-moon shape," and so on. In other words, an adept instructor needs a large vocabulary of alignment words and ideas for describing each exercise.

Did you come up with any image cues in the practice drill? Image cues are very common for detailing Pilates exercises. A common image cue for guiding students to curl-up or flex their spine, for example, is to ask them to curve into a half-moon shape or to form the letter C with their spine. Can you think of other image cues? Some instructors are quite creative, humorous, or fanciful with their cues. Remember that every student is unique. Some participants will respond better to image cues than to more straightforward cues. A skilled instructor is able to cue in a variety of ways in order to most effectively reach all participants.

The majority of participants learn best by visual cues. Be sure to demonstrate each exercise at least once before getting up and moving around your class so that your students know what the exercise is supposed to look like. Alternatively, try asking a very skilled partici-

■ **Practice Drill**

Using a piece of paper to record your responses, come up with as many ways as you can to cue the following:

- Neutral spine
- Head high
- Shoulders down
- Abdominal muscles in
- Neutral pelvis
- Spinal articulation

pant to model the exercise. When detailing an exercise, it is very helpful if you provide visual cues using your own body. For example, practice giving head to toe alignment cues while pointing to various joints on yourself. When you say, "Shoulders down and back," point to your own shoulders as you exaggerate pressing them down and back. When you say, "Abdominal muscles in," exaggerate pulling your own abdominal wall in, pressing inward with your hand. This type of cue is quite effective in helping your class perform an exercise correctly.

Be sure to include educational or informational cues throughout your class. Especially in Pilates, the rationale for doing a particular exercise is not always immediately obvious. Many students will want to know why they should do a move in a certain way or where they should feel their muscles working. Explaining the purpose of an exercise or the principles behind Pilates can enhance adherence and keep your class motivated. For example, when teaching single-leg circles you might explain, "The purpose of this exercise is to promote core stability, so keep your abdominal muscles hollowed, your shoulder blades grounded, and your core very still while limbering your hip joint and allowing your leg to move freely." You could even go on to explain why core stability work is important. With these cues, your students will become more educated and enthusiastic about Pilates.

A tactile cue is a hands-on touch cue. While tactile cueing is very common among Pilates instructors, it is not without controversy. Since some participants are uncomfortable being touched and may feel that touch violates their personal space, you must always ask permission before touching someone. Even if your student grants you permission, you should still avoid touching her if you detect any discomfort (such as drawing away or cringing from your touch). This is especially important for male instructors cueing female participants. However, when participants are comfortable with being touched, there are benefits to tactile cueing. These include improving your student's alignment to make Pilates exercises safer and more effective. Generally, a student will be much more focused and concentrated on the exercise, not letting the mind wander, when an instructor is providing tactile cueing. This student is more likely to get the optimal benefit from the exercise.

Many instructors opt to teach their Pilates classes without music, believing that silence allows participants to be more mindful and have better concentration and focus. When music is used, it is usually amorphous, meaning that it lacks a strong, rhythmic beat. Some instructors prefer mellow classical or jazz; others choose new age or soft world music. In any case, if you choose to use music when teaching Pilates, make sure it is in the background.

TECHNIQUE AND SAFETY

Like the yoga postures (discussed in chapter 13), Pilates exercises run the gamut from very easy to very hard, from extremely basic and safe to advanced and potentially risky. Pilates instructors must understand the potential mechanisms of injury to each joint and especially to the spine, since so much of Pilates concerns the core. Table 14.2 briefly reviews the common mechanisms of injury to the spine.

Since several Pilates exercises place the student in potentially injury-producing positions, conscientious instructors should provide appropriate modifications, carefully detail each exercise in such a way that participants perform it completely correctly, or avoid leading the class in the high-risk Pilates exercises entirely. Table 14.3 lists some of the more problematic Pilates exercises and their mechanisms of injury.

Once again, let's revisit the progressive functional training continuum, which is discussed in our book *Functional Exercise Progressions* (Yoke and Kennedy 2004) and in chapter 3 (see page 40). Remember that the continuum can be used to organize a variety of exercises or to organize different variations of one exercise from easiest to hardest. Figure 14.4 shows an example of the progressive functional training continuum for the hundred. When teaching Pilates to a mixed-level class, it is best to start with the easiest and most conservative variation of an exercise, such as the variation shown in figure 14.4a.

Table 14.2 Common Mechanisms of Injury to the Spine

Cause	Effect
Unsupported spinal flexion	Overstretches the long posterior ligaments of the spine, which can lead to a loss of spinal stability.
Unsupported spinal flexion with rotation	Overstretches the long posterior ligaments of the spine, which can lead to a loss of spinal stability, plus carries an additional risk of disk herniation.
Unsupported lateral flexion	Overstretches the long ligaments of the spine, leading to a loss of spinal stability.
Extreme lumbar hyperextension	Overstretches the long anterior ligaments of the spine, leading to a loss of spinal stability.
Long-lever traction	May produce a shearing force on the spine, leading to ligament overstretch or protruding (bulging) disks.
Weight bearing on the cervical spine	Causes undue stress on the small cervical vertebrae and may impinge nerves and blood vessels.

We strongly recommend that you get competent safety and technique instruction as well as certification if you decide to become a Pilates instructor.

BASIC MOVES

Joseph Pilates specified that his mat exercises be performed in a particular order, and there are still some Pilates organizations that scrupulously adhere to his original method. Other organizations tout a more contemporary approach, modifying Pilates' work when necessary to reflect a more scientifically correct practice. In this chapter we present a few Pilates mat exercises that are either more basic or that can be easily modified to enhance safety.

 See the DVD for a demonstration of the hundred, roll up, single leg circle, and rolling like a ball.

The Hundred

This classic Pilates exercise is intended to promote core stability while the body is in resisted spinal flexion. It is also meant to oxygenate the body and increase circulation through a vigorous and rhythmic breathing pattern. The traditional version of the hundred exerts a long-lever trac-

tion force on the spine and should be done only by participants who are able to fully stabilize the spine in flexion; the traditional version is *not* for beginners! Modify the traditional version by keeping the feet on the floor or by lifting the legs into the tabletop position.

To perform the hundred, lie supine with the spine imprinted and the abdominal muscles hollowed. Flex the hips and knees to 90°, placing the legs in tabletop position. Curl the spine into flexion, lifting the shoulder blades off the floor

---

■ **Technique and Safety Check**

To help keep your classes safe, observe the following recommendations:

- Provide an appropriate warm-up.
- Provide plenty of modifications for each exercise, always starting with the easiest variation (unless you are teaching an advanced students only class).
- Avoid high-risk or controversial exercises unless teaching an advanced class (even then, offer modifications).
- Give plenty of alignment cues and detail each exercise carefully.
- Keep reminding participants to breathe.

Table 14.3 Mechanisms of Injury in Pilates Exercises

Exercise	Mechanism of injury
Hundred, roll-up, double-leg stretch, teaser	Long-lever traction
Spine stretch forward, rolling down the wall	Unsupported spinal flexion
Full swan dive, rocking	Extreme lumbar hyperextension
Rollover, jackknife, bicycle	Weight bearing on cervical spine

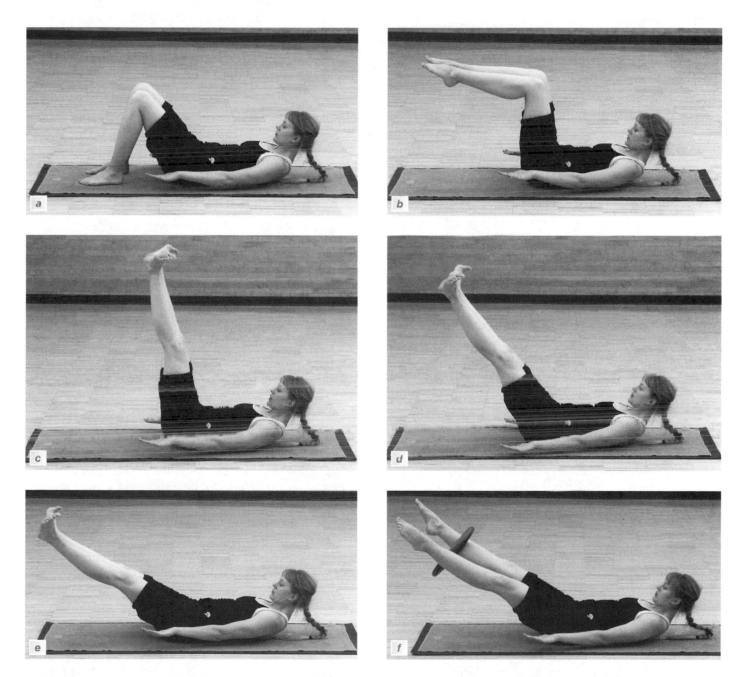

▶ **Figure 14.4** The hundred progression: *(a)* feet on floor, *(b)* legs in tabletop position, *(c)* legs straight up, *(d)* legs at 45°, *(e)* legs close to ground, and *(f)* legs close to ground with circle.

and allowing the head and neck to continue the line of the curved spine. Raise long, straight arms off the ground, keeping them parallel to the floor. Reach the fingers straight ahead. Inhale for 5 counts and exhale for 5 counts; continue this pattern 10 times (for a total of 100 counts). Keep pressing the abdominal muscles down and relaxing the neck and shoulders for the duration of the exercise (see figure 14.4b).

Roll-Up

Both core stability and core mobility are challenged in the roll up. The goal is to flex the spine as much as possible throughout the exercise, a feat that requires spinal suppleness. The rounder the spine, the more even and smooth the roll up and rolldown; if the spine is rigid and inflexible in places, rolling up or down smoothly will be impossible. Rectus abdominis strength and endurance are required to maintain a full contraction throughout the entire ROM of the exercise. If the abdominal muscles are weak and unable to maintain spinal flexion, the hip flexors may take over and create a long-lever traction force on the spine, causing the exercise to become unsafe. It is recommended that beginners practice a half roll-up (crunch) first, preferably with the knees bent, in order to develop a foundation of abdominal strength. A half roll-back (start in the seated position, round the spine and roll back halfway, and then return to sitting) can also prepare the beginner for the traditional roll-up. Yet another modification is to hold both ends of a strap secured around the feet; the strap allows participants (depending on their body segment lengths) to roll up and down more smoothly and safely.

To perform the roll-up, lie supine with the spine imprinted and abdominal muscles hollowed. Your legs are straight and long, toes are pointed, shoulders are flexed, and fingers are reaching toward the ceiling. Inhale and lift your head and neck off floor. Exhale and continue to curl up the rest of the spine, lifting it from the floor vertebra by vertebra. Keep your shoulder blades down and away from your ears throughout the movement. At the end of the exhale, your spine should be fully flexed as you reach your arms forward, keeping them parallel to your legs. Make certain your abdominal muscles are fully drawn in and your ribs are lifted up and over the belly. Inhale and begin to roll down, staying

in flexion. Exhale and continue rolling down, letting each vertebra independently lower onto the floor until the body is supine again, arms reaching toward the ceiling. Repeat 3 to 5 times (see figure 14.5).

Single-Leg Circle

The single-leg circle requires you to maintain spinal and pelvic stability in the neutral position while moving an extremity (the leg). When performing this exercise, you should feel as if the hip is moving effortlessly in its socket while the core is very stable. The single-leg circle may be troublesome for participants with tight hamstrings—because these students are unable to lift the leg to 90°, they may experience unnecessary hip flexor tension that pulls on the lumbar spine. Modifications include bending the bottom (support) leg and placing the foot on the floor; this will help relieve tension in the low back. Additionally, novice exercisers can be encouraged to make small circles instead of large ones or can even use a strap around the foot (holding the ends with the hands) to help the leg move in circles.

To perform the single-leg circle, lie supine with the spine imprinted and the abdominals hollowed. Your arms should be at your sides, your palms should face down, and your scapulae should be stabilized. Stretch the left leg out along the floor. Ideally with toes pointed. Reach the right leg up toward the ceiling (keep the toes pointed). Start the leg circle by bringing the leg across the midline of the body. Inhale. Move the leg down and around and back up to 90°. Exhale. Your torso and pelvis should remain motionless throughout the movement. The size of the leg circle will be determined by your ability to stabilize the torso. Beginners should start with small circles; they can increase the circle circumference as they become more adept. Repeat the circle 3 to 5 times in each direction. Then switch legs and repeat with the left leg circling (see figure 14.6).

Rolling Like a Ball

Rolling like a ball is similar to the roll-up in that the more supple and flexible the spine, the rounder the back and the easier it is to roll back and forth without any thumping or uneven movement. When performing rolling like a ball,

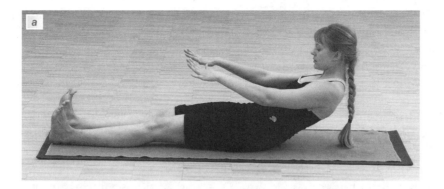

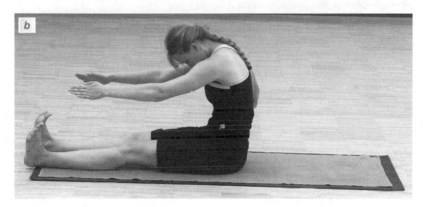

▶ **Figure 14.5** The roll-up: *(a)* halfway *(b)* full up position.

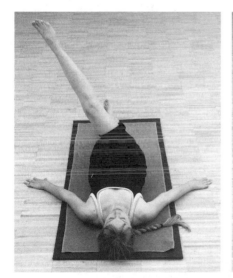
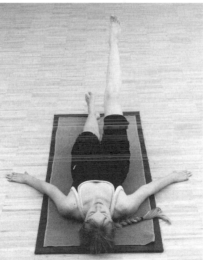
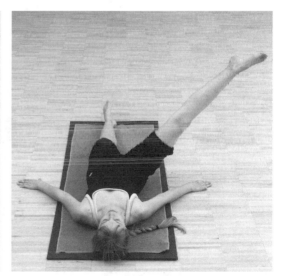

▶ **Figure 14.6** The single-leg circle.

you should maintain the spine in the best C curve possible; this is best accomplished by firmly hollowing the abdominal muscles throughout the exercise and maintaining core stability. In addition, rolling like a ball requires you to exert control when returning to the starting or balance point, a feat that is difficult without abdominal hollowing and mental focus. Rolling like a ball is a beginner exercise that can progress to a harder exercise such as the open-leg rocker.

To perform rolling like a ball, start in the up position, finding the balance point on your sitting bones. Your spine should be fully flexed and rounded into a C curve and your abdominal muscles should be drawn in. Hold the lower legs with your hands; your legs should be together and your toes should be pointed with the feet off the floor. Hollow the abdomen even further and allow yourself to roll back while you inhale. Be sure to maintain the distance between the abdomen and the thighs (in other words, do not change the angle of hip flexion). While exhaling, rock back up to the starting position. Avoid rolling so far back that you place weight onto the neck or head; keep your head off the floor. Roll back and forth 5 to 6 times (see figure 14.7).

Single-Heel Kick

The single-heel kick requires the spine to be maintained in slight extension, making this exercise a good counterbalance to all the flexion exercises found in Pilates. Throughout the kick the abdominal muscles are drawn up and in for support, which means this exercise helps promote core stability in spinal extension. Additionally, this exercise challenges the scapular depressors (lower trapezius and pectoralis minor) because

without concentration, gravity pulls the thoracic and cervical spine down and the scapulae ride up the back of the rib cage toward the ears. To prevent these effects, the participant must develop stamina and endurance in the upper body in order to maintain scapular depression against gravity for the duration of the exercise. A note of caution: Some participants may not be comfortable with the degree of spinal extension required by this exercise. If your participants report back discomfort, modify the exercise by allowing them to lie completely prone and rest their forehead on their hands. Then they can maintain spinal stability in the prone position throughout the exercise.

To perform the single-heel kick, start in the prone position and prop up the upper torso on the elbows. Rest the forearms on the floor. Press the shoulders down and away from the ears, lengthening the neck. Minimize spinal extension as much as possible by contracting the abdominal muscles to prevent the lower back from sagging toward the floor. Ideally, the belly is up and off the floor. Stabilize the shoulder blades, neck, torso, and pelvis while performing the leg movement. Energize and lengthen your legs and point your toes. Bend the right knee and exhale as you pulse the heel toward the body

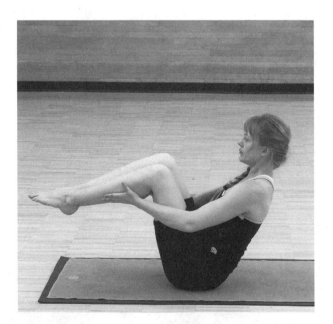
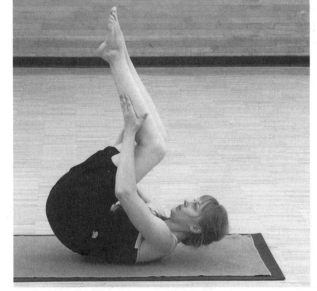

▶ **Figure 14.7** Rolling like a ball.

two times, attempting to kick the buttock. Inhale as you straighten the knee and return it to the mat. Switch sides and kick with the opposite leg. Repeat 5 to 10 times (see figure 14.8).

 See the DVD for a demonstration of the single heel kick, breast stroke, side-lying position, spine stretch forward, seated spine twist, plank, and leg pull front.

Breaststroke

The breaststroke emphasizes spinal extension and can serve as a preparatory exercise for harder Pilates extension moves such as swimming and the swan. If bringing the arms into full flexion overhead is too challenging or causes back or shoulder discomfort, you can modify the exercise by simply abducting the arms into a T position (90° angle to the torso) instead.

To perform the breast stroke, start in the prone position with the elbows bent, the hands under the shoulders, and the forearms on the floor. The spine, pelvis, and neck are all in neutral alignment; the legs are together and the toes are pointed. Keep the lower body energized by anchoring it to the floor throughout the exercise. Exhale and send the arms overhead and forward, hovering off the floor. Inhale and sweep the arms around to the sides while you simultaneously lift the chest and extend the spine, keeping the head and neck in line with the spine. Exhale and send the arms overhead again, as if performing a breaststroke; inhale and repeat the sweeping arm movement and spinal extension. Repeat 5 to 10 times (see figure 14.9).

Side-Lying Position

The side-lying position is slightly more challenging than the supine or prone position because in

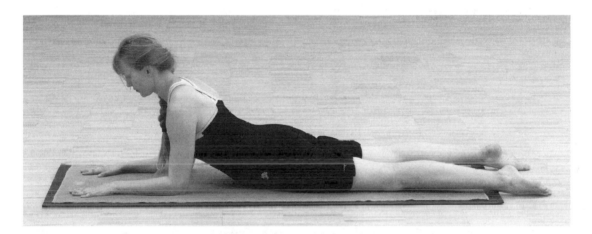

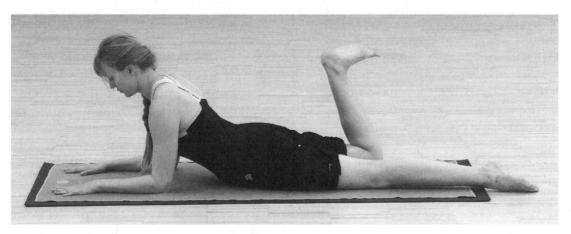

▶ **Figure 14.8** Single-heel kick.

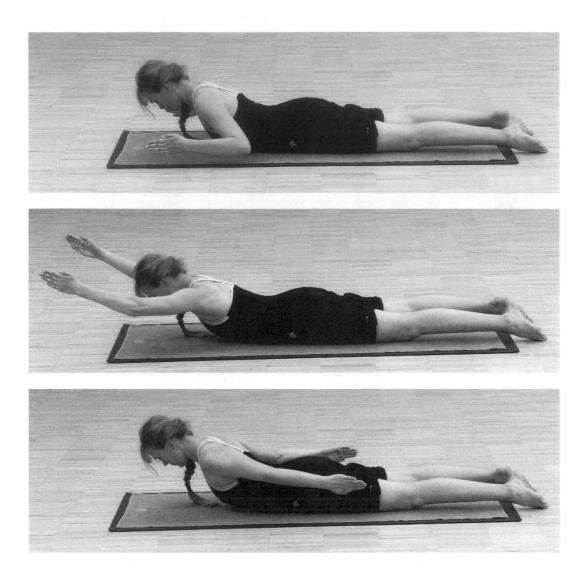

▶ **Figure 14.9** The breaststroke.

this position the body makes less contact with the floor and therefore the stabilizers must work harder to maintain good alignment. Although some Pilates' texts show more challenging variations such as resting the head on the hand or placing both hands behind the ears while propping up the upper body on the elbow, we suggest using the more basic and stable variation of resting the head on the arm, with the cervical spine in neutral. The goal is to keep the pelvis, spine, scapulae, neck, and head in neutral and to maintain abdominal hollowing throughout the exercise. To achieve this goal you must be particularly focused when bringing the leg back into extension, as during this motion the spine naturally tends to extend.

To perform the side-lying position front and back on your side with your hips and shoulders stacked, keep spine and pelvis in neutral, and your abdominal muscles contracted. Your bottom arm is stretched out under your head; your head and neck are in neutral. Bend your top arm and place your hand on the floor for stability. Dorsiflex your top ankle. Inhale and bring your top leg forward, flexing at the hip; pulse twice. Stay in control with abdominals securely contracted, as you exhale and bring the leg behind the body, pointing your toes. Be sure to keep the moving leg parallel to the floor. Repeat 8 to 10 times and then switch sides (see figure 14.10).

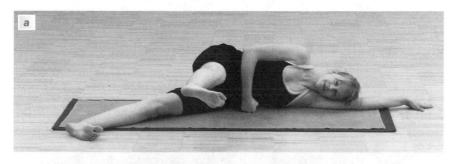

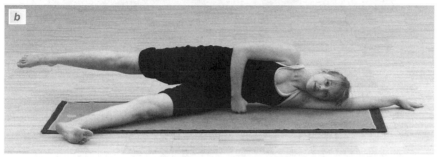

▷ **Figure 14.10** The side-lying for (a) front and (b) back.

Spine Stretch Forward

The spine stretch forward is very useful for improving sitting posture. Additionally, it teaches participants to automatically contract the abdominal muscles whenever the spine is rounded so that the spine is protected during unsupported forward flexion (technically, if the abdominal muscles are securely lifted and contracted, the spine is no longer unsupported). The ability to articulate the spine and keep the spine supple is a further benefit of this exercise.

To perform the spine stretch forward, sit with your legs straight out in front, your feet hip-width apart, and your ankles dorsiflexed. Lengthen your legs through your heels. Start with ideal, neutral sitting alignment, with your pelvis, spine, scapulae, and neck all in neutral. Your weight should be directly on the sitting bones (your tailbone should be slightly off the floor) and your hips should form a 90° angle. The shoulders are flexed, also at a 90° angle, parallel to the floor. Reach long in front with the fingers. Exhaling, start to move into spinal flexion, head and neck first, articulating the spine from the top down. Forcing the air out of the lungs, keep pulling in with the abdominal muscles, feeling as if they are lifting in and up behind the rib cage and as if you are curving over a bar without allowing your belly to touch it. Inhale and sequentially return the spine back to neutral, once again finding ideal sitting alignment. Repeat 5 to 8 times (see figure 14.11).

Seated Spine Twist

Most people in developed countries are sedentary, and it is ironic that very few of them actually sit correctly. The seated spine twist can help correct improper sitting, as it develops core stability and stamina in the seated position as well as promotes mobility in spinal rotation. Since this exercise requires a person to have adequate hamstring flexibility in order to sit in 90° of hip flexion, it will be difficult for some participants. Modifications include sitting on a pillow, a blanket, or the edge of a mat or simply sitting cross-legged or bending the knees.

To perform the seated spine twist, sit with the legs together and straight out in front and the ankles dorsiflexed. Lengthen the legs through the heels. Start with ideal sitting alignment, with the pelvis, spine, scapulae, and neck all in neutral. Your weight should be directly on your sitting

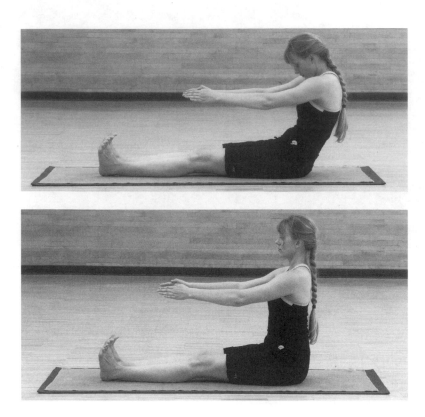

▶ **Figure 14.11** The spine stretch forward.

bones (your tailbone should be slightly off floor) and your hips should form a 90° angle. Lift up through the crown of the head and maintain the longest spine possible throughout the exercise. Abduct the shoulders out to the sides at a 90° angle so that your chest is open and lifted and your shoulder blades are down and back. Exhale and rotate your spine to the right; pulse to the right three times (perform a short exhale on each), sitting taller and taller with each pulse. Inhale and return to center. Exhale and repeat the twist to the left. Perform 3 to 5 repetitions per side (see figure 14.12).

Plank and Leg Pull Front

Participants may be familiar with the plank from traditional muscle conditioning because a full plank is required in order to do a proper push-up. The plank, push-up, and variations of the two such as the leg pull front are also part of Pilates' original repertoire of exercises. Obviously, these exercises require a considerable amount of core stability, as gravity tends to pull the spine, pelvis, and scapulae out of alignment. Dozens of variations of the plank and push-up exist. Two of the most common variations of the plank are the forearm plank (weight is on forearms and toes) and the knee-down plank (weight is on knees and hands). These are both good variations for novice exercisers since they are generally easier to perform correctly.

To perform the plank, start on your hands and knees. Place your pelvis, spine, scapulae, and neck in neutral and your hands directly below your shoulders. Maintaining the neutral position, extend the legs back into a full plank position; hollow the abdomen. Hold the position and take several even breaths (breathe with the rib cage) without letting the abdomen release. To perform the leg pull front, maintain the plank position while extending the right leg (knee straight and ankle dorsiflexed) up and away from the floor. Exhale and point the toes and slowly lower the leg to the floor. Repeat with the opposite leg, alternating legs 3 to 5 times (see figure 14.13).

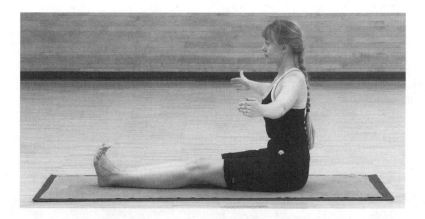

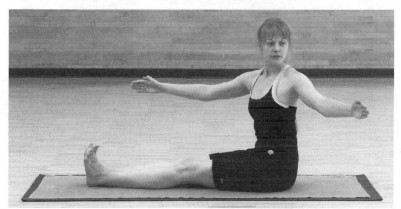

▶ **Figure 14.12** The seated spine twist.

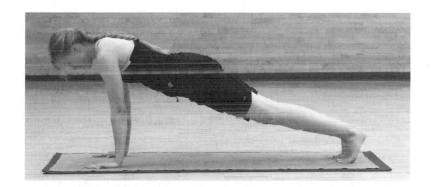

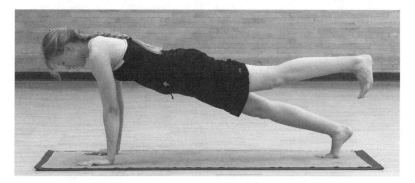

▶ **Figure 14.13** The plank and leg pull front.

■ **Practice Drill**

Start by performing a warm-up appropriate for a Pilates class. Then practice demonstrating and cueing five of the exercises described in this chapter. Pay special attention to incorporating the many alignment and image cues that are so important in teaching Pilates.

ENDING PILATES CLASS

Traditionally, a Pilates class ends with a plank or a push-up followed by walking the hands back to the feet to form a standing forward bend and rolling up to a standing finish. We recommend incorporating a flexibility and cool-down segment as discussed in chapter 7. Since the chest muscles, erector spinae, hip flexors, hamstrings, and calves are commonly tight, it's always a good idea to stretch these muscles.

CHAPTER WRAP-UP

The Pilates method of exercise has become very popular in both the group exercise and the personal training arenas. In this chapter we covered the basic principles of Pilates exercise, such as the powerhouse and the neutral spine as well as control, concentration, precision, proper breathing, imprinting, and abdominal hollowing. We also reviewed the major research findings on Pilates, provided suggestions for a warm-up, covered major technique and safety issues, and discussed elements of cueing that are unique to Pilates. We detailed 10 basic Pilates exercises and suggested drills for Pilates practice. It is our hope that this chapter motivates you to learn more about this valid method of exercise and to go on to become certified as a Pilates instructor.

▶ **Group Exercise Class Evaluation Form Key Points**

Pilates does not have a cardiorespiratory component. The evaluation form guidelines that apply to Pilates come from the warm-up, muscular conditioning and flexibility training, and cool-down sections of the form.

- Give rehearsal moves. Focus on postural symmetry, breath control, abdominal strength, and stabilization of the spine, pelvis, and shoulder. Rehearse any movements that you might introduce in class that day. Rather than warming up and stretching individual muscle groups, review and perform specific Pilates movements for the first 5 to 8 minutes of class. Concentrate on joint mobility and imprinting the spine. Teach neutral spine and breathing throughout the class and not just during the warm-up segment.

- Give verbal cues on posture and alignment. Every movement in Pilates requires appropriate cues on posture and alignment. Focus on lengthening the movements to increase flexibility.

- Encourage and demonstrate good body mechanics. Pilates movements require a visual demonstration by the instructor. Make sure all your demonstrations are appropriate and emphasize proper progressions.

- Observe participants' form and suggest modifications for participants with injuries or special needs as well as progressions for advanced participants. Walk around the room after giving a visual demonstration of the movement so you can observe participants and make sure they are performing the exercise appropriately with correct posture and alignment.

- Use music appropriately. Light background instrumental music or no music at all is appropriate for Pilates classes. Keep the volume low so you can also keep your voice low, calm, and soothing.

- Emphasize relaxation and stretching in the last few minutes of class. Stretch individual muscle groups and focus on relaxation at the end of a Pilates class.

▶ **Assignment**

Prepare to teach a short warm-up and five or more basic Pilates exercises to a small group of participants. Be prepared to use as many cues as possible.

Customizing Group Exercise Classes

CHAPTER OBJECTIVES

By the end of this chapter, you will

- be able to create client-centered group exercise classes;
- be able to design classes for niche markets;
- know how to develop lifestyle-based physical activity classes, such as walking, in-line skating, and pedometer programs;
- familiar with dance-style classes, such as ballet barre, NIA, Zumba, and hip-hop classes;
- know how to design equipment-based classes such as rebounding, treading, slide training, and BOSU balance training;
- understand how to develop fusion and mind–body group fitness classes; and
- be familiar with ethical practice guidelines for group fitness instructors.

Group exercise is constantly changing. Having the skills to update class formats both safely and effectively will be essential to group exercise leaders. In this chapter we detail how to create new formats for group exercise and then close with an overview of the ethical guidelines and standards for group fitness instructors. Group exercise is a diverse field with many teaching options. We recommend you become skilled in teaching at least one of the mainstream modalities such as basic cardio training, step, kickboxing, sport conditioning, functional training, yoga, Pilates, indoor cycling, or water exercise as well as be competent at instructing muscular conditioning and flexibility training. After you have achieved a secure foundation in these classes, you may want to expand your employment opportunities and increase your marketability by developing the skills to create and teach additional exercise modes such as some of the specialty classes that are described in this chapter. To lead specialty classes, you may need additional training and education or you may just need some creative

---

Group Exercise Class Evaluation Form Essentials

Key Points for Warm-Up Segment

- Includes appropriate amount of dynamic movement
- Provides rehearsal moves
- Stretches major muscle groups in a biomechanically sound manner with appropriate instructions
- Gives clear cues and verbal directions
- Uses an appropriate music tempo or motivating music that inspires movement

Key Points for the Cardiorespiratory Segment

- Gradually increases intensity
- Uses a variety of muscle groups (especially hamstrings and abductors)
- Minimizes repetitive movements
- Promotes participant interaction and encourages fun
- Demonstrates movement options and gives clear verbal cues
- Checks participants' intensity levels and gives modifications based on results
- Gradually decreases impact and intensity during cool-down following the cardiorespiratory session
- Uses music volume and tempo appropriate for biomechanical movement

Key Points for Muscle Strength and Endurance Segment

- Gives verbal cues on posture and alignment
- Encourages and demonstrates good body mechanics
- Observes participants' form and suggests modifications for participants with injuries or special needs as well as progressions for advanced participants
- Gives clear verbal directions and uses appropriate music volume
- Uses appropriate music tempo for biomechanical movement
- Chooses appropriate music for flexibility training
- Includes static stretching
- Appropriately emphasizes relaxation and visualization

energy to put a few class segments together. We refer to the group exercise class evaluation form both at the beginning and at the end of this chapter to remind you of the basic principles for teaching a safe and effective class. The main points on the group exercise class evaluation form are reviewed on page 290.

CREATING A CLIENT-CENTERED GROUP EXERCISE CLASS

As discussed in chapter 2, group exercise has evolved from just a few formats to a weekly offering of 20 to 30 different classes on a program schedule. What started out as aerobic dance has turned into an enjoyable movement experience utilizing group dynamics, music, and fun. Given the continual rise in obesity, intentional exercise is here to stay. As fitness professionals it is our job to keep people excited about exercising and to help them gain much more than fitness when they work out. People who have a sense of purpose for their exercise are much more likely to continue their physical activity. People are often busy and the movement experience often provides them a way to connect with others and to create a sense of community. Many of the modalities we will discuss in this chapter do not require a fitness center and are actually community outreach efforts. Everyone needs and seeks more fulfilling movement experiences in their lives. Group exercise classes that help participants meet others with similar interests and enable participants to discuss their lives and health create a unique exercise experience. For example, a group exercise class for breast cancer survivors has much more going on than just exercise. It allows its participants to connect with others who have experienced a life change due to breast cancer. Holmes and colleagues (2005) studied breast cancer survivors and found that walking 3 to 5 hours per week reduced death rates from the disease by almost 50%. Their study did not find that increasing the energy expenditure (i.e., increasing the exercise intensity) provided any additional benefits. Thus it was not a specific exercise progression or good technical information given by an exer-

■ Background Check

Before working your way through this chapter, you should do the following:

Read

- chapter 3 on core concepts in class design,
- chapter 5 on warming up,
- chapter 6 on cardiorespiratory training, and
- chapter 7 on muscular conditioning and flexibility training.

cise instructor that increased the survival rate in these participants. It was the regular exercise that helped these participants survive cancer. Now that is a sense of purpose for exercise! This is the type of client-centered exercise program that is simple to create but makes a huge difference in the lives of those who attend. Forming focus groups to discover the needs of your clients as well as keeping up on the research literature on the benefits of physical activity will help you get ideas for client-centered exercise groups you might like to form.

GROUP EXERCISE FOR NICHE MARKETS

Let's look at some other potential niche markets for group exercise. Many fitness professionals are targeting new mothers as exercise participants who could use camaraderie and support during their life transition into motherhood. Until 2000, classes for new moms were very hard to find, but today stroller-based exercise programs are on the rise (Asp 2006). Baby Boot Camp, StrollerFit, and Stroller Strides are only a few of the new group exercise classes that promote engaging in outdoor activity with your baby. These classes are held either indoors or outdoors in neighborhoods and provide a 60- to 75-minute workout combining all the health-related components of fitness. They average in size from 5 to 15 participants and are held in more than 150 locations in many different U.S. states. They are a wonderful way to get new mothers to interact with one another and enjoy a movement experience together. Most participants stay in the program until their kids are around 3 years old. These programs, which are franchises that can be started by any fitness professional, are listed in the resource guide at the end of this chapter (see page 301).

Another niche class that is popping up is a postpartum class in which the children are involved directly with the exercise experience. A recent article (Davies 2006) described a class named *Baby Steps* in which the mother and baby work out together. Some people call this type of class a *mommy and me* program (for more information, see the resource list on page 301). The format is usually strength based, with the new moms using their babies as weight rather than holding a dumbbell or a resistance tube. These types of classes are rich experiences in so many ways. The mothers avoid the guilt of leaving their child in order to go exercise. The families don't have to pay for day care. The baby loves the interaction and attention. The mothers get a wonderful interactive experience with their child and also get a good workout. And this form of exercise is definitely functional training since the mothers become fit using the weight they carry around all day—their baby.

Another very creative example of a niche market program is a class that combines the enjoyment of music with physical movement. This class, which is based on basic conducting techniques, is called *conductorcise.* The inventor is a retired conductor, David Dworkin, who played clarinet for the American Symphony Orchestra. He suggests that conductorcise is a very good workout, especially for the upper body (Gerard 2006). He also feels that it improves the listening skills of participants and teaches them about the lives and works of great composers. Many musicians are sedentary due to the nature of their activity. Yet they love listening to and learning about music. Thus this mode of exercise can bring a whole new group of participants— musicians—to the exercise experience.

As exercise instructors, we know that there are clients out there we are missing, and so we need to be creative and think outside of the box when coming up with new movement experiences. Keller (2008) outlines several ideas that

have brought energy to group exercise. There's drop-in dodgeball, a game that is held in a basketball court and resembles the dodgeball game played by children. Or there's stadium stompers, a class whose participants use the stairs of an outdoor football stadium to enhance their fitness. Finally, there is the breakfast club, a senior fitness class that combines all the components of fitness with an opportunity to eat breakfast and socialize at the facility's café. All of these programs are client centered and involve not only a fitness component but also a meaningful life experience. This is what creating niche markets in group exercise is all about.

LIFESTYLE-BASED PHYSICAL ACTIVITY CLASSES

Besides the outdoor classes just discussed (StrollerFit, stadium stompers, and so on), there are several lifestyle group exercise opportunities that focus on getting exercise into daily life as a means to help people accomplish their physical activity goals. Many experts believe that public health and fitness professionals need to work together to get people to be more active in their general lives and not just in fitness facilities. As Hooker (2003) states, "Collaboration between public health experts/fitness professionals is not new, but the opportunities for such collaboration are expanding, especially at the community level, and are essential to stem the rising tide of sedentary living and its associated risks for many chronic diseases and conditions."

Pedometer Walking Programs

Several fitness professionals have started group pedometer training. A pedometer is a device that is worn on the hip and measures how many steps people take in a day to give them an idea of how active they are. Some clubs give pedometers to their members, especially those members who are interested in weight loss. Working out in a facility builds fitness but does not expend enough energy to create a large caloric deficit. Everyday movement is needed to reach a healthy weight. This is an important concept for fitness professionals to model to their clients. We need to be active in our activities of daily living and provide programs that help participants measure their own activity levels outside of their fitness experiences. Online pedometer recording and a 6-week pedometer competition program are a group activity that allows participants to exercise on their own time but still support and talk to one another if desired. An online lifestyle-based physical activity program can provide a means for participants to record their activity, communicate with others, set up walking meetings, or just chat about walking opportunities. These types of programs are available and are easy to add to a group exercise schedule.

An example of a lifestyle-based physical activity program in the United States is the President's Challenge, which includes a Presidential Active Lifestyle Award that recognizes children for their regular participation in physical activity by giving them a presidential emblem and a certificate signed by the U.S. President. For this program, students must engage in physical activity for at least 60 minutes or take 11,000 steps (as shown on the pedometer in figure 15.1) each day for 5 days per week for 6 weeks. These types of lifestyle programs allow fitness instructors to demonstrate concern for their participants by educating them that physical activity happens not just in a facility or in a group exercise class but also in daily life.

Outdoor Walking and In-Line Skating

People often rank walking as their number one sport and recreational activity, and so leading a walking class can be a great way to expand your teaching options. A walking class should include a warm-up and cool-down with plenty of stretching. Many instructors also include drills such as walking backward or sideways or incorporate interval training. Some even provide strength training stations along the walking route for circuit-type muscular conditioning. It's ideal to lead a walking class with two instructors, one as the leader in front and one as the shepherd in back. This way the class can accommodate participants of varying fitness levels and the participants can walk at their appropriate speed.

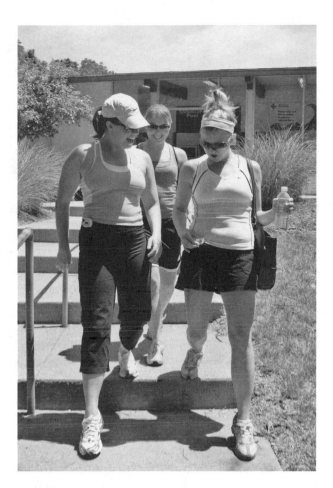

▶ **Figure 15.1** One of the most important lessons that we as group exercise instructors can teach our participants is that physical activity can happen all day long.

Various walking devices may be used to increase the intensity (Porcari 1999). These include weighted vests, hand weights or weighted gloves, walking poles, and power belts (a belt worn around the waist that provides resistance cords with handles). Another way to increase intensity is power walking or power striding, a high-intensity version of walking that uses more vigorous upper-body movements and some hip rotation (see figure 15.2). Encourage your class members to walk with good technique: head and neck in neutral, eyes looking ahead, arms and hands relaxed, each step rolling from heel to toe, knees soft, pelvis in neutral.

 See the DVD for a demonstration of a walking class.

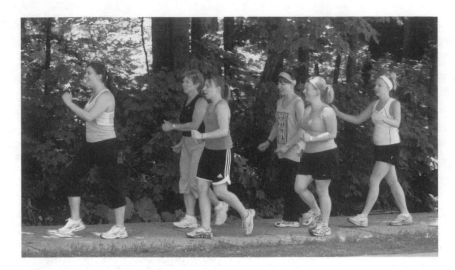

▶ **Figure 15.2** An outdoor walking class.

In-line skating is another lifestyle-based group exercise option. It has been shown to be an appropriate form of exercise for improving cardiorespiratory fitness (Melanson et al. 1996). However, instructors who wish to lead in-line skating classes must have the proper training, must use the appropriate locations (such as an empty parking lot), must require proper equipment (such as skates, helmets, wrist guards, and elbow and knee pads), and, as always, must promote safety and fun!

DANCE-BASED CLASSES

Several different dance-based classes are finding their way into the group exercise setting. Many people who once danced on their high school dance and drill team or took dance lessons as a child find that moving to music is what they enjoy doing for their daily physical activity. One example of such a program is a cheer-dance class we once had on our group exercise schedule. For this class, a cheerleader came to the facility to teach all the routines performed during the school fight song or during the half-time show. There was a huge response by participants wanting to learn these movements. Such a class is an example of using the client-centered approach to reach individuals who enjoy dance. There are several other dance formats used for dance-style group exercise that

we will review in this chapter. They are NIA, Latin dance, hip-hop, funk, country dancing, Zumba, and ballet barre.

NIA (neuromuscular integrative action) is a group exercise modality that incorporates free-style modern and ethnic dance, tai chi, martial arts, and yoga. It combines a cardiorespiratory stimulus with increased mind–body awareness, blending elements of Eastern and Western philosophies. According to Rosas and Rosas (2006), a typical NIA class is part choreographed movement, with students following the instructor's lead, and part freestyle movement, with participants dancing as if no one were watching. Dancing with partners or dancing in lines, circles, and rows may be used to vary the group dynamics. A variety of music styles are included—new age, funk, Latin, rock, rhythm and blues, and jazz— and the music tempo varies from song to song, depending on the instructor's plan. Shoes are off, impact is reduced, and participants are encouraged to express themselves. A major objective of NIA is to help participants become more internally directed in their physical expressions and to help them listen to their bodies and move in ways that are holistic, pleasurable, and joyful.

Many clubs offer specialty classes in a particular dance style such as Latin dance, funk, hip-hop, country, or Zumba. Kahn (2008) states that people are growing bored with traditional fitness classes and enjoy dancing and learning new movements they can use when they go out dancing for fun. Many of the dance styles used in group exercise classes come with specific moves or dance steps. Latin moves, for example, include the samba, rumba, merengue, cha-cha, lambada, salsa, calypso, and mambo. Country moves include the swivel, hip bump, tush push, and boot scoot; these moves are frequently arranged into line dances and can be readily adapted for cardiorespiratory classes (Lane 2000). Funk and hip-hop styles are performed to downbeat-centered music and combine upper-body isolations and many familiar dance moves such as the step touch, march, jazz square, and plié with African and street stylizations and complex rhythmic patterns. Zumba is a branded program that combines Latin moves and international music. It is an interval format that blends exercise and fun dancing into a positive movement experience that leaves people smiling when they work out.

 See the DVD for a demonstration of a hip-hop class.

 See the DVD for a demonstration of a Latin dance class.

A few clubs offer ballet barre or other dance-based classes fused with traditional fitness elements. These classes vary depending on the instructor's background and skills and can include muscular conditioning exercises performed at the bar, traditional cardio or jazz dance in the center of the room, Pilates exercises, and dance-based stretches. Barre work can consist of traditional fitness moves, such as standing hip abduction, hip adduction, extension work, lunges, and squats, or of ballet moves such as the plié, relevé, tendu, battement, frappé, rond de jambe, and port de bras. Center work might include traditional high-low impact moves or ballet moves such as turns, pirouettes, jumps, and choreographed routines. In these types of classes, care should be taken to modify the high-risk dance moves to make them appropriate for the general population. Moves such as the full port de bras, grand plié, and cervical hyperextension are risky for the neck, back, and knees and are not appropriate for deconditioned adults desiring health-related fitness. As always, a dance-based class should provide a proper warm-up and a sufficient cool-down, including flexibility work.

EQUIPMENT-BASED CARDIORESPIRATORY TRAINING

Equipment-based cardio programming involves classes that use traditional cardiorespiratory equipment such as treadmills, rowing machines, cross-country ski machines, and elliptical (cross-trainer) machines. Popular programs using one or more of these modalities have been developed by innovative instructors at several facilities (Nichols et al. 2000; Pillarella 1997). The steps involved in instructing an equipment-based cardio conditioning class are fairly simple:

1. Make certain you understand how to set up your machines, including how to use the instrument panel (if any) and how to adjust the machine to each individual.

2. Learn how to demonstrate and teach proper biomechanics, alignment, and technique on the machines.

3. Design a physiologically sound class format.

An appropriate class format adheres to the points outlined in the group exercise class evaluation form and includes a warm-up (usually performed on the machine itself), a cardio conditioning segment, and a postcardio cool-down. Some instructors move the class into another room for muscular conditioning or stretching after the cardio segment, although this is not necessary (see table 15.1). Many equipment-based classes use interval training, which can be adjusted to match all fitness levels. For interval training, participants need instruction regarding what intensity level to work at during the intervals. In general, you can encourage your class to work at a 12 or 13 on the RPE scale during the easier intervals and at a 14 or 15 during the harder intervals (see figure 6.3 from chapter 6).

In a treadmill (or treading) class, participants can walk or run, depending on their fitness level. If they wish to increase their intensity, participants can increase the treadmill speed or elevation or both. You can play motivating music in the background, or you can try putting on a song

Table 15.1 Sample Equipment-Based Class

Workout segment	Duration (min)	Intensity
Warm-up	5	Light
Stretch	3	Light
Flat road or easy paddle	5	Moderate
Interval training	5	Moderate to hard
Recovery	2	Light
Steady work	5	Moderate
Interval training	5	Hard
Steady work	5	Moderate
Interval training	5	Moderate to hard
Cool-down and stretch	5	Light

with an appropriate beat for movement, offering your class the option of walking or running on the beat (see figure 15.3).

 See the DVD for a demonstration of a treadmill class.

Slide Training

Another cardiorespiratory modality for group exercise is slide training, also known as *lateral movement training.* The slide workout provides an aerobic workout that compares with high-low impact, step, and cycling in terms of caloric expenditure (Frodge et al. 1993; Ludwig et al. 1994; Williford et al. 1993). Slide training involves lateral (side-to-side) motion and trains the body's systems in the frontal plane, which can be useful in many sports. Tennis, skating, skiing, basketball, and football all require the ability to move laterally and to maintain lateral stability around the joints. Slide training is low impact, enhances balance and agility, and injects variety into group exercise.

Specially designed boards, known as *slideboards,* and special booties that fit over the shoes are required for slide training. Most slideboards used in the fitness setting are 6 feet (1.8 m) long and have end ramps that stop the participant from sliding off the ends. The workouts can

resemble athletic training (performed without music or without following the beat) or can be choreographed to music with combinations and the 32-count phrase discussed in chapter 4. There are two basic stances on the slideboard: the upright stance and the athletic ready stance (which is more difficult and resembles the position of a speed skater). Possible moves on the slideboard include cross-country skiing and speed skating as well as the basic slide, slide touch, knee lift, hamstring curl, fencing slide, lunge, and slide squat. All of these can be accompanied by a variety of arm movements (see figure 15.4). Appropriate music speeds for slide training are 124 to 140 beats per minute. A warm-up that includes rehearsal moves on the slideboard and a cool-down that stretches the muscles used in lateral training (especially the hip abductors and adductors) are essential. Another form of slide training often used for muscular conditioning that is easier to incorporate into a group exercise class (because participants don't have to get out a lot of equipment) is a device called the *gliding disc.* Gliding discs are two round devices that you put under your feet to destabilize the lower body. The movements performed on gliding discs are similar to those performed on a slideboard. Gliding discs are portable and cost around $10.00 U.S. per pair. If slideboards are not in your budget, you

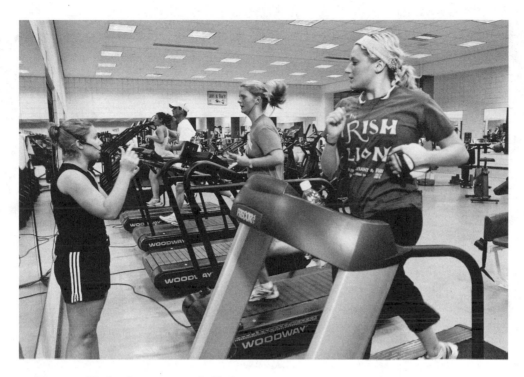

▶ **Figure 15.3** A group treadmill class.

can use these devices to accomplish some of the same fun, fitness, and core-stabilization exercises provided by a slideboard.

 See the DVD for a demonstration of slide training.

Rebounding

In rebounding, participants exercise on a rebounder, a device that looks like a minitrampoline. At least one study has shown that rebounding and treadmill exercise produce comparable cardiorespiratory results (McGlone et al. 2002). This finding indicates that rebounding meets ACSM criteria for the achievement of aerobic fitness. Rebounding is classified as a low-impact activity and appears to place minimal stress on the joints and connective tissues. Routines choreographed to music of approximately 126 beats per minute can be created with a variety of moves such as jumping jacks, twists, and alternating strides (all double-leg moves in which both feet contact the rebounder at the same time) and jogging, knee lifts, and kicks (one-leg moves in which only one foot contacts the rebounder

at a time). Rebounding is fun and playful and can provide a challenging workout.

BOSU Balance and Core Board Training

Chapter 7 discussed the appropriate use of the stability ball in a group exercise setting. Stability balls are a staple in most fitness facilities. They are so popular that many facilities place them on the floor so participants can utilize them when working out on their own. Two other destabilizing products have recently hit the fitness market. They are the core board made by Reebok and the BOSU balance trainer. The core board is sold for around $150.00 U.S. and is a bit more expensive than a stability ball, which generally sells for around $40.00 U.S. Still, some facilities have invested in core boards for their group exercise classes. The idea of these boards is that they destabilize the body so that the core does more work during a basic group exercise session. Some instructors use the board for a combination cardio and strength class, while others teach a strength-oriented class. The core board strives to incorporate balance and destabilization into

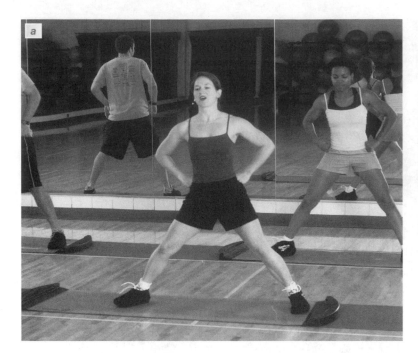
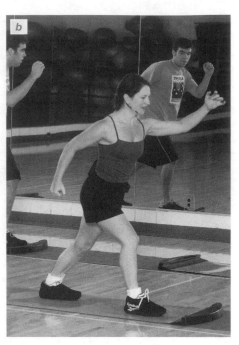

▶ **Figure 15.4** *(a)* Slide touch and *(b)* cross-country slide.

one equipment piece. Webb (2006) states that the board was designed to respond dynamically to the user's movements. Thus the core board adds a functional training aspect to a traditional stability ball workout. The core board may be ahead of its time, as balance and proprioception will most likely be the next health-related fitness components added to the ACSM guidelines.

The BOSU balance trainer is similar to the core board but is a lot less expensive, costing $100 to $120.00 U.S. Because it resembles half a stability ball, participants are a bit more familiar with this type of destabilization exercise. BOSU balance trainers have a flat base, and so they are easier for the participants to set up in a group class. Newcomers may find them intimidating because staying on them does require a great deal of balance (Webb 2005) and having to balance and move together can be overwhelming at first.·

Overall, the BOSU balance trainer and core board are very appropriate when used one on one in personal training. Utilizing them in a group setting is difficult because of the varying abilities of the participants. The fitness industry continually invents products that help the fit get fitter, and the BOSU balance trainer and core board are examples of such products. Instructors

who are interested in appreciating the beginner should focus more on products such as the pedometer, which can be sold to each participant for less than $15.00 U.S. and can make a huge difference in daily caloric expenditure.

MIND–BODY CLASSES

Two of the best examples of a mind–body experience are the old arts of tai chi and qigong. Both tai chi and qigong promote movement and meditation practices based on ancient Chinese philosophies. These philosophies are purported to promote mental and physical health, vitality, and functional well-being and are said to cultivate social and spiritual values. Several different versions of tai chi exist, but the Yang style is perhaps the most popular and accessible. It encompasses 24 forms, or series of movements. These forms are meant to be practiced daily and can be practiced anywhere. In terms of the health-related components of fitness, both tai chi and qigong promote flexibility, balance, muscle endurance, and coordination. They have been advocated as an ideal exercise for lifelong well-being, and they may especially appeal to seniors due to their gentle, nonimpact nature. In fact, several studies have shown that tai chi improves balance and reduces falls in the elderly (Lan et al. 1998; Li et al. 2005). Another study (Young et al. 1999) found that aerobic exercise and tai chi had similar effects on reducing blood pressure in older people. Tai chi and qigong encourage the integration of mind, body, and spirit, and, like yoga, focus on bringing the practitioner's attention into the present moment. This principle of mindfulness, as well as the focus on performing slow movements with complete awareness, is a concept that can be applied to other forms of group exercise. Chodzko-Zajko and colleagues (2006) published recommendations that can assist agencies and facilities seeking to develop and implement successful mind–body programs for their clients. These recommendations are worth reviewing before setting up such a program (see figure 15.5).

 See the DVD for a demonstration of a tai chi class.

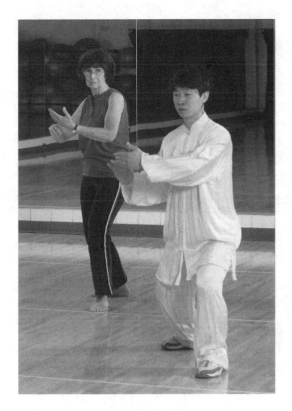

▶ **Figure 15.5** A group tai chi class.

FUSION CLASSES

These days, the latest buzzword in group exercise classes is *fusion*. A fusion class blends different components of exercise. For example, a cardio and core class is a fusion class is which 20 minutes of cardio is followed by 20 minutes of core strength training. Because people are busy, lack time, and bore easily, fusion classes were created to provide an exercise format that is more entertaining and efficient. The number and types of possible fusion classes are limited only by an instructor's imagination. Popular combinations include Yogilates (yoga plus Pilates), yoga tai chi, Spinning plus yoga, ballet and Pilates, outdoor walking followed by muscular conditioning on a stability ball, step intervals interspersed with intervals of Latin dance, and rebounding followed by 20 minutes of stretching. Some clubs offer jump and pump: intervals of jumping rope interspersed with intervals of muscular conditioning. Circuits are another great way to accomplish a lot of work in an hour. To devise a circuit, set up muscular conditioning stations around the room

and have participants rotate through the stations, either individually or in small groups (or pods). When designing fusion classes, be creative; you have an unlimited number of options and people like to have choices!

Some classes that combine many aspects of training do not like to be referred to as *fusion classes*. For example budokon is a blend of yoga, martial arts, and meditation that combines both the mental and the physical aspects of wellness into one group exercise offering. The inventor of budokon does not talk about the health benefits of exercise but rather the human potential and the art of movement (Anders 2006). The word *fusion* does not always mean the combining of two different modes of exercise; it can also be used to describe a combination of mind and body movements. This type of fusion brings us closer to calling our profession a *wellness profession* rather than an *exercise* or a *fitness profession*. In general, the fusion of various exercise modalities can have different interpretations for different professionals. Right now it is just the new buzzword in fitness programming.

ETHICAL PRACTICE GUIDELINES FOR GROUP FITNESS INSTRUCTORS

We wanted to take a moment to thank the IDEA Health and Fitness Association and AFAA for providing us with so much of the information collected in this book. Both organizations have led the way in setting practice guidelines and ethical standards for the field of group exercise. IDEA has outlined ethical practices for group fitness instructors (IDEA 2005), and AFAA has developed basic exercise standards and guidelines (AFAA 2002). If you keep these in mind along with the group exercise class evaluation form presented in this book, you will be well on your way to making a difference in the health and wellness of your participants.

Following are IDEA's ethical practice guidelines for group fitness instructors:

1. Always be guided by the best interests of the group, while still acknowledging individuals.
2. Provide a safe exercise environment.
3. Obtain the education and training necessary to lead group exercise.
4. Use truth, fairness, and integrity to guide all professional decisions and relationships.
5. Maintain appropriate professional boundaries.
6. Uphold a professional image through conduct and appearance.

The AFAA's basic exercise standards and guidelines make up the first 43 pages of AFAA's *Fitness Theory and Practice* (AFAA 2002). First formulated in 1983, they have been updated periodically based on new research findings. The AFAA standards and guidelines include basic fitness terminology, the AFAA 5 Questions (an excellent system of exercise analysis), lists and photographs of high-risk exercises and appropriate modifications, detailed descriptions and photographs of proper body alignment, and specific standards and guidelines for warm-up, cardiorespiratory training, muscular strength and endurance training, flexibility training, and the final class segment.

CHAPTER WRAP-UP

This chapter covered practical techniques for leading a wide variety of group exercise classes. When developing your original class, check yourself against the group exercise class evaluation form and the IDEA and AFAA practice guidelines and ethical standards to be sure your class meets the basic criteria for each segment. You will find helpful contact information for specific exercise formats in the resource list on page 301.

▶ **Group Exercise Class Evaluation Form Key Points**

■ Gradually increase intensity. This is especially important in cardiorespiratory classes such as treading, rowing, slide training, rebounding, and NIA.

■ Use a variety of muscle groups and minimize repetitive movements. This is especially important in classes such as sport conditioning, NIA, ballet barre, Zumba, hip-hop, and country dancing.

■ Demonstrate good form, alignment, and technique.

■ Use appropriate music. Some classes may be highly choreographed (NIA, Zumba, hip-hop, country dance) and may require you to be able to teach to the beat and use the phrasing of the music. Other classes such as treading, rowing, and BOSU balance training may require only background music, if any.

■ Give clear cues and verbal directions. Provide anticipatory cues, safety and alignment information, directional cues, and motivational cues.

■ Promote participant interaction and encourage fun. This is important in most classes; however, some classes such as tai chi and qigong are more meditative, in which case you may encourage participants to cultivate an inner awareness.

■ Gradually decrease intensity during cool-downs in all classes.

▶ **Assignment**

Using the group exercise class evaluation form in appendix A to record your observations, evaluate (but do not participate in) a unique group exercise class that uses any of the modalities mentioned in this chapter. See yourself as the supervisor of the class instructor and write a one-page paper describing any corrective feedback you would give this instructor to help improve the class. Start with the top three things you thought went well and then list the top three things you felt could use improvement. Staple together the completed evaluation form and the one-page analysis before handing them in.

Group Exercise Class Resource List for Other Modalities

The Indoor Rowing Institute, 800-245-5676, ext. 3022

United States Rowing Association, 317-237-5656

American Institute of Reboundology, www.healthbounce.com

Urban Rebounding, www.urbanrebounding.com

NIA, 800-762-5762, www.nianow.com

New York City Ballet, 212-870-4068, www.nycballet.com

International In-Line Skating Association, 407-368-9141

Baby Boot Camp, 888-990-BABY, www.babybootcamp.com

StrollerFit, 513-489-2920, www.strollerfit.com

Stroller Strides, 866-FIT-4MOM, www.strollerstrides.com

Mommy and Me, www.mommyandme.com

Conductorcise, www.conductorcise.com

Zumba, www.zumba.com

President's Challenge, www.fitness.gov/challenge

Budokon, www.budokon.com

National Qigong Association, www.nqa.org

Tai Chi Network, www.taichinetwork.org/index.html

Gliding, www.glidingdisc.com

Appendix A

GROUP EXERCISE CLASS EVALUATION FORM

Instructor: _____ Evaluator: _____

Date: _____ Class: _____

Time: _____

Scoring system: 2 = proficient, 1 = adequate, 0 = inadequate

Pre-Class Organization

Begins class on time . . . . □

Has equipment and music ready for use . . . . □

Acknowledges class . . . . □

Comments _____

_____

_____

Warm-Up

Includes appropriate amount of dynamic movement . . . . □

Provides rehearsal moves . . . . □

Stretches major muscle groups in a biomechanically sound manner with appropriate instructions . . . . □

Gives clear cues and verbal directions . . . . □

Uses an appropriate music tempo (120-136 beats per minute) or motivating music that inspires movement . . . . . □

Comments: _____

_____

_____

Warm-Up

Muscle groups	Warm-up	Stretch
Quadriceps and hip flexors		
Hamstrings		
Calves		
Shoulder joint muscles		
Low-back muscles		

Cardiorespiratory Training

Gradually increases intensity . . . . ☐

Uses a variety of muscle groups (especially hamstrings and abductors) . . . . ☐

Minimizes repetitive movements . . . . ☐

Promotes participant interaction and encourages fun . . . . ☐

Demonstrates movement options and gives clear verbal cues . . . . ☐

Gradually decreases impact and intensity during cool-down following the cardiorespiratory session . . . . ☐

Uses music volume and tempo (134-158 beats per minute) appropriate for biomechanical movement . . . . ☐

Comments: _____

_____

_____

Intensity Monitoring

Takes pulse rate (PR) or RPE at middle of activity . . . . ☐

Keeps participants moving during PR counts . . . . ☐

Suggests modifications based on PR or RPE results and encourages participants to work at their own levels . . . . . ☐

Comments: _____

_____

_____

Muscular Conditioning and Flexibility Training

Gives verbal cues on posture and alignment. . . . . □

Encourages and demonstrates good body mechanics. . . . . □

Observes participants' form and suggests modifications for participants with injuries
or special needs as well as progressions for advanced participants . . . . □

Gives clear verbal directions and uses appropriate music volume . . . . □

Uses appropriate music tempo for biomechanical movement . . . . □

Chooses appropriate music for flexibility training. . . . . □

Includes static stretching . . . . □

Appropriately emphasizes relaxation and visualization . . . . □

Comments: _____

_____

_____

Muscle group worked	Strengthening or flexibility exercise	Comments
Upper body		
Lower body		
Torso		

Overall Summary

From *Methods of Group Exercise Instruction, Second Edition,* by Carol Kennedy-Armbruster and Mary M. Yoke, 2009, Champaign, IL: Human Kinetics.

SHORT HEALTH HISTORY FORM

Name: _____   Date: _____

The following information will be kept strictly confidential and will be utilized only to help make your workout safe. Please check any conditions that may apply to you.

Have you ever been told by a physician that you have or have had any of the following?

	YES	NO
Heart attack.	☐	☐
Seizure	☐	☐
Stroke.	☐	☐
High cholesterol levels (>200)	☐	☐
High blood pressure.	☐	☐
Abnormal electrocardiogram (EKG)	☐	☐
Cancer	☐	☐
Diabetes.	☐	☐
Lung problems.	☐	☐
Arthritis	☐	☐
Osteoporosis	☐	☐
Gout.	☐	☐

If you are currently taking any prescription or over-the-counter medications, please list them here:

_____

_____

_____

	YES	NO
1. Do you smoke?	☐	☐
2. Can you swim?	☐	☐
3. Do you exercise aerobically three to four times per week?	☐	☐

Do you have any past or current injuries or problems with any of the following areas?

	YES	NO
Irregular heart beat	☐	☐
Cramping	☐	☐
Low back	☐	☐
Chest pain	☐	☐
Shin splints	☐	☐
Midback	☐	☐
Loss of coordination	☐	☐
Neck	☐	☐
Shoulders	☐	☐
Heat intolerance	☐	☐
Hands	☐	☐
Feet	☐	☐
Dizziness	☐	☐
Hips	☐	☐
Ankles	☐	☐
Fainting	☐	☐
Calves	☐	☐
Knees	☐	☐

I realize that there are risks, including injury and possible death, to all exercise. While every effort will be made to decrease any risk of injury, I take full responsibility for my participation in this class. Knowing that I may participate at my own pace and that I am free to discontinue participation at any time, I will inform the instructor of any problems—immediately.

Signature: _____ Date: _____

From *Methods of Group Exercise Instruction, Second Edition,* by Carol Kennedy-Armbruster and Mary M. Yoke, 2009, Champaign, IL: Human Kinetics.

Appendix C

LONG HEALTH HISTORY FORM

Name: _____

Street address: _____

City, state, zip code: _____

Home and work phone numbers: _____

Date of birth and age: _____

Physicians: _____

Date of last physical: _____

Date of last surgery: _____

Date of last electrocardiogram (EKG): _____

Please list any physician-prescribed drugs or dietary supplements you are taking now.

Drug: _____

Dosage: _____

For: _____

Reactions: _____

Drug: _____

Dosage: _____

For: _____

Reactions: _____

Please list any self-prescribed drugs or dietary supplements you are taking now.

Drug: _____

Dosage: _____

For: _____

Reactions: _____

Drug: _____

Dosage: _____

For: _____

Reactions: _____

If necessary, please list other medications on the back of this page.

Please indicate a yes response to the following questions by placing a check in the space provided.

Have you ever been told by a doctor that you have or have had the following?

	YES	NO
Rheumatic fever	☐	☐
Diabetes	☐	☐
Heart murmur	☐	☐
Lung or pulmonary conditions	☐	☐
Heart or vascular problems	☐	☐
Arthritis	☐	☐
Heart attack	☐	☐
Osteoporosis	☐	☐
Seizure or epilepsy	☐	☐
Gout or hyperuricemia	☐	☐
Stroke	☐	☐
Thyroid disorder	☐	☐
High cholesterol (>200)	☐	☐
Allergies	☐	☐
High blood pressure	☐	☐
Neck problems	☐	☐
High blood triglycerides	☐	☐
Midback problems	☐	☐
Abnormal electrocardiogram (EKG)	☐	☐
Low-back problems	☐	☐
Blood clots or thrombophlebitis	☐	☐
Varicose veins	☐	☐
Cancer	☐	☐

Has anyone in your immediate family (grandparents, parents, brothers, or sisters) had any of the following?

	YES	NO
Heart attack or stroke before the age of 55	☐	☐
High blood pressure	☐	☐
Heart surgery	☐	☐
High blood triglycerides	☐	☐
High cholesterol (>200)	☐	☐
Diabetes	☐	☐

Do you smoke?

Yes . . . . □

No . . . . □

If you smoke, how much?

Half a pack or less a day . . . . □

One pack a day . . . . □

Two or more packs a day . . . . □

If you smoke, for how long?

Less than 5 years . . . . □

Between 5 and 15 years . . . . □

More than 15 years . . . . □

What type of exercise do you participate in regularly?

None . . . . □

Competitive sports . . . . □

Walking . . . . □

Outdoor cycling . . . . □

Jogging . . . . □

Weightlifting . . . . □

Running . . . . □

Dancing . . . . □

Group exercise (step, kickboxing, indoor cycling) . . . . □

Rebounding . . . . □

Swimming or water exercise . . . . □

Stationary cycling . . . . □

Other: _____

How many times per week do you participate in the previously listed activities?

1. . . . . ☐

2. . . . . ☐

3. . . . . ☐

4. . . . . ☐

5. . . . . ☐

6. . . . . ☐

7. . . . . ☐

How much time do you spend at each session?

Less than 15 minutes . . . . ☐

30 to 45 minutes . . . . ☐

15 to 20 minutes . . . . ☐

45 to 60 minutes . . . . ☐

20 to 30 minutes . . . . ☐

More than 60 minutes. . . . . ☐

What word best describes the intensity of your average workout?

Very light . . . . ☐

Light. . . . . ☐

Moderate . . . . ☐

Hard . . . . ☐

Very hard . . . . ☐

Extremely hard . . . . ☐

During or after exertion, do you experience any of the following?

	YES	NO
Shortness of breath or wheezing	☐	☐
Vomiting	☐	☐
Side aches or side stitches	☐	☐
Swelling of ankles or hands	☐	☐
Extremely high heart rate	☐	☐
Cramping	☐	☐
Irregular heartbeat	☐	☐
Shin splints	☐	☐
Sharp chest pain	☐	☐
Arm or neck pain	☐	☐
Dull, aching chest pain	☐	☐
Hip pain	☐	☐
Overall or one-sided weakness	☐	☐
Calf pain	☐	☐
Loss of coordination	☐	☐
Low-back pain	☐	☐
Heat intolerance	☐	☐
Midback pain	☐	☐
Dizziness	☐	☐
Shoulder pain	☐	☐
Mental confusion	☐	☐
Foot or ankle pain	☐	☐
Fainting	☐	☐
Knee pain	☐	☐

What would you like to accomplish through exercise? _____

_____

I acknowledge that my answers to these questions are true and complete. I will immediately inform the exercise instructor of any changes in my health.

Signature: _____

Date: _____

From *Methods of Group Exercise Instruction, Second Edition,* by Carol Kennedy-Armbruster and Mary M. Yoke, 2009, Champaign, IL: Human Kinetics.

Appendix D

INFORMED CONSENT FORM

I desire to engage voluntarily in _____ (name of program, club, or agency) to improve my physical fitness.

I know that I am required to fill out a health and lifestyle questionnaire before I begin to exercise. The information obtained from the questionnaire will be used in the following ways:

- To indicate any cardiac risk or other reason why I should not exercise based on the ACSM guidelines
- To determine the need for a physician's evaluation and written approval before I enter the exercise program
- To recommend the types of exercise I should concentrate on to reach my fitness goals and the types of exercises I should avoid

I understand that my participation in the program may not benefit me directly in any way. I realize that the program may help me evaluate my lifestyle, choose the activities I may safely carry out, and increase my quality of life.

I also understand that the reaction of the body to activity cannot always be predicted with complete accuracy. The changes that may occur and are associated with physical activity include, but are not limited to, the following signs and symptoms:

- Abnormal blood pressure or heart rate responses
- Breathlessness
- Chest discomfort
- Muscular or skeletal injury
- Heart attack and death, in very rare instances

I realize my responsibility in recognizing these potential hazards; monitoring myself before, during, and after exercise; and seeking help in the event of injury, if possible. I will attend the orientation session and talk to my personal trainer or exercise instructor to learn how to minimize these potential hazards and what I should do in an emergency. I understand that I can minimize my risk during exercise by following these steps:

- I will give priority to regular attendance.
- I will not withhold any information pertinent to my health from the instructor or supervisor in charge of the program, and I will immediately update my health and lifestyle questionnaire if changes in my medication or status occur.
- I will report any unusual symptoms or problems that I experience before, during, or after exercise.
- I will follow the amounts and types of activities recommended during the orientation session.
- I will not exceed my target heart rate.
- I will not exercise when not feeling well or for 2 hours after eating, smoking a cigarette, drinking alcohol, or taking over-the-counter medications or street drugs.
- I will cool down slowly after exercise and will not take an extremely hot shower after exercise.
- I will not undertake isometric, straining, or any other exercises that I know by my experience or my physician's or therapist's recommendation to be painful or detrimental to me.
- I realize that unsupervised exercise done on my own is performed at my own risk, even though I may be following guidelines or recommendations established during this program.

The information obtained from this exercise program will be treated as privileged and confidential and will not be released to any person without my written consent. Information regarding my health and program may be shared with instructors involved in my instruction or physical training. The information obtained also may be used for statistical or scientific purposes, with my right to privacy retained.

I, the undersigned, waive and release _____ (name of program, club, or agency) and its employees, officers, or directors from any and all claims in any way connected with my participation in this program. This agreement is binding on my heirs and executors.

I acknowledge that I have read or heard this document in its entirety and that I fully understand it. I have asked any questions that may have occurred to me and have been answered to my satisfaction.

Signature: _____

Date: _____

Witness: _____

Date: _____

From *Methods of Group Exercise Instruction, Second Edition,* by Carol Kennedy-Armbruster and Mary M. Yoke, 2009, Champaign, IL: Human Kinetics.

Appendix E

PAR-Q & YOU

(A Questionnaire for People Aged 15 to 69)

Regular physical activity is fun and healthy, and increasingly more people are starting to become more active every day. Being more active is very safe for most people. However, some people should check with their doctor before they start becoming much more physically active.

If you are planning to become much more physically active than you are now, start by answering the seven questions in the box below. If you are between the ages of 15 and 69, the PAR-Q will tell you if you should check with your doctor before you start. If you are over 69 years of age, and you are not used to being very active, check with your doctor.

Common sense is your best guide when you answer these questions. Please read the questions carefully and answer each one honestly: check YES or NO.

YES	NO		
☐	☐	1.	**Has your doctor ever said that you have a heart condition <u>and</u> that you should only do physical activity recommended by a doctor?**
☐	☐	2.	**Do you feel pain in your chest when you do physical activity?**
☐	☐	3.	**In the past month, have you had chest pain when you were not doing physical activity?**
☐	☐	4.	**Do you lose your balance because of dizziness or do you ever lose consciousness?**
☐	☐	5.	**Do you have a bone or joint problem (for example, back, knee or hip) that could be made worse by a change in your physical activity?**
☐	☐	6.	**Is your doctor currently prescribing drugs (for example, water pills) for your blood pressure or heart condition?**
☐	☐	7.	**Do you know of <u>any other reason</u> why you should not do physical activity?**

If you answered

YES to one or more questions

Talk with your doctor by phone or in person BEFORE you start becoming much more physically active or BEFORE you have a fitness appraisal. Tell your doctor about the PAR-Q and which questions you answered YES.

- You may be able to do any activity you want — as long as you start slowly and build up gradually. Or, you may need to restrict your activities to those which are safe for you. Talk with your doctor about the kinds of activities you wish to participate in and follow his/her advice.
- Find out which community programs are safe and helpful for you.

NO to all questions

If you answered NO honestly to <u>all</u> PAR-Q questions, you can be reasonably sure that you can:

- start becoming much more physically active — begin slowly and build up gradually. This is the safest and easiest way to go.
- take part in a fitness appraisal — this is an excellent way to determine your basic fitness so that you can plan the best way for you to live actively. It is also highly recommended that you have your blood pressure evaluated. If your reading is over 144/94, talk with your doctor before you start becoming much more physically active.

DELAY BECOMING MUCH MORE ACTIVE:

- if you are not feeling well because of a temporary illness such as a cold or a fever — wait until you feel better; or
- if you are or may be pregnant — talk to your doctor before you start becoming more active.

PLEASE NOTE: If your health changes so that you then answer YES to any of the above questions, tell your fitness or health professional. Ask whether you should change your physical activity plan.

<u>Informed Use of the PAR-Q</u>: The Canadian Society for Exercise Physiology, Health Canada, and their agents assume no liability for persons who undertake physical activity, and if in doubt after completing this questionnaire, consult your doctor prior to physical activity.

No changes permitted. You are encouraged to photocopy the PAR-Q but only if you use the entire form.

NOTE: If the PAR-Q is being given to a person before he or she participates in a physical activity program or a fitness appraisal, this section may be used for legal or administrative purposes.

"I have read, understood and completed this questionnaire. Any questions I had were answered to my full satisfaction."

NAME _____

SIGNATURE _____   DATE _____

SIGNATURE OF PARENT _____   WITNESS _____
or GUARDIAN (for participants under the age of majority)

Note: This physical activity clearance is valid for a maximum of 12 months from the date it is completed and becomes invalid if your condition changes so that you would answer YES to any of the seven questions.

CSEP
SCPE
© Canadian Society for Exercise Physiology   Supported by:  Health Canada   Santé Canada

continued on other side...

From *Physical Activity Readiness Questionnaire* (PAR-Q) © 2002. Reprinted with permission for the Canadian Society for Exercise Physiology. http://www.csep.ca/forms.asp

PAR-Q & YOU

...continued from other side

Physical Activity Readiness
Questionnaire - PAR-Q
(revised 2002)

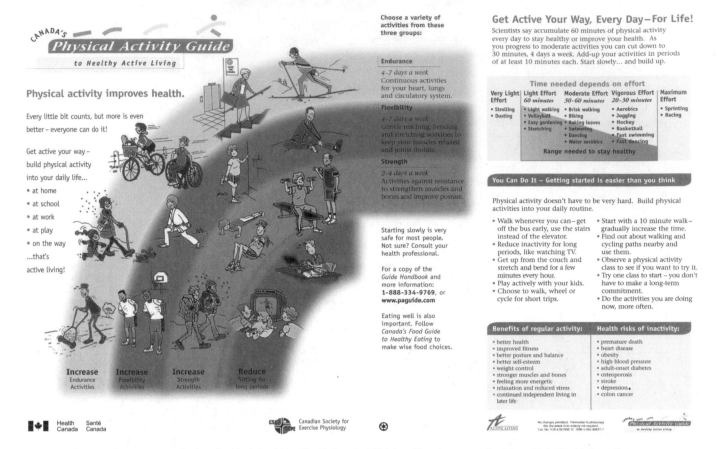

Canada's Physical Activity Guide to Healthy Active Living

Physical activity improves health.

Every little bit counts, but more is even better – everyone can do it!

Get active your way – build physical activity into your daily life...

• at home
• at school
• at work
• at play
• on the way
...that's active living!

Choose a variety of activities from these three groups:

Endurance
4-7 days a week
Continuous activities for your heart, lungs and circulatory system.

Flexibility
4-7 days a week
Gentle reaching, bending and stretching activities to keep your muscles relaxed and joints mobile.

Strength
2-4 days a week
Activities against resistance to strengthen muscles and bones and improve posture.

Starting slowly is very safe for most people. Not sure? Consult your health professional.

For a copy of the *Guide Handbook* and more information: **1-888-334-9769**, or **www.paguide.com**

Eating well is also important. Follow *Canada's Food Guide to Healthy Eating* to make wise food choices.

Increase Endurance Activities	Increase Flexibility Activities	Increase Strength Activities	Reduce Sitting for long periods

Get Active Your Way, Every Day – For Life!

Scientists say accumulate 60 minutes of physical activity every day to stay healthy or improve your health. As you progress to moderate activities you can cut down to 30 minutes, 4 days a week. Add-up your activities in periods of at least 10 minutes each. Start slowly... and build up.

Time needed depends on effort

Very Light Effort	Light Effort 60 minutes	Moderate Effort 30-60 minutes	Vigorous Effort 20-30 minutes	Maximum Effort
• Strolling • Dusting	• Light walking • Volleyball • Easy gardening • Stretching	• Brisk walking • Biking • Raking leaves • Swimming • Dancing • Water aerobics	• Aerobics • Jogging • Hockey • Basketball • Fast swimming • Fast dancing	• Sprinting • Racing

Range needed to stay healthy

You Can Do It – Getting started is easier than you think

Physical activity doesn't have to be very hard. Build physical activities into your daily routine.

• Walk whenever you can – get off the bus early, use the stairs instead of the elevator.
• Reduce inactivity for long periods, like watching TV.
• Get up from the couch and stretch and bend for a few minutes every hour.
• Play actively with your kids.
• Choose to walk, wheel or cycle for short trips.

• Start with a 10 minute walk – gradually increase the time.
• Find out about walking and cycling paths nearby and use them.
• Observe a physical activity class to see if you want to try it.
• Try one class to start – you don't have to make a long-term commitment.
• Do the activities you are doing now, more often.

Benefits of regular activity:	Health risks of inactivity:
• better health • improved fitness • better posture and balance • better self-esteem • weight control • stronger muscles and bones • feeling more energetic • relaxation and reduced stress • continued independent living in later life	• premature death • heart disease • obesity • high blood pressure • adult-onset diabetes • osteoporosis • stroke • depression • colon cancer

Health Canada / Santé Canada

Canadian Society for Exercise Physiology

Source: *Canada's Physical Activity Guide to Healthy Active Living*, Health Canada, 1998 http://www.hc-sc.gc.ca/hppb/paguide/pdf/guideEng.pdf

© Reproduced with permission from the Minister of Public Works and Government Services Canada, 2002.

FITNESS AND HEALTH PROFESSIONALS MAY BE INTERESTED IN THE INFORMATION BELOW:

The following companion forms are available for doctors' use by contacting the Canadian Society for Exercise Physiology (address below):

The **Physical Activity Readiness Medical Examination (PARmed-X)** — to be used by doctors with people who answer YES to one or more questions on the PAR-Q.

The **Physical Activity Readiness Medical Examination for Pregnancy (PARmed-X for Pregnancy)** — to be used by doctors with pregnant patients who wish to become more active.

References:
Arraix, G.A., Wigle, D.T., Mao, Y. (1992). Risk Assessment of Physical Activity and Physical Fitness in the Canada Health Survey Follow-Up Study. **J. Clin. Epidemiol.** 45:4 419-428.
Mottola, M., Wolfe, L.A. (1994). Active Living and Pregnancy, In: A. Quinney, L. Gauvin, T. Wall (eds.), **Toward Active Living: Proceedings of the International Conference on Physical Activity, Fitness and Health**. Champaign, IL: Human Kinetics.
PAR-Q Validation Report, British Columbia Ministry of Health, 1978.
Thomas, S., Reading, J., Shephard, R.J. (1992). Revision of the Physical Activity Readiness Questionnaire (PAR-Q). **Can. J. Spt. Sci.** 17:4 338-345.

To order multiple printed copies of the PAR-Q, please contact the:

Canadian Society for Exercise Physiology
202-185 Somerset Street West
Ottawa, ON K2P 0J2
Tel. 1-877-651-3755 • FAX (613) 234-3565
Online: www.csep.ca

The original PAR-Q was developed by the British Columbia Ministry of Health. It has been revised by an Expert Advisory Committee of the Canadian Society for Exercise Physiology chaired by Dr. N. Gledhill (2002).

Disponible en français sous le titre «Questionnaire sur l'aptitude à l'activité physique - Q-AAP (revisé 2002)».

 © Canadian Society for Exercise Physiology

Supported by: Health Canada / Santé Canada

From *Physical Activity Readiness Questionnaire* (PAR-Q) © 2002. Reprinted with permission for the Canadian Society for Exercise Physiology. http://www.csep.ca/forms.asp

Appendix F

SAMPLE STEP WARM-UP

The following is an outline of the sample step warm-up found on the accompanying DVD. This routine demonstrates

- the appropriate amount of dynamic movement for a step warm-up,
- appropriate rehearsal moves for step, and
- methods to limber and stretch the erector spinae, hamstrings, calves, hip flexors, chest muscles, and anterior shoulder muscles.

Table F.1   Teach Block 1

Move	Foot pattern	Number of counts
Grapevine	R, L, R, tap	4
Tap-up, tap-down	Up, tap, down, tap[a]	4
Grapevine	L, R, L, tap	4
Tap-up, tap-down	Up, tap, down, tap[b]	4
Repeat combination		16

R = right; L = left. Keep drilling the combination until participants know it. [a]Lead L off R end of step; [b]lead R off L end of step.

Table F.2   Teach Block 2

Move	Foot pattern	Number of counts
March on floor	R, L, R, L	4
March on step	R, L, R, L	4
March on floor	R, L, R, L	4
March on step	R, L, R, L	4

R = right; L = left. Repeat block, adding arms: Pump or shake hands down when marching on floor. Pump hands up, shaking R, L, R, L, when marching on step. Keep drilling this combination until participants know it.

Table F.3   Teach Block 3

Move	Foot pattern	Number of counts
Step touch on floor	R, tap, L, tap (repeat)	8
Step touch on step	R, tap, L, tap (repeat)	8
Step touch on floor	R, tap, L, tap (repeat)	8
Step touch on step	R, tap, L, tap (repeat)	8

R = right; L = left. Keep drilling this combination as necessary.

Table F.4 Combine Elements of the Blocks to Create a
Total Combination

Move	Foot pattern	Number of counts
March on floor	R, L, R, L	4
March on step	R, L, R, L	4
March on floor	R, L, R, L	4
March on step	R, L, R, L	4
Step touch on floor	R, tap, L, tap	4
Step touch on floor	R, tap, L, tap	4
Grapevine R	R, L, R, tap	4
Tap-up, tap-down on step	L, tap, R, tap	4

R = right; L = left.

Table F.5 Repeat All Leading Left

Move	Foot pattern	Number of counts
March on floor	L, R, L, R	4
March on step	L, R, L, R	4
March on floor	L, R, L, R	4
March on step	L, R, L, R	4
Step touch on floor	L, tap, R, tap	4
Step touch on floor	L, tap, R, tap	4
Grapevine L	L, R, L, tap	4
Tap-up, tap-down on step	R, tap, L, tap	4

R = right; L = left. Entire combination can be repeated with arms.

Table F.6 Incorporate Joint-Specific Limbering and
Static Stretches Near Left Corner

Move	Foot pattern	Number of counts
Tap-up, tap-down on step	R, tap, L, tap	4
Wide squat on floor, hands on thighs	Wide for 2, together for 2	4
Tap-up, tap-down on step	R, tap, L, tap	4
Wide squat on floor, hands on thighs	Wide for 2, together for 2	4
Stay in squat position with hands on thighs and rhythmically move in and out of spinal flexion (e.g., neutral spine, spinal flexion, neutral spine, spinal flexion)		16+
Hold in spinal flexion for erector spinae static stretch		8+
Move to L corner of bench; place R heel on bench and hinge at hips for R hamstring stretch; perform ankle dorsiflexion and plantar flexion		8+
Hold static R hamstring stretch		8+
Place R foot completely on step and move into calf-stretch position; perform L ankle limbering with dorsiflexion and plantar flexion (add arms reaching up and down)		8
Hold L calf stretch		8+
Bending L knee, roll L heel up and down, adding rhythmic pelvic tilting (add biceps curls)		8+
Hold L hip flexor stretch (pelvis is posteriorly tilted); simultaneously perform a static chest stretch		8+

R = right; L = left

Table F.7 Transition to Other Side by
Performing Initial Combo One Time

Move	Foot pattern	Number of counts
March on floor	R, L, R, L	4
March on step	R, L, R, L	4
March on floor	R, L, R, L	4
March on step	R, L, R, L	4
Step touch on floor	R, tap, L, tap	4
Step touch on floor	R, tap, L, tap	4
Grapevine R	R, L, R, tap	4
Tap-up, tap-down on step	L, tap, R, tap	4

R = right; L = left.

Table F.8 Incorporate Joint-Specific Limbering and Static Stretches Near Right Corner

Move	Foot pattern	Number of counts
Tap-up, tap-down on step	L, tap, R, tap	4
Wide squat on floor, hands on thighs	Wide for 2, together for 2	4
Tap-up, tap-down on step	L, tap, R, tap	4
Wide squat on floor, hands on thighs	Wide for 2, together for 2	4
Stay in squat position, alternately press shoulders down toward floor, rotating the upper spine		16
Hold R shoulder down for static stretch, turn head to L		8
Hold L shoulder down for static stretch, turn head to R		8
Move to R corner of bench; place L heel on bench and hinge at hips for L hamstring stretch; perform ankle dorsiflexion and plantar flexion		8+
Hold static L hamstring stretch		8+
Place L foot completely on step and move into calf-stretch position. Perform R ankle limbering with dorsiflexion and plantar flexion (add arms reaching up and down)		8
Move to R corner of bench; place L heel on bench and hinge at hips for L hamstring stretch; perform ankle dorsiflexion and plantar flexion		8+
Hold R calf stretch		8+
Bending R knee, roll R heel up and down, adding rhythmic pelvic tilting (add biceps curls)		8+
Hold R hip flexor stretch (pelvis is posteriorly tilted); simultaneously perform a static chest stretch		8+

R = right; L = left.

From *Methods of Group Exercise Instruction, Second Edition,* by Carol Kennedy-Armbruster and Mary M. Yoke, 2009, Champaign, IL: Human Kinetics.

Appendix G

SAMPLE WATER EXERCISE PLAN

Warm-Up—8 Minutes

- Play "Brilliant Disguise" and "Sneaker Pumps."
- Teach proper posture for using buoyancy belts.
- Review basic total-body movements such as the jog, mall walk, cross-country skier, and rock climber.
- Review the muscle groups and perform movements through full ROM.
- To work the upper back, lift hands in front, thumbs up.
- To work the chest, lift hands out to the sides and horizontally adduct toward the front; use different planes.
- To work the abdominal muscles, move side-to-side and perform the superman or lie in the sun.
- To work the latissimi dorsi, lift the arms out to the sides and adduct them toward the body, action and reaction, move up.
- To work the biceps and triceps, review movement.
- To work the abductors and adductors, perform jumping jacks with full ROM.
- To work the hamstrings and quadriceps, perform the sit kick and the straight-leg raise with the opposite hand and foot for hip flexion or extension.

Hip Joint Exercises—5 to 7 Minutes

- Play Afro Celtic music.
- To work the pectorals and adductors, move into the seated V-position with arms and legs; power the move.
- To work the rhomboids and abductors, stay in the seated V-position and work the arms and legs together.
- To work the pectorals and abductors, stay in the seated V-position (do little traveling).
- To work the rhomboids and adductors, stay in the seated V-position (do little traveling).
- To work the rhomboids and abductors, sit and scissor the arms, legs starting with arms, legs in front.
- To work the adductors and abdominal stabilizers, keep the legs straight and crisscross them with a small ROM.

Upper-Body Segment—7 Minutes

- Play "I Can See Clearly Now" and "Mixica."
- To work the pectorals, mark the movement, move backward, and run against the water resistance.
- To work the upper back, mark the movement, move forward, and flutter kick against the water resistance.
- To work the latissimi dorsi, take advantage of action and reaction and then overload the muscles by not moving the legs at all.

Quadriceps and Hamstrings Knee Flexion and Extension—8 Minutes

- Play "Beautiful Life" and "Born to Run."
- To work the quadriceps and hamstrings, perform sit kicks using knee flexion and extension.
- Lead the participants in the frustrated dolphin by performing upright double-leg curls.
- To work the hamstrings and gluteal muscles, bicycle in a circle and slice the arms out to the side.
- Bicycle in a circle and add overload by opening the hand while circling.
- To work the hamstrings and deltoids, sit in the V-position and flex the heel to the seat.

Interval Training Using Total-Body Movements and Abdominal Work—6 to 8 Minutes

- Perform 30 seconds work followed by 30 seconds rest—watch the big clock. Suggested movements include jogging, the mall walk, the cross-country skier, the rock climber, the latissimi dorsi leap frog, the straight-leg raise with opposite hand and foot, and the jumping jack. Perform all abdominal movements first.
- Depending on participants' feedback, perform 6 to 8 different intervals.

Inertia Current Work—4 Minutes

- Play "Turn Turn Turn."
- Form a circle and jog into the circle.
- Turn around and run against the inertia current.
- Use all four corners to move. Change the movement to a rock climber.

Wall Movements to Cool-Down—4 Minutes

- Play "Secret Garden."
- Perform standing hip rotation exercises.
- Perform standing stretches to stretch the total body.
- Put the feet on the wall for a hamstring and calf stretch.
- Hold the legs in a V-shape and walk side to side on the wall.
- Face into the pool and stretch the shoulders (Titanic move).

Thermal Rewarming—3 Minutes

- Play "Streets of Philadelphia."
- Perform flutter kick using belts on stomach and in front.
- Stand on the belt for balance training.
- Perform your favorite move and then put the equipment away.

From *Methods of Group Exercise Instruction, Second Edition*, by Carol Kennedy-Armbruster and Mary M. Yoke, 2009, Champaign, IL: Human Kinetics.

Bibliography

Adams, K.J., N.B. Allen, J.E. Schumm, and A.M. Swank. 1997. Oxygen cost of boxing exercise utilizing a heavy bag. Abstract. *Med Sci Sports Exerc* 29(5): S1067.

Aerobics and Fitness Association of America. 2002. *Exercise standards and guidelines manual.* 2nd ed. Sherman Oaks, CA: Aerobics and Fitness Association of America.

AFAA. 2002. *Fitness theory and practice.* 4th ed. Sherman Oaks, CA: Aerobics and Fitness Association of America.

Ahmed, C., W. Hilton, and K. Pituch. 2002. Relations of strength training to body image among a sample of female university students. *J Strength and Cond Res* 16(4): 645-8.

Alan, K. 2003. Building socialization into choreography. *IDEA Fitness Edge* September: 1-5.

Albano, C., and D.J. Terbizan. 2001. Heart rate and RPE difference between aerobic dance and cardio-kickboxing. Abstract. *Med Sci Sports Exerc* 33(5): S604.

Alter, M.J. 2004. *The science of flexibility.* 3rd ed. Champaign, IL: Human Kinetics.

American College of Sports Medicine. 1978. The recommended quantity and quality of exercise for developing and maintaining fitness in healthy adults. *Med Sci Sports Exerc* 10: vii-x.

American College of Sports Medicine. 1990. The recommended quantity and quality of exercise for developing and maintaining fitness in healthy adults. *Med Sci Sports Exerc* 22: 265-74.

American College of Sports Medicine. 1998. The recommended quantity and quality of exercise for developing and maintaining cardiorespiratory and muscular fitness, and flexibility in healthy adults. *Med Sci Sports Exerc* 30(6): 975-91.

American College of Sports Medicine. 2001. Exercise recommendations for flexibility and range of motion. In *ACSM's resource manual for guidelines for exercise testing and prescription,* 4th ed., 468. New York: Lippincott Williams & Wilkins.

American College of Sports Medicine. 2002. Position stand: Progression models in resistance training for healthy adults. *Med Sci Sports Exerc* 34(2): 364-80.

American College of Sports Medicine. 2005. *ACSM's resource manual for guidelines for exercise testing and prescription.* 5th ed. Baltimore: Lippincott Williams & Wilkins.

American College of Sports Medicine. 2006. *ACSM's guidelines for exercise testing and prescription.* 7th ed. Baltimore: Lippincott Williams & Wilkins.

American Council on Exercise. 2000. *Group exercise instructor manual.* San Diego: American Council on Exercise.

American Council on Exercise. 2005. What every fitness professional needs to know about the accreditation of certification programs. *Ace Certified News* October-November: 20-1.

American Heart Association. 2002. Automated external defibrillators in health/fitness facilities. *Circulation* 105(9): 1147-52.

Anders, M. 2006. Budokon: Beyond fusion. *ACE Fitness Matters* May-June: 6-9.

Andersen, J.C. 2005. Stretching before and after exercise: Effect on muscle soreness and injury risk. *J Athl Train* 40: 218-20.

Anderson, P. 2000. The active range warm-up: Getting hotter with time. *IDEA Fitness Edge* April: 6-10.

Anning, J.H., C. Armstrong, E. Mylona, S. Norkus, R. Sterner, and F. Andres. 1999. Physiological responses during cardiovascular kickboxing: A pilot study. Abstract. *Med Sci Sports Exerc* 31(5): S403.

Appel, A. 2007. The right rehearsal. *IDEA Fitness Journal* January: 94.

Aquatic Exercise Association. 1995. *Aquatic fitness professional manual.* Nokomis, FL: Aquatic Exercise Association.

Archer, S. 2005. Tai chi for me. *IDEA Fitness Journal* July-August: 46-51.

Archer, S. 2007. Fitness and wellness intertwine: A major industry arises. *IDEA Fitness Journal* July-August: 36-47.

Ariyoshi, M., K. Sonoda, K. Nagata, T. Mashima, M. Zenmyo, C. Paku, Y. Takamiya, H. Yoshimatsu, Y. Hirai, H. Yasunaga, H. Akashi, H. Imayama, T. Shimokobe, A. Inoue, and Y. Mutoh. 1999. Efficacy of aquatic exercise for patients with low-back pain. *Kurume Med J* 46(2): 91-6.

Arpita. 1990. Physiological and psychological effects of hatha yoga: A review. *J Int Assoc of Yoga Ther* 1(I & II): 1-28.

Astrand, P. 1992. Why exercise? *Med Sci Sports Exerc* 24(2): 153-62.

Astrand, P., and K. Rodahl. 1977. *Textbook of work physiology,* New York: McGraw Hill.

Asp, K. 2006. Group training servies, stroller-based exercise programs. *ACE Certified News* December-January: 6-8.

Asp, K. 2007. Looking back and looking forward: The group fitness instructor. *ACE Certified News* December-January: 6-7.

Baechle, T., and T. Earle. 2003. *Essentials of strength training and conditioning*. 3rd ed. Champaign, IL: Human Kinetics.

Bain, L., T. Wilson, and E. Chaikind. 1989. Participant perceptions of exercise programs for overweight women. *Res Q* 60(2): 134-43.

Baker, A. 1998. *Bicycling medicine: Cycling nutrition, physiology, and injury prevention and treatment for riders of all levels*. New York: Fireside.

Bandy, W.D., and J.M. Irion. 1994. The effect of time of static stretch on the flexibility of the hamstring muscles. *Phys Ther* 74: 845-52.

Bates, A., and N. Hanson. 1996. *Aquatic exercise therapy*. Philadelphia: Saunders.

Beals, K. 2003. Mirror, mirror on the wall, who is the most muscular one of all? *ACSM Health and Fitness Journal* March-April: 6-11.

Beckham, S.G., and C.P. Earnest. 2000. Metabolic cost of free weight circuit weight training. *J Sports Med Phys Fitness* 40: 118-25.

Bednarski, K. 1993. Convincing male managers to target women customers. *Working Woman* June: 23-8.

Begley, S. 2006. How to keep your aging brain fit: Aerobics. *Wall Street Journal.* November 16.

Bellinger, B., G.A. St. Clair, A. Oelofse, and M. Lambert. 1997. Energy expenditure of a noncontact boxing training session compared with submaximal treadmill running. *Med Sci Sports Exerc* 29(12): 1653-6.

Bemben, M.G., S.R. Clary, C. Barnes, D.A. Bemben, and A.W. Knehans. 2006. Effects of ballates, step aerobics, and walking on balance in women aged 50-75 years. *Med Sci Sports Exerc* 38(5): S445.

Benson, H. 1980. *The relaxation response*. New York: Avon.

Bernardo, L.M. 2007. The effectiveness of Pilates training in healthy adults: An appraisal of the research literature. *Journal of Bodywork Movement Therapies* 11(2): 106-10.

Bijlani, R.L, R.P. Vempati, R.K. Yadav, R.B. Ray, V. Gupta, R. Sharma, N. Mehta, and S.C. Mahapatra. 2005. A brief but comprehensive lifestyle education program based on yoga reduces risk factors for cardiovascular disease and diabetes mellitus. *J Alt Comp Med* 11(2): 267-74.

Birkel, D.A., and L. Edgren. 2000. Hatha yoga: Improved vital capacity of college students. *Altern Ther Health Med* 6(6): 55-63.

Bissonnette, D., N. Guzman, L. McMillan, S. Catalano, M. Giroux, K. Greenlaw, S. Vivolo, R.M. Otto, and J. Wygand. 1994. The energy requirements of karate aerobic exercise versus low impact aerobic dance. Abstract. *Med Sci Sports Exerc* 26(5): S58.

Blahnik, J., and P. Anderson. 1996. Wake up your warm up. *IDEA Today* June: 46-52.

Blessing, D., G. Wilson, J. Puckett, and H. Ford. 1987. The physiologic effects of 8 weeks of aerobic dance with and without hand-held weights. *Am J Sports Med* 15(5): 508-10.

Borg, G. 1982. Psychophysical bases of perceived exertion. *Med Sci Sports Exerc* 14: 377-81.

Bortz, W. 2003. Prevention: A solution to combat rising health care costs. *ACSM Health and Fitness Journal* November-December: 6-8.

Bottomley, J. 1997. *T'ai-chi: Choreography of body and mind. Complementary therapies in rehabilitation: Holistic approaches for prevention and wellness*. Thorofare, NY: Slack.

Bowman, A.J., R. Clayton, A. Murray, J. Reed, M. Subhan, and G. Ford. 1997. Effects of aerobic exercise training and yoga on the baroreflex in healthy elderly persons. *Eur J Clin Invest* 27(5): 443-9.

Bradford, A., M. Scharff-Olson, H.N. Williford, S. Walker, and S. Crumpton. 1999. Cardiorespiratory responses to traditional and advanced group cycling techniques. Abstract. *Med Sci Sports Exerc* 31(5): S422.

Brathwaite, A., D. Davidson, and J. Eickhoff-Shemek. 2006. Recruiting, training, and retaining qualified group exercise leaders: Part 1. *ACSM Health and Fitness Journal* 10(2): 14-8.

Bravo, G., P. Gauthier, P.M. Roy, H. Payette, and P. Gaulin. 1997. A weight bearing, water-based exercise program for orthopedic women: Its impact on bone, functional fitness, and well being. *Arch Phys Med Rehabil* 78(12): 1375-80.

Bray, S., N. Gyurcsik, S. Culos-Reed, K. Dawson, and K. Martin. 2001. An exploratory investigation of the relationship between proxy efficacy, self-efficacy and exercise attendance. *J Health Psychol* 6(4): 425-34.

Brooks, D. 1995. *Resist-a-Ball, programming guide for professionals*. Mammoth Lakes, CA: Moves International.

Brown, P., and M. O'Neill. 1990. A retrospective survey of the incidence and pattern of aerobics-related injuries in Victoria, 1987-1988. *Aust J Sci Med Sport* 22(3): 77-81.

Brown, S., L. Chitwood, K. Beason, and D. McLemore. 1997. Male and female physiologic responses to treadmill and deep water running at matched running cadences. *J Strength Cond Res* 11(2): 107-14.

Burke, E.R. 1994. Proper fit of the bicycle. *Clin Sports Med* 13: 1-14.

Burnette, K., K. Johnson, and P. Kolber. 1999. *Reebok martial arts training: Trainer manual*. Canton, MA: Reebok.

Buschbacher, R.M., and T. Shay. 1999. Martial arts. *Phys Med Rehabil Clin N Am* 10(1): 35-47.

Bushman, B., M. Flynn, F. Andres, C. Lambert, M. Taylor, and W. Braunl. 1997. Effect of 4 weeks of deep water run training on running performance. *Med Sci Sports Exerc* 29(5): 694-9.

Byrnes, W. 1985. Muscle soreness following resistance exercise with and without eccentric contractions. *Res Q Exerc Sport* 56: 283.

Calarco, L., R. Otto, J. Wygand, J. Kramer, M. Yoke, and F. D'Zamko. 1991. The metabolic cost of six common movement patterns of bench-step aerobic dance. Abstract. *Med Sci Sports Exerc* 23(4): S839.

Cappo, B.M., and D.S. Homes. 1984. The utility of prolonged respiratory exhalation for reducing physiological and psychological arousal in non-threatening and threatening situations. *J Psychosom Res* 28: 263-73.

Capra, F. 1982. *The turning point.* New York: Bantam Books.

Carmichael, M. 2007. Stronger, faster, smarter. *Newsweek* March 26: 38-46.

Carriere, B. 1998. *The Swiss ball: Theory, basic exercises and clinical application.* Berlin: Springer-Verlag.

Carroll, J., A. Blansit, R.M. Otto, and J.W. Wygand. 2003. The metabolic requirements of Vinyasa yoga. *Med Sci Sports Exer* 35(5): S155.

Carron, A., H. Hausenblas, and D. Mack. 1996. Social influence and exercise: A meta-analysis. *J Sport Exerc Psychol* 18: 1-16.

Carron, A., W. Widmeyer, and L. Brawley. 1988. Group cohesion and individual adherence to physical activity. *J Sport Exerc Psychol* 10: 127-38.

Chapman, A., B. Vicenzino, P. Blanch, and P. Hodges. 2004. Do muscle recruitment patterns differ between trained and novice cyclists? *Med Sci Sports Exerc* 36(5): S169.

Chinsky, A., J. DeFrancisco, K. Flanagan, R.M. Otto, and J. Wygand. 1998. A comparison of two types of spin exercise classes. Abstract. *Med Sci Sports Exerc* 30(5): S954.

Chodzko-Zajko, W., L. Beattie, R. Chow, J. Firman, R. Jahnke, C. Park, K. Rosengren, L. Sheppard, and Y. Yang. 2006. Qi gong and tai chi: Promoting practices that promote healthy aging. *Journal on Active Aging* September-October: 50-6.

Choi, P., J. Van Horn, D. Picker, and H. Roberts. 1993. Mood changes in women after an aerobics class: A preliminary study. *Health Care Women Int* 14(2): 167-77.

Cholewicki, J., M.M. Panjabi, and A. Khachatryan. 1997. Stabilizing function of trunk flexor-extensor muscles around a neutral spine posture. *Spine* 22(19): 2207-12.

Chu, D.A. 1992. *Jumping into plyometrics.* Champaign, IL: Human Kinetics.

Cinque, C. 1989. Back pain prescription: Out of bed and into the gym. *Phys Sportsmed* 17(9): 185-8.

Clapp, J., and K. Little. 1994. The physiological response of instructors and participants to three aerobics regimens. *Med Sci Sports Exerc* 26(8): 1041-6.

Clark, M., and C. Romani-Ruby. 2001. *The Pilates reformer: A manual for instructors.* Tarentum, PA: Word Association.

Clary, S., C. Barnes, D. Bemben, A. Knehans, and M. Bemben. 2006. Effects of ballates, step aerobics, and walking on balance in women aged 50-75 years. *J Sports Sci Med* 5: 390-9.

Claxton, C., and A. Lacy. 1991. Pedagogy: The missing link in aerobic dance. *J Phys Educ Rec Dance* August: 49-52.

Cooper, S., J. Oberne, S. Newton, V. Harrison, J. Coon, S. Lewis, & A. Tattersfield. 2003. Effect of two breathing exercises (Buteyko and pranayama) in asthma, a randomized controlled trial. *Thorax* 58: 674-9.

Copeland-Brooks, C., and D. Brooks. 1995. Guide to slide. *IDEA Today* 13(3): 33-40.

Cosio-Lima, L.M., M.T. Jones, V.J. Paolone, and C.R. Winter. 2001. Effects of a physioball training program on trunk and abdominal strength and static balance measures. Abstract. *Med Sci Sports Exerc* 33(5): S1825.

Craig, A.B., and A.M. Dvorak. 1968. Thermal regulation of man exercising during water immersion. *J Appl Physiol* 25: 23-35.

Cress, M., D. Buchner, K. Questad, P. Esselman, B. deLateur, and R. Schwartz. 1999. Exercise: Effects of physical functional performance in independent older adults. *J Gerontol* 54(5): 242-8.

Crumpton, S., M. Scharff Olson, H.N. Williford, A. Bradford, and S. Walker. 1999. The effects of a commercially-produced "spinning" video: Aerobic responses and caloric expenditure. Abstract. *Med Sci Sports Exerc* 31(5): S415.

D'Acquisto, L., D. D'Acquisto, and D. Renne. 2001. Metabolic and cardiovascular responses in older women during shallow water exercise. *J Strength Cond Res* 15(1): 12-9.

Darby, L.A., K.D. Browder, and B.D. Reeves. 1995. The effects of cadence, impact, and step on physiological responses to aerobic dance exercise. *Res Q Exerc Sport* 66: 231-8.

Darby, L.A., W.A. Skelly, B. Durbin, R.P. Heitkamp, C.J. Hansen, and A.C. Stillman. 2002. Physiological responses to bench stepping on three different landing surfaces. Abstract. *Med Sci Sports Exerc* 34(5): S1651.

Darling, J., J. Linderman, and L. Laubach. 2005. Energy expenditure of continuous and intermittent exercise in college aged males. *J Exerc Physiol-Online.* [Online]. 8(4): 1-8.

Davidson, D., A. Brathwaite, and J. Eickhoff-Shemek. 2006. Recruiting, training, and retaining qualified group exercise leaders: Part II. *ACSM Health and Fitness Journal* 10(3): 22-6.

Davidson, K., and L. McNaughton. 2000. Deep water running training and road running training improve $\dot{V}O_2$max in untrained women. *J Strength Cond Res* 14(2): 191-5.

Davies, A. 2006. Baby steps. *IDEA Fitness Journal* November-December: 86-8.

Davis, C. 1994. The role of physical activity in the development and maintenance of eating disorders. *Psychol Med* 24: 957-67.

Davis, S.E., L.J. Romaine, K. Casebolt, and K. Harrison. 2002. Incidence of injury in kickboxing. Abstract. *Med Sci Sports Exerc* 34(5): S1438.

DeMaere, J.M., and B C. Ruby. 1997. Effects of deep water and treadmill running on oxygen uptake and energy expenditure in seasonally trained cross country runners. *J Sports Med Phys Fitness* 37(3): 175-81.

DeVreede, P., M. Samson, and N. VanMeeteren. 2005. Functional-task exercise vs. resistance strength exercise to improve daily tasks in older women: A randomized, controlled trial. *J Am Geriatr Soc* 53: 2-10.

DiCarlo, L.J., P.B. Sparling, B.T. Hinson, T. Snow, and L. Rosskopf. 1995. Cardiovascular, metabolic and perceptual responses to hatha yoga standing poses. *Med Exerc Nutr Health* 4: 107-12.

Dunbar, C., R. Robertson, R. Baun, M. Blandin, K. Metz, R. Burdett, and R. Goss. 1992. The validity of regulating exercise intensity by ratings of perceived exertion. *Med Sci Sports Exerc* 24(1): 94-9.

Dwyer, J. 1995. Effect of perceived choice of music on exercise intrinsic motivation. *Health Values* 19(2): 18-26.

Edmundson, A. 2007. *Globalized e-learning cultural challenges.* Hershey, PA: Information Science.

Eickhoff-Shemek, J., and S. Selde. 2006. Evaluating group exercise leader performance: An easy and helpful tool. *ACSM Health and Fitness Journal* 10(1): 20-3.

Eklund, R., and S. Crawford. 1994. Social physique anxiety, reasons for exercise, and attitudes toward exercise settings. *J Sport Exerc Psychol* 16: 70-82.

Eller, D. 1996. News + views: Is aerobics dead? *Women's Sports and Fitness* January-February: 19-20.

Esco, M.R., M.S. Olson, R. St. Martin, E. Woollen, M. Ellis, and H.N. Williford. 2004. Abdominal EMG of selected Pilates' mat exercises. *Med Sci Sports Exerc* 36(Suppl. no. 5): S357.

Ergun, A.T., P.A. Plato, and C.J. Cisar. 2006. Cardiovascular and metabolic responses to noncontact kickboxing in females. *Med Sci Sports Exerc* 38(5): S497.

Estabrooks, P. 2000. Sustaining exercise participation through group cohesion. *Exerc Sport Sci Rev* 28(2): 63-7.

Estabrooks, P., and A. Carron. 1999. The influence of the group with elderly exercisers. *Small Group Research* 30(4): 438-52.

Estivill, M. 1995. Therapeutic aspects of aerobic dance participation. *Health Care Women Int* 16(4): 341-50.

Evans, E. 1993. Body image: Programming for a healthy perspective. *NIRSA Journal* Fall: 46-51.

Evans, E., and P. Connor. 1995. Body image of water aerobic instructors. Abstract. *Med Sci Sports Exerc* 27(5): 852.

Evans, E., and K. Cureton. 1998. Metabolic, circulatory and perceptual responses to bench stepping in water. *J Strength Cond Res* 12(2): 95-100.

Evans, E., and C. Kennedy. 1993. The body image problem in the fitness industry. *IDEA Today* May: 50-6.

Eyestone, E., G. Fellingham, J. George, and G. Fisher. 1993. Effect of water running and cycling on maximum oxygen consumption and 2-mile run performance. *Am J Sports Med* 21(1): 41-4.

Falsetti, H., S. Blau, E. Burke, and K. Smith. 1995. Heart rate response and caloric expenditure during a Spinning class. In *Spinning Instructor Manual,* ed. Johnny Goldberg, 4.15-4.18. Venice, CA: Johnny Goldberg Publications.

Faulds, R. 2006. *Kripalu Yoga: A guide to practice on and off the mat.* New York: Bantam Dell.

Feigenbaum, M., and M. Pollock. 1997. Strength training. *Phys Sportsmed* 25(2): 44-64.

Feigenbaum, M.S., and M.L. Pollock. 1999. Prescription of resistance training for health and disease. *Med Sci Sports Exerc* 31: 38-45.

Feland, J.B. 2000. The effect of stretch duration on hamstring flexibility in an elderly population. Abstract. *Med Sci Sports Exerc* 32(5): S354.

Fischer, M.E., B.W. Evans, J.E. Edwards, and J.S. Kuhlman. 1998. Changes in fitness after a twelve week step aerobic program in women 50 to 65 years. Abstract. *Med Sci Sports Exerc* 30(5): S951.

Fitt, S., J. Sturman, and S. McClain-Smith. 1993/1994. Effects of Pilates-based conditioning on strength, alignment, and range of motion in university ballet and modern dance majors. *Kinesiology in Medicine and Dance* 16(1): 36-51.

Flanagan, K., J. DeFrancisco, A. Chinsky, J. Wygand, and R.M. Otto. 1998. The metabolic and cardiovascular response to select positions and resistances during Spinning exercise. Abstract. *Med Sci Sports Exerc* 30(5): S944.

Flegal, K., B. Graubard, D. Williamson, and M. Gail. 2005. Excess deaths associated with underweight, overweight, and obesity. *JAMA* 293(15): 1861-7.

Fonda, J. 1981. *Jane Fonda's workout book.* New York: Simon & Schuster.

Foss, O., and J. Hallen. 2004. The most economical cadence increases with increasing workload. *Eur J Appl Physiol* 92: 443-51.

Fox, L., J. Rejeski, and L. Gauvin. 2000. Effects of leadership style and group dynamics on enjoyment of physical activity. *Am J Health Promot* 15(5): 277-83.

Francis, L. 1991. Improving aerobic dance programs: The key role of colleges and universities. *J Phys Educ Rec Dance* September: 59-62.

Francis, P. 1990. In step with science. *Fitness Management* 6(6): 37-8.

Francis, P., and L. Francis. 1988. *If it hurts, don't do it.* Rocklin, CA: Prima.

Francis, P.R., L. Francis, G. Miller, K. Tichenor, and B. Rich. 1994. *Introduction to Step Reebok.* San Diego: San Diego University.

Francis, P.R., J. Poliner, M.J. Buono, and L.L. Francis. 1992. Effects of choreography, step height, fatigue and gender on metabolic cost of step training. Abstract. *Med Sci Sports Exerc* 24(5): S69.

Francis, P.R., A.S. Witucki, and M.J. Buono. 1999. Physiological response to a typical studio cycling session. *ACSM Health and Fitness Journal* 3(1): 30-6.

Franco, O., C. deLaet, A. Peters, J. Jonker, J. Mackenbach, and W. Nusselder. 2005. Effects of physical activity on life expectancy with cardiovascular disease. *Arch Intern Med* 165: 2363-9.

Frangolias, D., and E. Rhodes. 1995. Maximal and ventilatory threshold responses to treadmill and water immersion running. *Med Sci Sports Exerc* 27(7): 1007-13.

Frangolias, D., E. Rhodes, and J. Taunton. 1996. The effects of familiarity with deep water running on maximal oxygen consumption. *J Strength Cond Res* 10(4): 215-9.

Frangolias, D.D., E.C. Rhodes, J.E. Taunton, A.N. Belcastro, and K. D. Coutts. 2000. Metabolic responses to prolonged work during treadmill and water immersion running. *J Sci Med Sport* 3(4): 476-92.

Franzese, P., T. Taglione, C. Flynn, J. Wygand, and R.M. Otto. 2000. The metabolic cost of specific Taebo exercise movements. Abstract. *Med Sci Sports Exerc* 32(5): S150.

Freeman, R. 1988. *Bodylove: Learning to like our looks and ourselves*. New York: Harper-Collins.

Frodge, S., A. Kunz, R. Liebman, J. Wygand, A. VanGelder, and R.M. Otto. 1993. A metabolic comparison of treadmill walking versus slideboard exercise. Abstract. *Med Sci Sports Exerc* 25(5): S622.

Frymoyer, J.W., and W.L. Cats-Baril. 1991. An overview of the incidences and costs of low back pain. *Orthop Clin North Am* 22: 263.

Gaesser, G. 1999. Thinness and weight loss: Beneficial or detrimental to longevity? *Med Sci Sports Exerc* 31(8): 1118-28.

Galantino, M.L., T.M. Bzdewka, J.L. Eissler-Russo, M.L. Holbrook, E.P. Mogck, P. Geigle, and J.T. Farrar. 2004. The impact of modified hatha yoga on chronic low back pain: A pilot study. *Altern Ther Health Med* 10: 56-9.

Gallagher, S., and R. Kryzanowska. 2000. *The Joseph H. Pilates archive collection: Photographs, writings and designs*. Philadelphia: Bainbridge Books.

Gallagher, S.P., and R. Kryzanowska. 1999. *The Pilates method of body conditioning*. Philadelphia: TransAtlantic.

Garber, C.E., J.S. McKinney, and R.A. Carleton. 1992. Is aerobic dance an effective alternative to walk–jog exercise training? *J Sports Med Phys Fitness* 32(2): 136-41.

Gavin, J. 2007. IDEA fitness industry compensation survey 2006. *IDEA Fitness Journal* June: 45-55.

Gehring, M., B. Keller, and B. Brehm. 1997. Water running with and without a flotation vest in competitive and recreational runners. *Med Sci Sports Exerc* 29(10): 1374-8.

Gerard, J. 2006. Shake, lead and other new ways to get fit. *ACE Fitness Matters* July-August: 6-8.

Ginis, M., M. Jung, and L. Gauvin. 2003. To see or not to see: Effects of exercising in mirrored environments on sedentary women's feeling states and self-efficacy. *Health Psychol* 22(4): 354-61.

Girouard, C., and B. Hurley. 1995. Does strength training inhibit gains in range of motion from flexibility training in older adults? *Med Sci Sports Exerc* 27(10): 1444-9.

Gladwell, M. 2005. *Blink: The power of thinking without thinking*. New York: Time Warner Book Group.

Gladwell, V., S. Head, M. Haggar, and R. Beneke. 2006. Does a program of Pilates improve chronic non-specific low back pain? *J Sport Rehabil* 15(4): 338-50.

Goldenberg, L., and P. Twist. 2002. *Strength ball training*. Champaign, IL: Human Kinetics.

Goleman, D. 1998. *Working with emotional intelligence*. New York: Bantam Books.

Goleman, D. 2006. *Social Intelligence: The new science of social intelligence*. New York: Bantam Dell Pub Group.

Goodman, S. 1997. The care and feeding of your sound system. *IDEA Today* June: 43-50.

Goss, F.L., R.J. Robertson, R.J. Spina, T.E. Auble, D.A. Cassinelli, R.M. Silberman, R.W. Galbreath, and K.F. Metz. 1989. Energy cost of bench stepping and pumping light handweights in trained subjects. *Res Q Exerc Sport* 60(4): 369-72.

Gotchalk, L., R. Berger, and W. Kraemer. 2004. Cardiovascular responses to a high-volume continuous circuit resistance training protocol. *J Strength and Cond Res* 18(4): 760-4.

Grant, S., K. Corbett, K. Todd, C. Davies, T. Aitchison, N. Mutrie, J. Byrne, E. Henderson, and H. Dargie. 2002. A comparison of physiological response and rating of perceived exertion in two modes of aerobic exercise in men and women over 50 years of age. *Br J Sports Med* 36: 276-81.

Grant, S., K. Todd, T. Aitchison, P. Kelly, and D. Stoddart. 2004. The effects of a 12-week group exercise programme on physiological and psychological variables and function in overweight women. *Public Health* 118(1): 31-42.

Graves, B.S., J.V. Quinn, J.A. O'Kroy, and D.J. Torok. 2005. Influence of Pilates-based mat exercise on chronic lower back pain. *Med Sci Sports Exerc* 37(Suppl. no. 5): S27.

Greendale, G.A., A. McDivit, A. Carpenter, L. Seegar, and M. Huang. 2002. Yoga for women with hyperkyphosis: Pilot study. *Am J Pub Health* 92(10): 1611-14.

Greene, L., L. Kravitz, J. Wongsathikun, and T. Kemerly. 1999. Metabolic effect of punching tempo. Abstract. *Med Sci Sports Exerc* 31(5): S674.

Greenlaw, K., L. McMillan, S. Catalano, S. Vivolo, M. Giroux, J. Wygand, and R.M. Otto. 1995. The energy cost of traditional versus power bench step exercise at heights of 4, 6, and 8 inches. Abstract. *Med Sci Sports Exerc* 27(5): S1343.

Gregor, P. 2006. Screening with meaning. *IDEA Fitness Journal* October: 82-6.

Grier, T.D., L.K. Lloyd, J.L. Walker, and T.D. Murray. 2001. Metabolic cost of aerobic dance bench stepping at varying cadences and bench heights. Abstract. *Med Sci Sports Exerc* 33(5): S123.

Griffith, S. 2005. Integrate to elevate. *IDEA Fitness Journal* July-August: 39-44.

Hagan, M. 2005. Group fitness takes center stage: 10 tips for creating a scheduling masterpiece. *IDEA Fitness Manager* March: 12-4.

Hahn, S., D. Stanforth, P.R. Stanforth, and A. Phillips. 1998. A 10 week training study comparing Resistaball and traditional trunk training. *Med Sci Sports Exerc* 30(5): S1128.

Hale, B.S., and J.S. Raglin. 2002. State anxiety responses to acute resistance training and step aerobic exercise across eight weeks of training. *J Sports Med Phys Fitness* 42(1): 108-12.

Hallam, S. 2001. *The power of music.* London: The Performing Rights Society.

Hawks, S.R., N. Harmon, and L. Kravitz. 2007. The effects of music on exercise. *IDEA Fitness Journal* September: 73-7.

Hawks, S.R., M.L. Hull, R.L. Thalman, and P.M. Richins. 1995. Review of spiritual health: Definition, role, and intervention strategies in health promotion. *Am J Health Promot* 9(5): 371-8.

Hedley, A., C. Ogden, C. Johnson, M. Carroll, L. Curtin, and K. Flegal. 2004. Prevalence of overweight and obesity among US children, adolescents, and adults, 1999-2002. *J Am Med Assoc* 23(291): 2847-50.

Heidel, S., and J. Torgerson. 1993. Vocal problems among aerobic instructors and aerobic participants. *J Commun Disord* 26(3): 179-91.

Heinzelmann, F., and P. Bagley. 1970. Response to physical activity programs and their effects on health behavior. *Public Health Rep* 86: 905-11.

Helgerud, J., K. Hoydal, E. Wang, T. Karlsen, P. Berg, M. Bjerkaas, T. Simonsen, and C. Helgensen. 2007. Aerobic high-intensity intervals improve $\dot{V}O_2$max more than moderate training. *Med Sci Sports Exerc* 39(4): 665-71.

Herbert, R.D., and M. de Noronha. 2007. Stretching to prevent or reduce muscle soreness after exercise. *Cochrane Database of Systematic Reviews,* 4: 1.

Hodges, P., C. Richardson, and G. Jull. 1996. Evaluation of the relationship between laboratory and clinical tests of transverse abdominis function. *Physiother Res Int* 1(4): 269.

Hoeger, W., J. Warner, and G. Fahleson. 1995. Physiologic responses to self-paced water aerobics and treadmill running. Abstract. *Med Sci Sports Exerc* 27(5): 83.

Holmes, M., W. Chen, D. Feskanich, C. Kroecke, and G. Colditz. 2005. Physical activity and survival after breast cancer diagnosis. *JAMA* 293(20): 2479-86.

Hooker, S. 2003. The exercise/fitness professional's expanding role in promoting physical activity and the public's health. *ACSM Health and Fitness Journal* May-June: 7-11.

Hostler, D., C.I. Schwirian, F.C. Hagerman, R.S. Staron, G. Campos, K. Toma, M.T. Crill, and G. Hagerman. 1999. Skeletal muscle adaptations in elastic resistance trained young men and women. Abstract. *Med Sci Sports Exerc* 31(5): S1632.

Howley, E., D. Bassett, and D. Thompson. 2005. Get them moving: Balancing weight with physical activity part II. *ACSM Health and Fitness Journal* January-February: 19-24.

Howley, E., and B. Franks. 2007. Health fitness instructor's handbook. 5th ed. Champaign, IL: Human Kinetics.

Howley, E., and S. Powers. 2006. Exercise physiology: Theory and application to fitness and performance. 6th ed. New York: McGraw-Hill.

Hudson, S. 1998. Yoga aids in pain. *Aust Nurs J* 5(9): 27.

Hutton, R.S. 1992. Neuromuscular basis of stretching exercises. In *Strength and power in sports,* ed. P.V. Komi, 29-38. Boston: Blackwell Scientific.

Ibbetson, J. 1996. Body image and self-esteem: Factors that affect each and recommendations for fitness professionals. *NIRSA Journal* Fall 22-7.

IDEA. 2005. Group fitness instructor code of ethics. *IDEA Fitness Journal* February: 67.

IDEA. 2007. Spanning 25 years: IDEA and fitness industry milestones 1982-2007. *IDEA Fitness Journal* July-August: 24-35.

Immel, D.D., T. Tripplett-McBride, D.C.W. Fater, and C. Foster. 2000. Physiological responses to cardio kickboxing in females. Abstract. *Med Sci Sports Exerc* 32(5): S1557.

Impett, E., J. Daubenmier, and A. Hirschman. 2006. Minding the body: Yoga, embodiment, and well-being. *Sexuality Research and Social Policy: Journal of NSRC* 3(4): 39-48.

Innes, K.E., C. Bourguignon, and A.G. Taylor. 2005. Risk indices associated with insulin resistance syndrome, cardiovascular disease, and possible protection with yoga: A systematic review. *J Am Board Fam Med* 18(6): 491-519.

Isacowitz, R. 2006. *Pilates.* Champaign, IL: Human Kinetics.

Iyengar, B.K.S. 1996. *Light on yoga.* New York: Schocken Books.

Jacobs, B.P., W. Mehling, A.L. Avins, H.A. Goldberg, M. Acree, J.H. Lasater, R.J. Cole, D.S. Riley, S. Mauer. 2004. Feasibility of conducting a clinical trial on hatha yoga for chronic low back pain: Methodological lesson. 10: 80-3.

Jakicic, J.M., B.H. Marcus, K.I. Gallagher, M. Napolitano, and W. Lang. 2003. Effect of exercise duration and intensity on weight loss in overweight, sedentary women. *JAMA* 290(10): 1323-30.

Jakicic, J., and A. Otto. 2005. Physical activity considerations for the treatment and prevention of obesity. *Am J Clin Nutr* 82(1): 2265-95.

Janot, J. 2005. Comparing intensity monitoring methods. *IDEA Health and Fitness Journal* April: 38-41.

Jazzercise. 2008. Jazzercise company info. www.jazzercise.com/companyinfo.htm.

Jentoft, E., A. Kvalvik, and A. Mengshoel. 2001. Effects of pool-based and land-based aerobic exercise on women with fibromyalgia/chronic widespread muscle pain. *Arthritis Care and Research* 45(1): 42-7.

Jevning, R., R.K. Wallace, and M. Beidebach. 1992. The physiology of meditation: A review. *Neurosci Biobehav Rev* 16(3): 415-24.

John, D.H., and P. Schuler. 1999. Accuracy of using RPE to monitor intensity of group indoor stationary cycling. Abstract. *Med Sci Sports Exerc* 31(5): S643.

Johnson, B.F., K.D. Johnston, and S.A. Winnier. 1993. Bench-step aerobic ground forces for two steps at variable bench heights. Abstract. *Med Sci Sports Exerc* 25(5): S1100.

Johnson, E.G., A. Larsen, H. Ozawa, C.A. Wilson, and K.L. Kennedy. 2007. The effect of Pilates-based exercise on dynamic balance in healthy adults. *Journal of Bodywork Movement Therapies* 11(3): 238-42.

Kabat-Zinn, J., L. Lipworth, R. Burney, and W. Sellers. 1986. Four year follow-up of a meditation based program for the self-regulation of chronic pain: Treatment outcomes and compliance. *Clin J Pain.* 2(3): 159-73.

Kahlkoetter, J. 2002. Respect your body. *Triathlete* February: 48-9.

Kahn, J. 2008. What's shaking. *Boston Globe.* January 8.

Kandarian, M. 2006. Seven secrets for totally outrageous teaching. *IDEA Fitness Journal* September: 86-8.

Keller, J. 2008. Group energy. *IDEA Fitness Journal* January: 87.

Kellett, K., D. Kellett, and L. Nordholm. 1991. Effects of an exercise program on sick leave due to back pain. *Phys Ther* 71: 283-93.

Kennedy, C. 1997. Exercise analysis. *IDEA Today* January: 70-3.

Kennedy, C. 2003. Functional exercise progression. *IDEA Personal Trainer* February: 36-43.

Kennedy, C. 2004. Making a real difference. *IDEA Health and Fitness Source* January: 40-4.

Kennedy, C., and D. Legel. 1992. *Anatomy of an exercise class: An exercise educators' handbook.* Champaign, IL: Sagamore.

Kennedy, C., and M. Sanders. 1995. Strength training gets wet. *IDEA Today* May: 25-30.

Kennedy, J.E., R.A. Abbott, and B.S. Rosenberg. 2002. Changes in spirituality and well-being in a retreat program for cardiac patients. *Altern Ther Health Med* 8(4): 64-73.

Kennedy, M.M., and M. Newton. 1997. Effect of exercise intensity on mood in step aerobics. *J Sports Med Phys Fitness* 37: 3.

Kernodle, R. 1992. Space: The unexplored frontier of aerobic dance. *J Phys Educ Rec Dance* May-June: 65-9.

Khalsa, S.B. 2004. Yoga as a therapeutic intervention: A bibliometric analysis of published research studies. *Indian J Physiol Pharmacol* 48(3): 269-85.

Kiesling, S. 1990. *The complete recreational rower and racer: From indoor rowing machines to outdoor shells.* New York: Crown.

Kin Isler, A., S.N. Kosar, and F. Korkusuz. 2001. Effects of step aerobics and aerobic dancing on serum lipids and lipoproteins. *J Sports Med Phys Fitness* 41(3): 380-5.

King, R., and A. Brownstone. 1999. Neurophysiology of yoga meditation. *Int J Yoga Ther* 9: 9-17.

Klein, D., L. Burr, and W. Stone. 2005. Making physical activity stick: What can we learn from regular exercisers? *ACSM Health and Fitness Journal* 9(4): 19-25.

Knudson, D. 1995. A review of stretching research. *AHPERD Journal* October: 16-8.

Kory, K., and T. Seabourne. 1999. *Power pacing for indoor cycling.* Champaign, IL: Human Kinetics.

Koszuta, L. 1986. Low-impact aerobics: Better than traditional aerobic dance? *Phys Sportsmed* 14(7): 156-61.

Kraemer, W.J., M. Keuning, N.A. Ratamess, J.S. Volek, M. McCormick, J.A. Bush, B.C. Nindl, S.W. Gordon, S.A. Mazzetti, R.U. Newton, A.L. Gomez, R.B. Wickham, M.R. Rubin, and K. Hakkinen. 2001. Resistance training combined with bench step aerobics enhances women's health profile. *Med Sci Sports Exerc* 33(2): 259-69.

Kraftsow, G. 1999. *Yoga for wellness: Healing with the timeless teachings of viniyoga.* New York: Penguin Books.

Krane, V., S. Shipley, J. Waldron, and J. Michalenok. 2001. Relationships among body satisfaction, social physique anxiety, and eating behaviors in female athletes and exercisers. *J Sport Behav* 24(3): 247-64.

Kravitz, L. 1994. The effects of music on exercise. *IDEA Today* October: 56-61.

Kravitz, L. 2007. The 25 most significant health benefits of physical activity and exercise. *IDEA Fitness Journal* October: 55-63.

Kravitz, L., L. Greene, and J. Wongsathikun. 2000. The physiological responses to kick-boxing exercise. Abstract. *Med Sci Sports Exerc* 32(5): S148.

Kravitz, L., V.H. Heyward, L.M. Stolarczyk, and M.V. Wilmerding. 1995. Effects of step training with and without handweights on physiological and lipid profiles of women. Abstract. *Med Sci Sports Exerc* 27(5): S1012.

Kravitz, L., V. Heyward, L. Stolarczyk, and V. Wilmerding. 1997. Does step exercise with handweights enhance training effects? *J Strength Cond Res* 11(3): 194-9.

Kristal, A., A. Littman, D. Benitez, and E. White. 2005. Yoga practice is associated with attenuated weight gain in healthy middle-aged men and women. *Altern Ther Health Med* 11(4): 28-33.

Kunz, A., R. Liebman, J.W. Wygand, R.M. Otto, A. Van-Gelder, J. Meegan, and J. Ludwig. 1993. The effects of body position and slide technique on the metabolic response of slideboard exercise. Abstract. *Med Sci Sports Exerc* 25(5): S623.

LaForge, R. 1997. Mind body fitness: Encouraging prospects for primary and secondary prevention. *J Cardiovasc Nurs* 11(3): 53-65.

Lally, D. 1994. Stretching and injury in distance runners. *Med Sci Sports Exerc* 26(5): S84.

Lamb, T. 2004. Psychophysiological effects of yoga. International Association of Yoga Therapists. www.iayt.org.

Lan, C., J. Lai, S. Chen, and M. Wong. 1998. 12-month tai chi training in the elderly: Its effect on health fitness. *Med Sci Sports Exerc* 39(3): 345-51.

Lane, C. 2000. *Christy Lane's complete book of line dancing.* 2nd ed. Champaign, IL: Human Kinetics.

Larkin, M. 2007. Should your facility have an AED? *Journal on Active Aging* May-June: 57-61.

Lessen, D. 2005. *The PMA Pilates certification exam study guide.* Miami, FL: Pilates Method Alliance.

Li, F., P. Harmer, E. McAuley, N. Chaumeton, E. Eckstrom, and N. Wilson. 2005. Tai chi and fall reductions in older adults: A randomized controlled trial. *J Geront Med Sci* 60A: 66-74.

Liemohn, W., and G. Pariser. 2002. Core strength: Implications for fitness and low back pain. *ACSM Health and Fitness Journal* 6(5): 10-6.

Liggett, C.S. 1999. The Swiss ball: An overview of applications in sports medicine. *J Man Manip Ther* 7(4): 190-6.

Lofshult, D. 2002. Group fitness trend watch 2002. *IDEA Health and Fitness Source* July-August: 69-76.

Long, J., H. Williford, M. Olson, and V. Wolfe. 1998. Voice problems and risk factors among aerobics instructors. *J Voice* 12(2): 197-207.

Loupias, J., and L. Golding. 2004. Deep water conditioning: A conditioning alternative. *ACSM Health and Fitness Journal.* September-October: 5-8.

Lucia, A., A. San Juan, M. Montilla, S. Canete, A. Santalla, C. Earnest, and M. Perez. 2004. In professional road cyclists, low pedaling cadences are less efficient. *Med Sci Sports Exerc* 36: 1048-54.

Ludwig, J., A. VanGelder, J.W. Wygand, and R.M. Otto. 1994. The metabolic cost of fixed slideboard exercise at two different board lengths. Abstract. *Med Sci Sports Exerc* 26(5): S55.

Luskin, F., K. Newell, M. Griffith, M. Holmes, S. Telles, F. Marvasti, K. Pelletier, and W. Haskell. 1998. A review of mind-body therapies in the treatment of cardiovascular disease. *Altern Ther Health Med* 4(3): 46-61.

MacAuley, D. 1995. *A guide to cycling injuries: Prevention and treatment.* San Francisco: Bicycle Books.

Malek, M., D. Nalbone, D. Berger, and J. Coburn. 2002. Importance of health science education for personal fitness trainers. *J Strength Cond Res* 16(1): 19-24.

Manchanda, S.C., R. Narang, K.D. Reddy, U. Sachdeva, D. Prabhakaran, S. Dharmanand, M. Rajani, and R. Bijlani. 2000. Retardation of coronary atherosclerosis with yogic lifestyle intervention. *J Assoc Physicians India* 48: 687-94.

Marshall, P.W., and B.A. Murphy. 2006. Increased deltoid and abdominal muscle activity during Swiss ball bench press. *J Strength Cond Res* 20(4): 745-50.

Massie, J., and R. Sheperd. 1971. Physiological and psychological effects of training: A comparison of individual and gymnasium programs, with a characterization of the exercise "drop-out." *Med Sci Sports* 3: 110-7.

Mayo, J. 2000. Practical guidelines for the use of deep water running. *J Strength Cond Res* 22(1): 26-9.

McArdle, W.D., F.I. Katch, and V.L. Katch. 2006. *Exercise physiology: Energy, nutrition, and human performance.* 6th ed. Philadelphia: Lippincott Williams & Wilkins.

McCarberg, B., and J. Wolf. 1999. Chronic pain management in a health maintenance organization. *Clin J Pain* 15(1): 50-7.

McGill, S. 2002. *Low back disorders.* Champaign, IL: Human Kinetics.

McGlone, C., L. Kravitz, and J. Janot. 2002. Rebounding: A low-impact exercise alternative. *ACSM Health and Fitness Journal* 6(2): 11-5.

McGonigal, K. 2007. Facilitating fellowship. *IDEA Health and Fitness Journal* June: 73-9.

McKinney-Vialpando, K. 1999. *Cardio TKO: Aerobic kickboxing for the fitness professional.* 2nd ed. Idaho Falls, ID: Safax Fitness Training.

McLain, S. 2005. Boot camp Ohio style. *IDEA Fitness Journal* May: 31-3. (cited under Ornish)

McMillan, A., L. Proteau, and R. Lebe. 1998. The effect of Pilates-based training on dancers' dynamic posture. *J Dance Med Sci* 2(3): 101-7.

McMillan, S. 2005. Sample class: Sport step. *IDEA Fitness Journal* November-December: 79-80.

Melanson, E.L., P.S. Freedson, R. Webb, S. Jungbluth, and N. Kozlowski. 1996. Exercise responses to running and in-line skating at self-selected paces. *Med Sci Sports Exerc* 28(2): 247-50.

Menezes, A. 1998. *The complete guide to Joseph H. Pilates' techniques of physical conditioning.* Alameda, CA: Hunter House.

Meyers, C. 1992. *Walking: A complete guide to a complete exercise.* New York: Random House.

Michaud, T., D. Brennan, R. Wilder, and N. Sherman. 1995. Aquarunning and gains in cardiorespiratory fitness. *J Strength Cond Res* 9(2): 78-84.

Michaud, T., J. Rodriguez-Zayas, F. Andres, M. Flynn, and C. Lambert. 1995. Comparative exercise responses of deep-water and treadmill running. *J Strength Cond Res* 9(2): 104-9.

Miller, J.M., M.D. Rossi, H. Schurr, L.E. Brown, and M. Whitehurst. 2001. Force production in healthy males during a horizontal press that uses elastics for resistance. Abstract. *Med Sci Sports Exerc* 33(5): S139.

Miller, W. 1999. How effective are traditional dietary and exercise interventions for weight loss? *Med Sci Sports Exerc* 31(8): 1129-34.

Miller, W., J. Wallace, and K. Eggert. 1993. Predicting max HR and the HR-VO_2 relationship for exercise prescription in obesity. *Med Sci Sports Exerc* 25: 1007-81.

Monroe, M. 1999. And the beat goes on. *IDEA Health and Fitness Source* October: 31-7.

Monroe, R., R. Nagarathma, and H.R. Nagendra. 1990. *Yoga for common ailments.* New York: Simon & Schuster.

Mookadam, F., and H. Arthur. 2004. Social support and its relationship to morbidity and mortality after acute myocardial infarction: Systematic overview. *Arch Intern Med* 164(14): 1514-18.

Mora-Rodriguez, R., and R. Aguado-Jimenez. 2004. Performance at high pedaling cadences in well-trained cyclists. *Med Sci Sports Exerc* 38(5): 953-7.

Moses, R.D. 1993. Ground reaction forces in bench aerobics. Abstract 49. Paper presented at the 22nd Annual Meeting of the Southeast Regional Chapter of the American College of Sports Medicine, Greensboro, NC.

Mosher, P.E., M.A. Ferguson, and R.O. Arnold. 2005. Lipid and lipoprotein changes in premenstrual women following step aerobics dance training. *Int J Sports Med* 26: 669-74.

Mutoh, Y., S. Sawai, Y. Takanashi, and L. Skurko. 1988. Aerobic dance injuries among instructors and students. *Phys Sportsmed* 16(12): 81-6.

Myers, M.J., and P. Boyd. 2001. Metabolic cost of stepping: Effects of cadence and load. Abstract. *Med Sci Sports Exerc* 33(5): S501.

Nagle, E., R. Robertson, J. Jakicic, A. Otto, J. Ranalli, and L. Chiapetta. 2007. Effects of aquatic exercise and walking in sedentary obese women undergoing a behavioral weight-loss intervention. *IJARE* 1: 43-56.

Nardini, M., J. Raglin, and C. Kennedy. 1999. Body image, disordered eating, obligatory exercise and body composition among women fitness instructors. Abstract. *Med Sci Sports Exerc* 31(Suppl. no. 5): S297.

Neiman, D. 2003. *Exercise testing and prescription.* 5th ed. New York: McGraw-Hill.

Nelson, M., W. Rejeski, S. Blair, P. Duncan, J. Judge, A. King, C. Macera, and C. Castenada-Sceppa. 2007. Physical activity and public health in older adults: Recommendation from the American College of Sports Medicine and the American Heart Association. *Med Sci Sports Exer* 39(8): 1435-45.

Nichols, J.F., C.L. Sherman, and E. Abbott. 2000. Treading is new and hot. *ACSM Health and Fitness Journal* 4(2): 12-7.

Nobrega, A.C.L., K.C. Paula, and A.C.G. Carvalho. 2005. Interaction between resistance training and flexibility training in healthy young adults. *J Strength Cond Res* 19(4): 842-6.

Nogawa-Wasman, D. 2002. How to make group fitness profitable with fee-based programming. *IDEA Health and Fitness Source* May: 29-35.

Norris, C. M. 2000. *Back stability.* Champaign, IL: Human Kinetics.

Norton, C., K. Hoobler, A. Welding, and G.M. Jensen. 1997. Effectiveness of aquatic exercise in the treatment of women with osteoarthritis. *J Phys Ther* 5(3): 8-15.

O'Driscoll, E., J. Steele, H.R. Perez, S. Yreys, N. Snowkroft, and F. Locasio. 1999. The metabolic cost of two trials of boxing exercise utilizing a heavy bag. Abstract. *Med Sci Sports Exerc* 31(5): S676.

Ogden, C., K. Flegal, M. Carroll, and C. Johnson. 2002. Prevalence and trends in overweight among US children and adolescents, 1999-2000. *JAMA* 288(14): 1728-32.

Olson, M., H. Williford, D. Blessing, and R. Greathouse. 1991. The cardiovascular and metabolic effects of bench-stepping exercise in females. *Med Sci Sports Exerc* 23(11): 1311-8.

Olson, M., L. Williford, R. Brown, and S. Pugh. 1996. Self-reports on the Eating Disorder Inventory by female aerobic instructors. *Percept Mot Skills* 82: 1051-8.

Olson, M.S. 2005. Lessons from the lab. *IDEA Fitness Journal* 11(12): 38-43.

Olson, M.S., H.N. Williford, R. St. Martin, M. Ellis, E. Woollen, and M.R. Esco. 2004. The energy cost of a basic, intermediate, and advanced Pilates' mat workout. *Med Sci Sports Exerc* 36 (Suppl. no. 5): S357.

Ornish, D. 1998. *Love and survival.* New York: Harper Collins.

Ornish, D., S.E. Brown, L.W. Scherwitz, J.H. Billings, W.T. Armstrong, T.A. Ports, S.M. McLanahan, R. Kirkeeide, R. Brand, and K. Gould. 1990. Can lifestyle changes reverse coronary heart disease? The Lifestyle Heart Trial. *Lancet* 336: 129-33.

Osthye, T., J. Dement, and K. Krause. 2007. Obesity and workers compensation: Results from the Duke Health and Safety Surveillance System. *Arch Intern Med* 167: 766-73.

Otto, R., C. Parker, T. Smith, J. Wygand, and H. Perez. 1986. The energy cost of low impact and high impact aerobic exercise. Abstract. *Med Sci Sports Exerc* 18: S523.

Otto, R., M. Yoke, J. Wygand, and P. Larsen. 1988. The metabolic cost of multidirectional low impact and high impact aerobic dance. Abstract. *Med Sci Sports Exerc* 20(2): S525.

Otto, R.M., M. Yoke, K. McLaughlin, J. Morrill, A. Viola, A. Lail, M. Lagomarsine, and J. Wygand. 2004. The effect of twelve weeks of Pilates vs. resistance training on trained females. *Med Sci Sports Exerc* 36(Suppl. no. 5): S357.

Page, P., and T. Ellenbecker. 2003. *The scientific and clinical application of elastic resistance.* Champaign, IL: Human Kinetics.

Parker, S., B. Hurley, D. Hanlon, and P. Vaccaro. 1989. Failure of target heart rate to accurately monitor intensity during aerobic dance. *Med Sci Sports Exerc* 21(2): 230-4.

Pate, R.R., M. Pratt, S.N. Blair, W.L. Haskell, C.A. Macera, C. Bouchard, D. Buchner, W. Ettinger, G.W. Heath, and A.C. King. 1995. Physical activity and public health: A recommendation from the Centers for Disease Control and Prevention and the American College of Sports Medicine. *JAMA* 273(5): 402-7.

Pearson, D., A. Faigenbaum, M. Conley, and W. Kraemer. 2000. The National Strength and Conditioning Association's basic guidelines for resistance training of athletes. *J Strength Cond Res* 22(4): 14-27.

Perez, H.R., E. O'Driscoll, J. Steele, S. Yreys, N. Snowkroft, C. Steizinger, and F. Locasio. 1999. Physiological responses to two forms of boxing aerobics exercise. Abstract. *Med Sci Sports Exerc* 31(5): S673.

Peterson, T., D. Verstraete, W. Schultz, and J. Stray-Gundersen. 1993. Metabolic demands of step aerobics. Abstract. *Med Sci Sports Exerc* 25(5): S448.

Pilates, J.H. 1945. *Pilates' return to life through contrology.* Available from Balanced Body: 800-PILATES.

Pilates, J.H., W.J. Miller, S.P. Gallagher, and R. Kryzanowska, eds. 2000. *The complete writings of Joseph H. Pilates: Return to life through contrology and your health—the authorized editions.* Philadelphia: Bainbridge Books.

Pilates Method Alliance. 2006. *PMA position statement: On Pilates.* Miami, FL: Pilates Method Alliance.

Pillarella, D. 1997. Ready, set, row! *IDEA Today* 15(8): 36-43.

Popowych, K. 2005. A studio society. Creating a positive program experience by fostering and developing participant relationships. *IDEA Health and Fitness Journal* November-December: 72-3.

Porcari, J., and D. Boehde. 2005. Does yoga really do the body good? *ACE Fitness Matters* 9-10: 7-9.

Porcari, J.P. 1999. Pump up your walk. *ACSM Health and Fitness Journal* 3(1): 25-9.

Posner-Mayer, J. 1995. *Swiss ball applications for orthopedic and sports medicine.* Denver: Ball Dynamics International.

Pratt, M.C., C. Macera, and G. Wang. 2000. Higher direct medical costs associated with physical inactivity. *Phys Sportsmed* 28(10): 63-70.

Prins, J., and D. Cutner. 1999. Aquatic therapy in the rehabilitation of athletic injuries. *Clin. Sports Med* 18(2): 427-35.

Public Health Service, U.S. Department of Health and Human Services. 2004. *Healthy people 2010: National health promotion and disease prevention objectives.* Washington, DC: U.S. Government Printing Office, 2: 22.

Quinn, T., D. Sedory, and B. Fisher. 1994. Physiological effects of deep water running following a land-based training program. *Res Q Exerc Sport* 65: 386-9.

Raju, R.S., K. Prasad, R. Venkata, K. Murthy, and M. Reddy. 1997. Influence of intensive yoga training on physiological changes in 6 adult women: A case report. *J Altern Comp Med* 3(3): 291-5.

Ratey, J. 2008. *Spark.* New York: Little Brown and Company.

Raub, J.A. 2002. Psychophysiologic effects of yoga on musculoskeletal and cardiorespiratory function: A review. *J Altern Comp Med* 8(6): 797-812.

Ray, U.S., S. Mukhopadhyaya, S. Purkayastha, V. Asnani, O. Tomer, R. Prashad, L. Thakur, and W. Selvamurthy. 2001. Effect of yogic exercises on physical and mental health of young fellowship course trainees. *Indian J Physiol Pharmacol* 45(1): 37-53.

Reebok University. 1993. *Reebok training manuals: Slide Reebok basic training and Slide Reebok endurance training.* Canton, MA: Reebok University Press.

Reese, S. 1991. Slideboards: A conditioning and rehabilitative tool. *J Strength Cond Res* 13(5): 22-4.

Rhea, M., B. Alvar, L. Burkett, and S. Ball. 2003. A meta-analysis to determine the dose response for strength development. *Med Sci Sports Exerc* 35(3): 456-64.

Richey, R.M., R.M. Zabik, and M.L. Dawson. 1999. Effect of bicycle spinning on heart rate, oxygen consumption, respiratory exchange ratio, and caloric expenditure. Abstract. *Med Sci Sports Exerc* 31(5): S692.

Richie, D., S. Kelso, and P. Bellucci. 1985. Aerobic dance injuries: A retrospective study of instructors and participants. *Phys Sportsmed* 13(2): 130-40.

Riker, H.A., R.M. Zabik, M.L. Dawson, and P.A. Frye. 1998. The effect of step height and upper body involvement on oxygen consumption and energy expenditure during step aerobics. Abstract. *Med Sci Sports Exerc* 30(5): S945.

Riley, S. 2005. The pros and cons of automated external defibrillators. *IDEA Health and Fitness Manager* July-August: 10-1.

Roach, B., P. Croisant, and J. Emmett. 1994. The appropriateness of heart rate and RPE measures of intensity during three variations of aerobic dance. Abstract. *Med Sci Sports Exerc* 26(Suppl. no. 5): 24.

Robergs, R., and R. Landwehr. 2002. The surprising history of the "HRmax = 220 – age" equation. *J Exerc Physiol-Online.* [Online]. 5(2): 1-10.

Robertson, R., F. Goss, T. Auble, D. Cassinelli, R. Spina, E. Glickman, R. Galbreath, R. Silberman, and K. Metz. 1990. Cross-modal exercise prescription at absolute and relative oxygen uptake using perceived exertion. *Med Sci Sports Exerc* 22(5): 653-9.

Rodgers, C.D., C.E. Bjorkquist-Bearding, L.C. Forsblom, and M.E. Ewing. 1994. Comparison of high impact and controlled eccentric aerobic dance routines on cardio-respiratory parameters during exercise and recovery in college-aged women. Abstract. *Med Sci Sports Exerc* 26(5): S585.

Rogers, K., and A. Gibson. 2006. Effects of an 8-week mat Pilates training program on body composition, flexibility, and muscular endurance. *Med Sci Sports Exerc* 38(5): S279-80.

Rosas, D., and C. Rosas. 2006. NIA: The body's way. *IDEA Fitness Journal* February: 89-91.

Rupp, J.C., B.F. Johnson, and D.A. Rupp. 1992. Bench step activity: Effects of bench height and hand held weights. Abstract. *Med Sci Sports Exerc* 24(5): S12.

Ryan, P. 2006. Group exercise class participation. *IDEA Fitness Manager* 5: 14-5.

Ryan, P. 2007. 2007 IDEA fitness programs and equipment survey. *IDEA Fitness Manager* July-August: 7-15.

Rydeard, R., A. Leger, and D. Smith. 2006. Pilates-based therapeutic exercise: Effect on subjects with nonspecific chronic low back pain and functional disability: A randomized controlled trial. *J Orthop Sports Phys Ther* 36(7): 472-84.

Sanders, M., ed. 2000. *YMCA water fitness for health.* Champaign, IL: Human Kinetics.

Sanders, M., and D. Lawson. 2006. Use water's accommodating properties to help clients recovering from knee injuries return to sports. *IDEA Fitness Journal* September: 40-7.

Sanders, M.E., N. Constantino, and N. Rippee. 1997. A comparison of results of functional water training on field and laboratory measures in older women. *Med Sci Sports Exerc* 29(5): ixx-ixx.

Santana, J. 2002. The four pillars of human movement. *IDEA Personal Trainer* February: 22-8.

Schaller, K. 1996. Tai chi chih: An exercise option for older adults. *J Gerontol Nurs* 22(10): 12-7.

Scharff-Olson, M., and H.N. Williford. 1996. The energy cost associated with selected step training exercise techniques. *Res Q Exerc Sport* 67: 465-8.

Scharff-Olson, M., H.N. Williford, D.L. Blessing, R. Moses, and T. Wang. 1997. Vertical impact forces during bench-step aerobics: Exercise rate and experience. *Percept Mot Skills* 84(1): 267-74.

Scharff-Olson, M., H.N. Williford, A. Bradford, S. Walker, and S. Crumpton. 1999. Physiological and subjective psychological responses to group cycling exercise. Abstract. *Med Sci Sports Exerc* 31(5): S418.

Scharff-Olson, M., H.N. Williford, W.J. Duey, J. Barber, and S. Baldwin. 1997. Physiological responses of males and females to bench step exercise at two different rates. Abstract. *Med Sci Sports Exerc* 29(5): S160.

Scharff-Olson, M., H.N. Williford, W.J. Duey, S. Walker, S. Crumpton, and J. Sanders. 2000. The energy cost of martial arts aerobic exercise. Abstract. *Med Sci Sports Exerc* 32(5): S149.

Schell, F.J., B. Allolio, and O.W. Schonecke. 1994. Physiological and psychological effects of hatha-yoga exercise in healthy women. *Int J Psychosom* 41(1-4): 46-52.

Schroeder, J., and K. Friesen. 2007. Programs and equipment survey. *IDEA Fitness Journal* July 7-12..

Schroeder, J.M., J.A. Crussemeyer, and S.J. Newton. 2002. Flexibility and heart rate response to an acute Pilates reformer session. *Med Sci Sports Exerc* 34 (5): S258.

Schuster, K. 1979. Aerobic dance: A step to fitness. *Phys Sportsmed* 7(8): 98-103.

Segal, N.A., J. Hein, and J.R. Basford. 2004. The effects of Pilates training on flexibility and body composition: An observational study. *Arch Phys Med Rehabil* 85(12): 1977-81.

Sherman, K.J., D.C. Cherkin, et al. 2005. Comparing yoga, exercise, and a self-care book for chronic low back pain. *Ann Intern Med* 143(12): 849-56.

Shrier, I. 1999. Stretching before exercise does not reduce the risk of local muscle injury: A critical review of the clinical and basic science literature. *Clin J Sports Med* 9: 221-7.

Shrier, I., and K. Gossal. 2000. Myths and truths of stretching. *Phys Sportsmed* 28(8): 57-63.

Shyba, L. 1990. Finding the elusive downbeat. *IDEA Today* June: 23-30.

Silberstein, L., R. Striegel-Moore, and J. Rodin. 1987. *Feeling fat: A woman's shame.* Hillsdale, NJ: Erlbaum.

Siler, B. 2000. *The Pilates body.* New York: Broadway Books.

Simmons, V., and P. Hansen. 1996. Effectiveness of water exercise on postural mobility in the well elderly: An experimental study on balance enhancement. *J Gerontol Med Sci* 51A(5): M233-8.

Spilde, S., and J.P. Porcari. 2005. Can Pilates do it all? *ACE Fitness Matters* 11(6): 10-1.

Sorace, P., and T. LaFontaine. 2005. Resistance training muscle power: Design programs that work! *ACSM Health and Fitness Journal* 9(2): 6-12.

Sorenson, J., and B. Bruns. 1983. *Jacki Sorensen's aerobic lifestyle book.* New York: Poseidon Press.

Sovik, R. 2000. The science of breathing—the yogic view. *Prog Brain Res* 122: 491-505.

Spink, K., and A. Carron. 1992. Group cohesion and adherence in exercise classes. *J Sport Exerc Psychol* 14: 78-86.

Spink, K., and A. Carron. 1993. The effects of team building on the adherence patterns of female exercise participants. *J Sport Exerc Psychol* 15: 39-49.

Spink, K., and A. Carron. 1994. Group cohesion effects in exercise classes. *Small Group Research* 25(1): 26-42.

Stanforth, D., and P. Stanforth. 1993. The effect of adding external weight on the aerobic requirements of bench stepping. Abstract. *Med Sci Sports Exerc* 25(5): S470.

Stanforth, D., P.R. Stanforth, and K.S. Velasquez. 1993. Aerobic requirement of bench stepping. *Int J Sports Med* 14(3): 129-33.

Stanforth, D., K. Velasquez, and P. Stanforth. 1991. The effect of bench height and rate of stepping on the metabolic cost of bench stepping. Abstract. *Med Sci Sports Exerc* 23(4): S143.

Stanforth, P.R., and D. Stanforth. 1996. The effect of adding external weight on the aerobic requirement of bench stepping. *Res Q Exerc Sport* 67: 469-72.

Step Reebok. 1997. *1997 revised guidelines for Step Reebok.* Canton, MA: Reebok University Press.

Stephens, T., and S. Craig. 1990. *The well-being of Canadians: Highlights of the 1988 Campbell's survey.* Ottawa: Canadian Fitness and Lifestyle Research Institute.

Stoppani, J. 2005. *Encyclopedia of muscle strength.* Champaign, IL: Human Kinetics.

Sullivan, M.G., J.J. Dejulia, and T.W. Worrell. 1992. Effect of pelvic position and stretching method on hamstring muscle flexibility. *Med Sci Sports Exerc* 24(12): 1383-9.

Suomi, R., and D.M. Koceja. 2000. Postural sway characteristics in women with lower extremity arthritis before and after an aquatic exercise intervention. *Arch Phys Med Rehabil* 8(6): 780-5.

Sutherland, R., J. Wilson, T. Aitchison, and S. Grant. 1999. Physiological responses and perceptions of exertion in a step aerobics session. *J Sports Sci* 17(6): 495-503.

Svedenhag, J., and J. Seger. 1992. Running on land and in water: Comparative exercise physiology. *Med Sci Sports Exerc* 24: 1155-60.

Takeshima, N., M. Rogers, E. Watanabe, W. Brechue, A. Okada, T. Yamada, M. Islam, and J. Hayano. 2002. Water-based exercise improves health-related aspects of fitness in older women. *Med Sci Sports Exerc* 33(3): 544-51.

Taylor, D., J. Dalton, A. Seaber, and W. Garrett. 1990. Viscoelastic properties of muscle-tendon units: The biomechanical effects of stretching. *Am J Sports Med* 18: 300-9.

Telles, S., R.S. Kumar, and H.R. Nagendra. 2000. Oxygen consumption and respiration following two yoga relaxation techniques. *Appl Psychophysiol Biofeedback* 25(4): 221-7.

Thacker, S., J. Gilcrest, D. Stroup, and C. Kimsey. 2004. The impact of stretching on sports injury risk: A systematic review of the literature. *Med Sci Sports Exerc* 36(3): 371-8.

Tharrett, S. 2008. *Fitness management.* 2nd ed. Monterey, CA: Healthy Learning.

Thompson, C., K. Cobb, and J. Blackwell. 2007. Functional training improves club head speed and functional fitness in older golfers. *J Strength Cond Res* 21(1): 131-7.

Thompson, W. 2007. Worldwide survey reveals fitness trends for 2008. *ACSM Health and Fitness Journal* 11(6): 7-13.

Tran, M.D., R.G. Holly, J. Lashbrook, and E.A. Amsterdam. 2001. Effects of yoga practice on the health-related aspects of physical fitness. *Prev Cardiol* 4(4): 165-70.

Templeton, M.S., D.L. Booth, and W.D. O'Kelly. 1996. Effects of aquatic therapy on joint flexibility and functional ability in subjects with rheumatic disease. *J Orthop Sports Phys Ther* 23(6): 376-81.

Tsourlou, T., A. Benik, K. Dipla, A. Zafeiridis, and S. Kellis. 2006. The effects of a twenty-four week aquatic training program on muscular strength performance in healthy elderly women. *J Strength Cond Res* 20(4): 811-8.

Tuosto, C.W., and R.P. Tobin. 1997. The effect of board length and cadence on cardiorespiratory and metabolic responses to slideboard exercise. Abstract. *Med Sci Sports Exerc* 29(5): S1064.

Twist, P. 2004. Sports conditioning fast track. *IDEA Personal Trainer* January: 21-6.

Uchino, B. 2006. Social support and health: A review of physiological processes potentially underlying links to disease outcomes. *J Behav Med* 29(4): 377-87.

U.S. Department of Health and Human Resources. 2000. *Healthy people 2010.* www.healthypeople.gov.

U.S. Department of Health and Huamn Services. 2008. *Guidelines for Physical Activity.* www.health.gov/paguidelines.

Van Mechelen, W., H. Hlobil, C. Kemper, W. Voorn, and H. deJongh. 1993. Prevention of running injuries by warm-up, cool-down, and stretching exercises. *Am J Sports Med* 21: 711-9.

Velasquez, K., and J.H. Wilmore. 1992. Changes in cardiorespiratory fitness and body composition after a 12 week bench step training program. Abstract. *Med Sci Sports Exerc* 24(5): S464.

Vogel, A. 2006. How to create a profitable boot camp program. *ACE Certified News* December-January: 11-3.

Vogel, A. 2006. What's hot in H_2O? *IDEA Fitness Journal* July-August: 53-9.

Walker, M. 1989. *Jumping for health.* Garden City, NY: Avery.

Wallace, A. 2002. True thighs. *More* September: 90-5.

Wallin, D., B. Ekblom, R. Grahn, and T. Nordenborg. 1985. Improvement of muscle flexibility. A comparison between two techniques. *Am J Sports Med* 13(4): 263-8.

Walter, J., F. Figoni, and F. Andres. 1995. Effect of stretching intensity and duration on hamstring flexibility. Abstract. *Med Sci Sports Exerc* 27(5): S240.

Wang, N., M. Scharff-Olson, and H.N. Williford. 1993. Energy cost and fuel utilization during step aerobics exercise. Abstract. *Med Sci Sports Exerc* 25(5): S630.

Watts, J.H. 1996. Sport-specific conditioning for anaerobic athletes. *J Strength Cond Res* 18(4): 33-5.

Webb, M. 2005. Group training series: BOSU. *ACE Certified News* October-November: 6-8.

Webb, M. 2006. Group training series: Reebok core board. *ACE Certified News* February-March: 6-8.

Webb, T. 1989. Aerobic Q signs. *IDEA Today* 10: 30-1.

Weir, T. 2004. "New PE" objective: Get kids in shape. *USA Today.* [Online]. www.usatoday.com/sports/2004-12-15-phys-ed-cover_x.htm.

Weltman, A. 1995. *The blood lactate response to exercise.* Champaign, IL: Human Kinetics.

Wen, H., K. Tsai, S. Maiw, C. Lee, and C. Fang. 2007. The effects of step-aerobics and resistance training on BMD and immune functioning in postmenopausal women. *Med Sci Sports Exerc* 39(5): S229.

Westcott, W. 1991. Role-model instructors. *Fitness Management* March: 48-50.

Westcott, W. 2000. Strength training frequency. *Fitness Management* November: 50-4.

Westcott, W., and T. Baechle. 2007. *Strength training past 50.* 2nd ed. Champaign, IL: Human Kinetics.

Whaley, M. 2003. ACSM credentialing: The more towards formal education. *Health and Fitness Journal* July-August: 31-2.

Whaley, M., L. Kaminsky, and G. Dwyer. 1992. Predictions of over- and underachievement of age-predicted maximal heart rate. *Med Sci Sports Exerc* 24: 1173-9.

Whitmer, R. 2005. Obesity in middle age and future risk of dementia: A 27 year longitudinal population based study. *Br Med J* 22(330): 1360.

Whitney, C., J.P. Porcari, W. Floyd, and L.A. Chase. 1993. Step aerobics: The influence of different arm movements and step heights. Abstract. *Med Sci Sports Exerc* 25(5): S453.

Wilbur, R., R. Moffatt, B. Scott, K. Biggerstaff, and K. Hayes. 1995. Comparison of physiological responses during submaximal deep water and treadmill running. Abstract. *Med Sci Sports Exerc* 27(5): 1352.

Wilbur, R., R. Moffatt, B. Scott, D. Lee, and N. Cucuzzo. 1996. Influence of water run training on the maintenance of aerobic performance. *Med Sci Sports Exerc* 28(8): 1056-62.

Willardson, J.M. 2004. The effectiveness of resistance exercises performed on unstable equipment. *J Strength Cond Res* 26(3): 70-4.

Williams, K.A., J. Petronis, D. Smith, D. Goodrich, J. Wu, N. Ravi, R. Doyle, G. Jeckett, M. Kolar, and R. Gross. 2005. Effect of Iyengar yoga therapy for chronic low back pain. *Pain* 115: 107-17.

Williams, K., L. Steinberg, and J. Petronis. 2003. Therapeutic application of Iyengar yoga for healing chronic low back pain. *Int J Yoga Ther* 13: 55-67.

Williford, H., D. Blessing, M. Olson, and F. Smith. 1989. Is low impact aerobic dance an effective cardiovascular workout? *Phys Sportsmed* 17(3): 95-109.

Williford, H.N., M. Scharff-Olson, and D.L. Blessing. 1989. The physiological effects of aerobic dance, a review. *Sports Med* 8(6): 335-45.

Williford, H.N., M. Scharff-Olson, A. Bradford, S. Walker, and S. Crumpton. 1999. Maximum cycle ergometry and group cycle exercise: A comparison of physiological responses. Abstract. *Med Sci Sports Exerc* 31(5): S423.

Williford, H.N., N. Wang, M. Scharff-Olson, D.L. Blessing, and J. Buzbee. 1993. Energy expenditure of slideboard exercise training. Abstract. *Med Sci Sports Exerc* 25(5): S621.

Wilmore, J.H., and D.L. Costill. 2004. *Physiology of sports and exercise.* Champaign, IL: Human Kinetics.

Wingfield, L.D., E.A. Dowling, J.D. Branch, S.R. Colberg, and D.P. Swain. 2006. Differences in VO_2 between kickboxing and treadmill exercise at similar heart rates. *Med Sci Sports Exerc* 38(5): S497.

Wininger, S. 2002. Instructors' and classroom characteristics associated with exercise enjoyment by females. *Percept Mot Skills* 94(2): 395-8.

Wisloff, U., A. Stoylan, J. Loennechen, M. Bruvold, O. Rognmo, P. Haram, A. Tjonna, J. Helgerud, S. Slordahl, S. Lee, V. Videm, A. Bye, G. Smith, S. Najjar, O. Ellingsen, and R. Skjaerpe. 2007. Superior cardiovascular effect of aerobic interval training versus moderate continuous training in heart failure patients. *Circulation* 115: 3086-94.

Witvrouv, E., N. Mahieu, L. Danneels, and P. McNair. 2004. Stretching and injury prevention: An obscure relationship. *Sports Med* 34(7): 443-9.

Wolf, C. 2001. Moving the body. *IDEA Personal Trainer* June: 23-31.

Wolfe, B.L., L.M. Lemura, and P.J. Cole. 2004. Quantitative analysis of single vs. multiple-set programs in resistance training. *J Strength Cond Res* 18(1): 35-47.

Woodby-Brown, S., K. Berg, and R.W. Latin. 1993. Oxygen cost of aerobic dance bench stepping at three heights. *J Strength Cond Res* 7(3): 163-7.

Workman, D., D. Kern, and C. Earnest. 1993. Cardiorespiratory responses of isolated arm movements and hand weighting during bench stepping aerobic dance in women. Abstract. *Med Sci Sports Exerc* 25(5): S466.

Yager, Z., and A. Jennifer. 2005. The role of teachers and educators in the prevention of eating disorders and child obesity: What are the issues? *Eat Disord* 13(3): 261-78.

Yamashita, S., K. Iwai, T. Akimoto, J. Sugawara, and I. Kono. 2006. Effects of music during exercise on RPE, heart rate and the autonomic nervous system. *J Sports Med Phys Fitness* 46(3): 425-30.

Yoke, M.M. 2006. *Personal fitness training: Theory and practice.* Sherman Oaks, CA: Aerobics and Fitness Association of America.

Yoke, M., and C. Kennedy. 2004. *Functional exercise progressions.* Monterey, CA: Healthy Learning.

Yoke, M., R. Otto, P. Larsen, C. Kamimukai, and J. Wygand. 1989. The metabolic cost of instructors' low impact and high impact aerobic dance sequences. In *IDEA 1989 research symposium manual.* San Diego: IDEA.

Yoke, M., R. Otto, J. Wygand, and C. Kamimukai. 1988. The metabolic cost of two differing low impact aerobic dance exercise modes. Abstract. *Med Sci Sports Exerc* 20(2): S527.

Young, D., L. Appel, S. Jee, and E. Miller. 1999. The effects of aerobic exercise and t'ai chi on blood pressure in older people: Results of a randomized trial. *J Am Geriatr Soc* 47(3): 277-84.

Zabukovec, R., and P.M. Tiidus. 1998. Physiological and anthropometric profile of elite kickboxers. *J Strength Cond Res* 9(4): 240-2.

Zeni, A., M.D. Hoffman, and P.S. Clifford. 1996. Energy expenditure with indoor exercise machines. *JAMA* 275(18): 1424-7.

Index

NOTE: Page numbers followed by an italicized *f* or *t* indicate figures or tables will be found on those pages, respectively. Italicized *ff* or *tt* indicate multiple figures or tables, respectively.

About the Authors

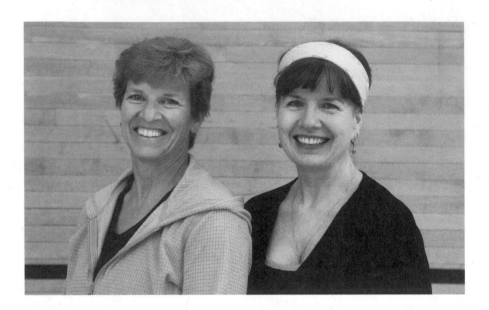

Carol Kennedy-Armbruster, MS, is a lecturer in the fitness specialist program within the department of kinesiology at Indiana University at Bloomington. During her more than 25 years of teaching and training fitness leaders, she has served on the American Council on Exercise (ACE) National Advisory Board and the American College of Sports Medicine (ACSM) credentialing committee, and she chaired the IDEA Water Fitness Committee.

She is certified by ACSM as a Health Fitness Instructor and ACE as a group exercise instructor. She is currently working on her PhD in Human Performance with a Health Minor at Indiana University where she was awarded a trustees teaching award. Her research interests are in the area of group exercise and college students.

Kennedy-Armbruster resides in Indianapolis, Indiana with her husband, Marty. She enjoys outdoor activities, biking, exercising, traveling, and supporting her kids (Tony and Jessica) in their life activities.

Mary M. Yoke, MA, MM, has more than 23 years of experience teaching and training group exercise leaders. In addition to working as a clinical exercise physiologist and leading group exercise classes (including yoga and Pilates) on a regular basis, she is an adjunct professor at Adelphi University in New York, where she teaches a graduate course in exercise leadership. She is an associate board member and master trainer for the Aerobics and Fitness Association of America (AFAA) and served on the American College of Sports Medicine (ACSM) credentialing committee for six years.

Yoke has led seminars for fitness professionals in Europe, Asia, Africa, and South America. She gives numerous presentations throughout the United States to both fitness professionals and the general public. She is the author of three other books on fitness, as well as three videos.

Having obtained more than 20 certifications from organizations such as the ACSM, AFAA, American Council on Exercise (ACE), National Academy of Sports Medicine (NASM), Johnny G. Spinning, Stott Pilates, and the Pilates Method Alliance (PMA), Yoke received her master's degree in exercise physiology from Adelphi University, where she has authored several research studies on group exercise. She also holds two degrees in music performance.

Mary Yoke lives in New York with her two sons. She is a Classical pianist, former opera singer, dancer, linguist, avid naturalist, hiker, backpacker, skier, gardener, cook, traveler, and adventurer.

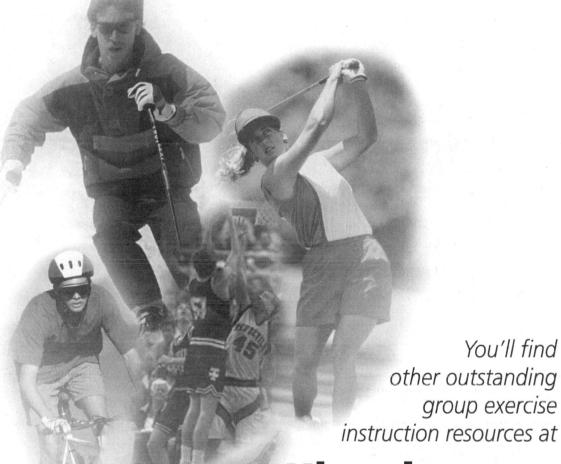

*You'll find
other outstanding
group exercise
instruction resources at*

www.HumanKinetics.com

In the U.S. call

1-800-747-4457

Australia...08 8372 0999
Canada 1-800-465-7301
Europe...+44 (0) 113 255 5665
New Zealand..0064 9 448 1207

HUMAN KINETICS
The Premier Publisher for Sports & Fitness
P.O. Box 5076 • Champaign, IL 61825-5076 USA

DVD Instructions

The enclosed DVD includes video clips that demonstrate techniques for a variety of group exercise formats discussed in this book.

You can view the video content either on a television set with a DVD player or on a computer with a DVD-ROM drive.

The DVD includes a chapter selections menu. When you select a chapter you'll be taken to a menu with a list of the specific video clips for that chapter. After you have viewed one video clip, the DVD will automatically return to the chapter menu, where you can select another video clip.

To use the DVD, place it in your DVD player or DVD-ROM drive. A title screen will welcome you to the program. Then the main menu with buttons for each chapter will appear. When you click on one of the clip titles within the chapter list, the video will play.

Select the HK Running Man logo on the main menu to access production credits and information on contacting Human Kinetics to order other products.